Malignant Bone Lesions and Beyond

Claudio Pusceddu • Salvatore Marsico
Editors

Malignant Bone Lesions and Beyond

Practical Guide to Interventional Radiological Procedures

Springer

Editors
Claudio Pusceddu
Department of Radiology
Mater Olbia Hospital
Olbia, Cagliari, Italy

Interventional Oncology Institute
Barcelona, Spain

Salvatore Marsico
Department of Radiology
Hospital del Mar
Barcelona, Spain

Interventional Oncology Institute
Barcelona, Spain

ISBN 978-3-032-00017-0 ISBN 978-3-032-00018-7 (eBook)
https://doi.org/10.1007/978-3-032-00018-7

This Springer imprint is published by the registered company Springer Nature Switzerland AG
The registered company address is: Gewerbestrasse 11, 6330 Cham, Switzerland

Preface

When we embarked on the writing of this book, we did so with a clear and shared vision: to create a practical, image-based, and clinically oriented guide that would help interventional radiologists and clinicians approach complex oncologic bone lesions with confidence and precision.

This work was born from the idea that the key to effective treatment in interventional oncology lies not only in mastering the techniques but in deeply understanding the oncologic disease itself—its biology, its progression, and its therapeutic context. For this reason, every chapter of the book is conceived as a synthesis between clinical rationale, technical possibilities, and real-world applicability, enriched by illustrative cases, procedural details, and decision-making strategies.

Our aim has been to offer not only a technical manual but a tool that reflects the experience of those who deal daily with patients suffering from bone tumors—often fragile, complex, and in urgent need of a rapid yet thoughtful therapeutic response. The selection of topics has been carefully made to cover the most critical and frequent scenarios in the oncologic interventional practice, with a focus on how to tailor the approach based on lesion location, biomechanics, imaging findings, and overall clinical strategy.

This book brings together the perspectives of multiple experts from different institutions, with the goal of providing a wide-ranging yet coherent overview of the current possibilities in interventional radiology. It is our belief that the future of this field lies in a multidisciplinary, integrated, and creative approach—where knowing the full arsenal of available techniques is as essential as having the flexibility and insight to adapt them to the most challenging situations.

We are deeply grateful to all the contributors who enthusiastically accepted our invitation and shared their expertise. Our heartfelt thanks go also to the patients who, often in very delicate moments of their life, have allowed us to grow professionally and contribute to the advancement of care through their stories.

Special thanks go to the medical, technical, and administrative teams of our respective institutions, whose constant support has made possible the development of this clinical and scientific journey.

We would also like to thank Springer for believing in this project and supporting it throughout its development.

But above all, this book is dedicated to our families. To Marta and Gaia, for their boundless patience, love, and encouragement throughout the long days (and nights) of writing, reviewing, and revising. Without their understanding and strength, this book would simply not exist.

We hope that this work may serve not only as a guide but also as an inspiration for those who, like us, believe in the value of combining clinical rigor with creative thinking in the service of patients.

Olbia, Cagliari, Italy Claudio Pusceddu
Barcelona, Spain Salvatore Marsico

Contents

Abbreviations

ABC	Aneurysmal Bone Cyst
ADP	Adenosine Diphosphate
AR	Augmented Reality
ASA	American Society of Anesthesiologists
ATP	Adenosine Triphosphate
BMD	Bone Mineral Density
BMI	Body Mass Index
BPI	Brief Pain Inventory
BT	Bone Tumor
CAD	Computer-Aided Design
CBCT	Cone-Beam Computed Tomography
CIRSE	Cardiovascular and Interventional Radiological Society of Europe
CLB	Capo Lungo del Bicipite
CO	Cryoablation
CP	Cementoplasty
CPN	Celiac Plexus Neurolysis
CR	Complete Response
CRAB	HyperCalcemia, Renal insufficiency, Anemia, Bone lesions
CS	Chondrosarcoma
CT	Computed Tomography
CTCAE	Common Terminology Criteria for Adverse Events
CTC	Circulating Tumor Cells
DMWA	Directional Microwave Ablation
DRG	Dorsal Root Ganglion
DWI	Diffusion-Weighted Imaging
EA	Embolic Agent
EANM	European Association of Nuclear Medicine
EAU	European Association of Urology
ECOG	Eastern Cooperative Oncology Group
EMG	Electromyography
EMR	Electronic Medical Record
EORTC	European Organisation for Research and Treatment of Cancer
ES	Ewing's Sarcoma
ESMO	European Society for Medical Oncology

ESUR	European Society of Urogenital Radiology
FDA	Food and Drug Administration
FCC	Federal Communications Commission
FDG	Fluorodeoxyglucose
FMS	Functional Mobility Scale
GCTB	Giant Cell Tumor of Bone
HCC	Hepatocellular Carcinoma
HIFU	High-Intensity Focused Ultrasound
IRE	Irreversible Electroporation
IO	Interventional Oncology
IR	Interventional Radiology
ISUP	International Society of Urological Pathology
IV	Intravenous
LAPC	Locally Advanced Pancreatic Cancer
MEDD	Morphine Equivalent Daily Dose
MIP	Maximum Intensity Projection
MM	Multiple Myeloma
MRI	Magnetic Resonance Imaging
MR-HIFU	Magnetic Resonance-guided High-Intensity Focused Ultrasound
MWA	Microwave Ablation
NCCN	National Comprehensive Cancer Network
NICE	National Institute for Health and Care Excellence
NSAIDs	Non-Steroidal Anti-Inflammatory Drugs
ODI	Oswestry Disability Index
OO	Osteoid Osteoma
OR	Operating Room
ORIF	Open Reduction and Internal Fixation
OS	Osteosarcoma
PBL	Primary Bone Lymphoma
PET	Positron Emission Tomography
PET/CT	Positron Emission Tomography/Computed Tomography
Pi	Inorganic Phosphate
PMBT	Primary Malignant Bone Tumors
PMMA	Polymethylmethacrylate
PNS	Peripheral Nerve Stimulation
PR	Partial Response
PRF	Pulsed Radiofrequency
PSF	Percutaneous Screw Fixation
PSMA	Prostate-Specific Membrane Antigen
PSN	Peripheral Somatic Neurolysis
QoL	Quality of Life
RECIST	Response Evaluation Criteria In Solid Tumors
RFA	Radiofrequency Ablation
ROI	Region of Interest
S11	Reflection Coefficient

SAIF	Stent-Assisted Internal Fixation
SBRT	Stereotactic Body Radiotherapy
SD	Stable Disease
SIJ	Sacroiliac Joint
SINS	Spinal Instability Neoplastic Score
SIOG	International Society of Geriatric Oncology
SREs	Skeletal-Related Events
SUV	Standardized Uptake Value
SUVmax	Maximum Standardized Uptake Value
TENS	Transcutaneous Electrical Nerve Stimulation
US-HIFU	Ultrasound-Guided High-Intensity Focused Ultrasound
VAS	Visual Analog Scale
VR	Volume Rendering
WB-MRI	Whole-Body Magnetic Resonance Imaging
WHO	World Health Organization
X-ray	Radiography

Introduction to Malignant Bone Tumors: Clinical Presentation and Diagnostic Imaging

1

Giacomo Vignati, Giulia Zantonelli, Domenico Albano, Salvatore Gitto, and Luca Maria Sconfienza

1.1 Introduction

Malignant bone tumors (BTs), though relatively rare compared to benign BTs, present significant diagnostic challenges. They can arise as primary malignancies originating within the bone or, more commonly, as secondary lesions resulting from metastatic disease from other sites, such as breast, prostate, and lung cancer.

Primary malignant BTs are infrequently encountered in clinical practice, comprising less than 0.2% of all malignancies [1]. The clinical presentation of BTs can vary significantly based on the type of lesion, its location, and expansion; it is also influenced by the age of the patient, with certain tumors being more prevalent in specific age groups. For instance, osteosarcoma typically occurs in adolescents and young adults, while metastatic lesions are more common in older individuals.

Common clinical symptoms include pain, which may worsen at night (a red flag) and after sports activities, swelling, loss of function, systemic symptoms (such as fever, night sweats, weight loss, and malaise), or less common neurological symptoms due to peripheral nerve involvement. BT can be discovered by chance in an acute trauma setting when a patient presents with a pathological fracture, or it may be an incidental finding on radiological investigations performed for unrelated

G. Vignati
University of Milano, Milan, Italy

G. Zantonelli
IRCCS Ospedale Galeazzi – Sant'Ambrogio, Milan, Italy
e-mail: giulia.zantonelli@grupposandonato.it

D. Albano · S. Gitto · L. M. Sconfienza (✉)
University of Milano, Milan, Italy

IRCCS Ospedale Galeazzi – Sant'Ambrogio, Milan, Italy
e-mail: domenico.albano@unibs.it; salvatore.gitto@unimi.it; io@lucasconfienza.it

C. Pusceddu, S. Marsico (eds.), *Malignant Bone Lesions and Beyond*,
https://doi.org/10.1007/978-3-032-00018-7_1

reasons. A detailed clinical history, along with clinical examination, is essential and should be followed by appropriate radiological investigations [2].

Imaging plays a pivotal role in the detection, characterization, assessment of treatment response, and follow-up of musculoskeletal tumors. It is also critical for defining tumor extent and determining marrow, soft tissue, and adjacent joint involvement, as well as the presence of skip lesions and possible metastases. Each imaging modality—whether X-ray, CT, magnetic resonance imaging (MRI), or positron emission tomography (PET)—has distinct advantages and limitations that must be understood to avoid potential pitfalls.

Conventional radiography is generally recommended as the initial imaging modality for evaluating suspected BT. It can provide valuable information on the morphologic characteristics of a lesion, its location and size, and soft tissue involvement, subsequently providing initial information about the aggressiveness of the lesion [3]. The radiographic pattern and the zone of transition between the tumor and surrounding normal bone are essential to differentiate aggressive from nonaggressive lesions. A permeative or moth-eaten pattern with ill-defined margins and a wide zone of transition is typical of malignant BT (e.g., Ewing sarcoma, osteosarcoma), while a geographic pattern with well-defined margins is generally associated with benign and slow-growing lesions (e.g., bone cyst, nonossifying fibroma, enchondroma).

Another crucial feature that should be evaluated is the periosteal reaction, which results from any insult to the periosteum (e.g., BT, trauma, infection). The periosteal reaction depends on the intensity, aggressiveness, and duration of the insult, and it should be evaluated correctly. Conditions like infection (osteomyelitis), especially in children, can manifest as an aggressive reaction that mimics a BT. Malignant BT may present with lamellated ("onion skin"), spiculated, sunburst, and/or disorganized periosteal reactions, with the typical "Codman's Triangle" observed when the periosteum has insufficient time to ossify and cover the lesion spreading into the soft tissues. In contrast, in benign bone lesions, when a periosteal reaction is present, it generally appears thin, solid, and homogeneous.

Thus, the age of the patient, location and size of the lesion, and characteristic features such as radiographic pattern, zone of transition, and periosteal reaction can help categorize malignant BT. CT provides more anatomical detail and is particularly useful in anatomically challenging areas, such as the spine and the pelvis. Also, it helps to better assess subtle periosteal reaction and cortical disruption.

Magnetic resonance imaging (MRI) plays a central role in the detection, characterization, and monitoring of BT due to its excellent contrast resolution and ability to evaluate soft tissues. MRI is essential for detecting intramedullary and periosteal involvement, evaluating extension to contiguous structures such as physes, joints, muscles, and neural structures, monitoring the response after surgery or chemo/radiotherapy, and performing follow-up over time [4].

This imaging modality has limited value in evaluating lytic versus sclerotic lesions, for which CT imaging is preferred. Despite developments in metal artifact reduction sequences, MRI performance can suffer from susceptibility artifacts when BTs are close to orthopedic implants. Tumor protocols may vary between institutions but should generally include a preoperative MRI with a coronal or sagittal T1-weighted and fluid-sensitive sequence in addition to the standard protocol, in order to identify skip lesions [5].

Peri-tumoral bone marrow edema is generally regarded as a sign of malignancy; however, the greater the extent of bone edema, the higher the probability of an underlying benign lesion [6]. Gadolinium-based contrast agents improve the visibility of tumor blood vessels and cellularity and help identify cystic and necrotic components of a bone tumor.

Diffusion-weighted imaging (DWI) can assist in differentiating between benign and malignant tumors by providing insight into the cellularity of a lesion. Malignant tumors typically exhibit markedly increased cellularity, which can lead to a more restricted diffusion, as reflected by a high DWI signal and a low apparent diffusion coefficient (ADC) value. However, DWI has a limited role in the characterization of BT due to the wide overlap of ADC values between benign and malignant lesions, particularly with chondrosarcoma presenting high ADC values and giant cell tumors, solitary fibrous tumors, and osteoblastomas exhibiting low ADC values [3, 7].

Bone scintigraphy is indicated when multifocal bone lesions are suspected and to rule out bone metastases in high-risk patients (e.g., breast carcinoma, prostate cancer) [3]. Increased osteoblastic activity may suggest tumor activity; however, since the assay measures bone deposition rather than tumor-specific proliferation, scintigraphy can result in both false positives and false negatives.

Other limitations of bone scintigraphy include its inability to detect osteoclastic metastatic lesions and its limited value in spinal lesions, as degenerative disease may also lead to increased uptake. Nonetheless, this imaging modality lacks specificity and often cannot distinguish between benign and malignant BT.

The role of planar bone scintigraphy is evolving with the increasing use of positron emission tomography (PET). Fluorodeoxyglucose-Positron Emission Tomography (FDG-PET)/CT produces images that facilitate the diagnosis of BT, initial staging, selection of biopsy sites, evaluation of treatment response, and assessment for tumor recurrence. The coregistration of CT images significantly improves the localization of metabolic abnormalities [8].

FDG-PET/CT is not routinely used for most BT but proves to be highly useful for initial evaluation, staging, and prognostic purposes in certain primary BT, such as Ewing sarcoma and osteosarcoma [9].

1.2 Malignant Bone Tumors

1.2.1 Metastasis

Bone is the third most common site of distant metastasis, surpassed only by the lungs and liver. Bone metastases are the most frequent malignant entity observed in the bone, primarily due to the spread of breast, prostate, lung, and renal cancers, in that order of frequency [10].

Metastatic bone disease can occur at the time of presentation of the primary malignancy (metasynchronous) or years after treatment (metachronous) [11]. Bone metastases cause considerable morbidity, and clinical symptoms can vary widely, including pain, impaired mobility, hypercalcemia, pathological fractures, spinal cord or nerve root compression, and bone marrow infiltration [12].

Malignant cells disrupt the normal turnover of bone cells by releasing local cytokines and growth factors, which can upregulate osteoclastic activity in osteolytic lesions or osteoblastic activity in osteosclerotic lesions, or both, as occurs in most cases. Therefore, the imaging appearance of bone metastases is often variable and unpredictable. Metastases are generally mixed (lytic and sclerotic) in breast cancer, sclerotic in prostate cancer, and lytic in lung, renal, and thyroid cancers [10].

Bone metastases preferentially spread to bones with a high content of red marrow, such as the spine and pelvis (the most common sites), but also involve the ribs, skull, and the proximal third of the femur and humerus. Early diagnosis of bone metastases is essential to undertake personalized and minimally invasive treatments, improve survival rates, and reduce local complications (e.g., pathological fractures or hypercalcemia).

Plain radiography is the first-level imaging technique to evaluate patients with suspected bone metastases or those in cancer follow-up. However, diagnostic accuracy is low, especially in areas where bone metastases are most common, such as the spine, ribs, and pelvis, due to complex anatomy. Computed Tomography (CT) has higher diagnostic performance than plain radiography in detecting bone metastases and allows precise differentiation between cortical and trabecular bone (Fig. 1.1). It is particularly useful for characterizing both osteolytic lesions, with erosion and bone remodeling, and osteosclerotic metastases. In the latter, evaluating the attenuation values of bone metastases has proven to be a useful feature for assessing the response to chemotherapy and radiation therapy [13]. CT is also helpful for

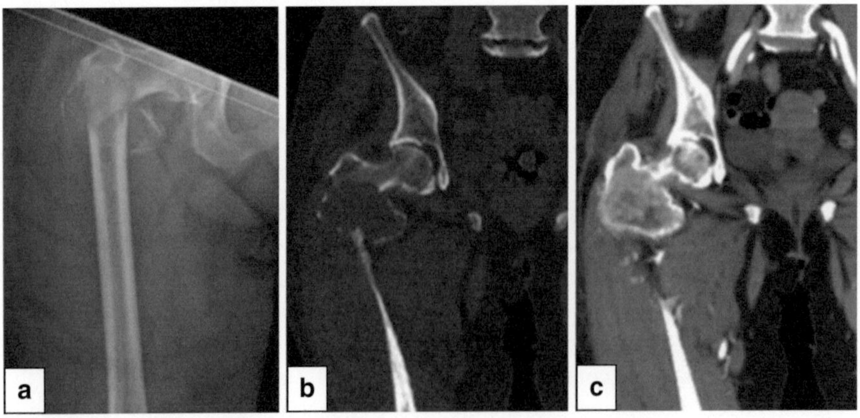

Fig. 1.1 X-ray (**a**) and CT coronal images (**b**, **c**) of a pathological fracture of the proximal femur secondary to bone metastasis from breast cancer in a 59-year-old woman

evaluating the risk of pathological fracture and can effectively monitor reossification that is evident following therapeutic response [11].

MRI is considered the best imaging modality for assessing bone metastases due to its superior contrast resolution in the bone marrow and accurate evaluation of the disease extent. In bone metastases, the bone marrow is infiltrated by pathologic tissue, leading to a subsequent decrease in T1 signal in the affected area. The appearance on T2-weighted images is extremely variable and depends on the type of metastases. However, a restricted pattern of diffusion on DWI and contrast enhancement following gadolinium-based contrast administration is invariably observed [14].

The introduction of whole-body MRI (WB-MRI) with DWI for oncologic purposes in clinical practice is promising; it is a radiation-free modality that allows not only the detection of metastatic disease but also the evaluation of treatment response [15].

Regarding nuclear medicine imaging, bone scintigraphy is widely used to detect skeletal metastases, particularly in breast and prostate cancer. Its sensitivity (almost 90%) is higher than that of CT, although it is inferior to both MRI and FDG-PET/CT [14].

PET offers several advantages compared to bone scintigraphy: PET tracers can be selected based on the primary tumor type (e.g., Prostate-Specific Membrane Antigen (PSMA) in prostate cancer), improving the specificity of the examination. Additionally, the simultaneous acquisition of CT images provides anatomical detail and reduces the number of false-positive findings. Lastly, PET can also detect extraskeletal locations of disease [16].

1.2.2 Lymphoma

Lymphoma primarily involves the bone as a secondary site of disease. Primary bone lymphoma (PBL), which can manifest as a unique localization, is a rare malignant entity, accounting for 2% of all BT and approximately 5% of all extranodal lymphomas [17]. Non-Hodgkin lymphoma is the most frequent histotype in both cases.

Primary bone lymphoma has a peak incidence between 50 and 70 years and predominantly affects the metaphyses of long bones (femur, humerus, and tibia) and the pelvis [18]. Clinical presentations are generally nonspecific and may include pain and symptoms related to local structure compression. Less common manifestations include soft tissue edema, palpable masses, pathological fractures, reduced mobility, and classic "B" symptoms, namely fever, night sweats, and unintentional weight loss.

The imaging appearance of PBL is highly variable and nonspecific. Radiographic findings are often equivocal, leading to diagnostic delays. X-rays may show a permeative radiographic pattern with a wide zone of transition, but identification can be particularly challenging in the pelvis and spine. Periosteal reactions commonly present as lamellar, multilamellar ("onion skin"), or discontinuous.

CT is the modality of choice for managing PBL, as it can effectively depict periosteal reactions, cortical disruption, bone marrow involvement, and soft tissue extension. Notably, the cortical bone is preserved while lymphomatous cells spread to soft tissues through the vascular channels of the cortex. CT is also used for radiologically guided biopsy, which is essential for the definitive diagnosis of PBL [19, 20].

MRI is superior to other imaging techniques, allowing for the evaluation of bone marrow involvement and soft tissue extension (Fig. 1.2). Lymphoma is characterized by very high cellularity, resulting in an intermediate T2 signal and a high DWI signal with very low ADC values. Typically, there are areas of moderate enhancement after contrast injection, usually without significant cortical disruption [21–23].

FDG-PET/CT is the preferred modality for imaging lymphoma and is recommended for initial staging, interim assessment, treatment response evaluation, and recurrence detection. Although bone scintigraphy could be used to image bone lymphoma, FDG-PET/CT offers higher sensitivity and specificity and provides valuable prognostic information. A rapid decrease in FDG uptake compared to initial imaging indicates a successful response, while newly depicted FDG-avid lesions can be assumed to represent recurrences. An SUVmax of 2.5 is used as a cutoff to differentiate between residual and metabolically inactive disease. However, a high false-positive rate has been reported, mainly due to post-therapeutic osteonecrosis [24].

1.2.3 Osteosarcoma

Osteosarcoma (OS) is a malignant bone tumor characterized by the production of osteoid matrix along with variable amounts of cartilage and fibrous tissue [25]. It is the most common malignant primary bone tumor in individuals under 20 years of age, with a second peak of incidence reported in elderly patients due to factors such as Paget's disease, prior radiation exposure, or dedifferentiated chondrosarcomas [26].

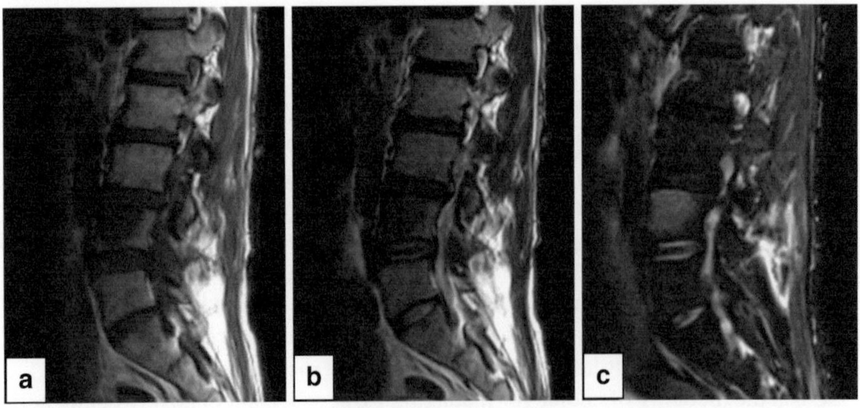

Fig. 1.2 T1 (**a**), T2 (**b**), and Short Tau Inversion Recovery (STIR) (**c**) sagittal images show an example of a rare primary vertebral lymphoma of L4

Pain and swelling are the most common symptoms of osteosarcoma; pain typically arises after exercise or trauma and usually presents 2–4 months before diagnosis. Chronic knee pain in a child should not be easily dismissed [27, 28].

OS can occur in various bones, but the preferred locations are areas of rapid bone growth or turnover, particularly the meta-diaphyseal regions of long bones. It predominantly affects the lower limbs, with the femur involved in almost half of cases, followed by the tibia and humerus (both approximately 15%). Involvement of the spine is rare (less than 5%), primarily affecting the neural arch of thoracic and lumbar segments [27, 29, 30].

OS comprises different subtypes based on histology as well as gross morphological findings, the latter of which can be recognized through appropriate imaging examinations. Conventional osteosarcoma typically starts intramedullary and grows toward the cortex; less frequently, it can grow on the surface (including parosteal, periosteal, and high-grade surface osteosarcoma) or, rarely, intracortically. Telangiectatic osteosarcoma is a rare variant characterized by hemorrhagic, cystic, or necrotic spaces that should be distinguished from benign lesions such as aneurysmal bone cysts [25].

Plain radiography typically displays aggressive features, including a wide zone of transition, ill-defined margins, a permeative or moth-eaten appearance, and aggressive periosteal reactions (such as onion skin, Codman's Triangle, and sunburst patterns) along with a variable amount of ossified and calcified matrix [31].

CT is superior for assessing bone matrix and soft tissue involvement, making it useful during the preoperative period as an anatomical guide and for detecting skip lesions [32, 33]. MRI findings in osteosarcoma can vary based on the specific subtype and the extent of ossification/calcification of the tumor matrix, primarily affecting the T2 signal (with T2 hyperintensity in nonmineralized lesions and T2 hypointensity in highly mineralized ones).

Reactive peritumoral edema is generally observed on fluid-sensitive sequences, which makes assessing the true margins of the tumor challenging; these margins are best defined on T1 fat-saturated sequences before and after contrast agent administration. Osteosarcoma typically shows heterogeneous enhancement and restricted diffusion due to its high cellularity, which correlates with low ADC values [33, 34].

Evaluating atypical subtypes such as telangiectatic osteosarcoma can be particularly challenging due to their cystic appearance, fluid levels (due to hemorrhage), and high ADC values. Bone scintigraphy using technetium-99-methylene diphosphonate can be useful for suspecting skeletal metastases, which typically present with strong radiotracer uptake, further confirmed by CT or MRI (Fig. 1.3).

FDG-PET/CT is valuable for staging, detecting local recurrence, and identifying distant metastases, demonstrating approximately 100% sensitivity in detecting lesions and over 90% sensitivity and specificity in identifying local recurrences and distant metastases. Both bone scintigraphy and FDG-PET/CT can also predict responses to neoadjuvant chemotherapy in patients with osteosarcoma [35, 36].

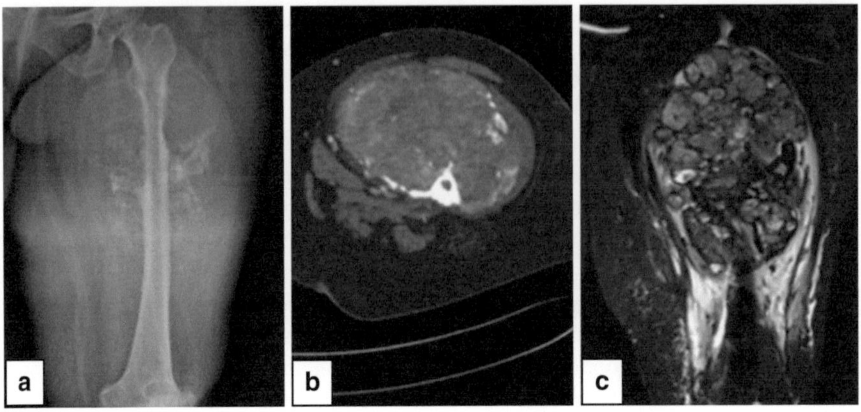

Fig. 1.3 X-ray (**a**), axial CT (**b**) and STIR coronal MRI (**c**) images of a left femur osteosarcoma with extraskeletal involvement

1.2.4 Ewing Sarcoma

Ewing sarcoma is the second most common primary malignant tumor of bone in children and adolescents, following osteosarcoma. It is an aggressive bone tumor composed of small blue round cells and belongs to a family of sarcomas characterized by a specific genetic abnormality, namely a translocation between chromosomes 11 and 22.

Ewing sarcoma exhibits a wide skeletal distribution, with the most commonly affected sites (in order of frequency) being the femur, pelvis, tibia, humerus, fibula, ribs, and sacrum. Spinal involvement is rare, often affecting the posterior elements [37, 38]. At the time of diagnosis, 20–30% of patients have pulmonary and skeletal metastases.

The clinical presentation of Ewing sarcoma is nonspecific; patients may experience pain, swelling, or a palpable mass, but symptoms are often present for more than six months before diagnosis. Pathological fractures are uncommon as an initial clinical presentation; fever and elevated erythrocyte sedimentation rate are common features associated with advanced disease.

Imaging findings for Ewing sarcoma are similar to those of osteosarcoma, with the exception of the absence of matrix ossification. Plain radiography typically reveals aggressive features that reflect the high-grade nature of this malignant lesion; these include a permeative or moth-eaten pattern with a wide zone of transition and aggressive periosteal reactions. Common features also include cortical destruction accompanied by an associated soft tissue mass and sclerotic components. Atypical and rare radiographic findings may include cortical thickening, pathological fractures, and expansile bone remodeling.

CT is more sensitive than radiographs for the detection of early bone lesions and the delineation of associated circumferential soft tissue masses. It is particularly useful for identifying subtle pathological fractures, extraosseous tumor extension, and the relationship between intraosseous and soft tissue components [37, 39].

MRI is essential for evaluating intramedullary and soft tissue extension of Ewing sarcoma. The MRI signal characteristics are similar to those of lymphoma, as both conditions present elevated cellularity that results in low T1 signal intensity, intermediate T2 signal intensity, and restricted diffusion on DWI, along with homogeneous contrast enhancement (Fig. 1.4) [39, 40].

FDG-PET is the standard for initial staging, as well as for detecting recurrence or metastatic disease. It is more sensitive in detecting metastases than conventional bone scintigraphy because increased glucose uptake by the tumor typically precedes any osteoblastic response, allowing for the identification of non-osseous metastases as well.

The initial standardized uptake value (SUV) of the tumor has been correlated with tumor aggressiveness, with an SUVmax of ≥ 2.5 used as a cutoff for indicating increased pathological uptake in the tumor lesions [41].

1.2.5 Chordoma

Chordoma is the second most common primary spinal tumor, accounting for about 4% of all primary BT. It primarily affects middle-aged patients, with a male predominance, and is most often located at the base of the skull (spheno-occipital region) and in the sacrococcygeal region.

Chordomas arise from notochord remnants that persist in the axial skeleton throughout life and may undergo malignant transformation into chordoma at any age [42, 43].

The most common signs and symptoms of chordoma are location-dependent and may include a combination of pain, weakness, sensory abnormalities, or bowel,

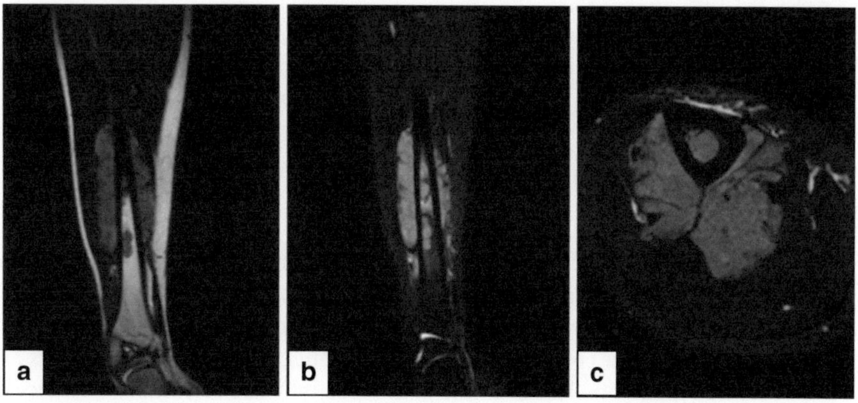

Fig. 1.4 T2 images in the coronal plane (**a**) and STIR images in the coronal (**b**) and axial planes (**c**) of an Ewing sarcoma with a voluminous extraskeletal mass of the right diaphysis of the tibia in a 23-year-old boy

bladder, and sexual dysfunction. For example, in the sacral region, patients may experience lower back pain, constipation (due to rectal compression), neurological compromise (attributable to sacral plexus involvement), and the presence of a gluteal mass.

On radiography, when visible, chordomas appear as geographic osteolytic and expansile lesions with well-defined margins. On CT examination, chordomas typically present as lobulated, hypoattenuating, heterogeneous lesions with extensive lytic bone destruction, periskeletal extension, and common intra-lesional calcifications, which represent small bone sequestra [44].

On MRI, chordomas usually appear hypointense on T1-weighted images, with occasional small foci of hyperintensity (indicative of proteinaceous or hemorrhagic content) and T2 hyperintensity due to their high water content, similar to that of chondrosarcomas. Moderate to marked contrast enhancement is observed after the administration of contrast media (Fig. 1.5).

Post-contrast dynamic perfusion imaging can be used to monitor chordomas after radiotherapy, as a decrease in contrast enhancement is generally associated with a good response [45].

Nuclear medicine modalities are not typically utilized for chordoma diagnosis. FDG-PET/CT can show heterogeneous increased uptake of FDG and allows for whole-body staging, although chordomas have a low rate of metastasis [46].

1.2.6 Chondrosarcoma

Chondrosarcoma is a malignant tumor that produces a cartilage matrix. Primary chondrosarcoma, which arises de novo, is the third most common primary malignant bone tumor (after myeloma and osteosarcoma), with a male predominance and a peak incidence in the fourth to fifth decade of life. Secondary chondrosarcoma is associated with preexisting cartilaginous lesions, such as enchondromas or osteochondromas [47].

The most common skeletal locations for chondrosarcomas are the long tubular bones (femur, humerus, and tibia), followed by the pelvis, ribs, and spine, where it can arise from the vertebral body and neural arch [48]. Involvement of the hands and feet is rare.

Clinical symptoms often include pain and tenderness with or without a palpable mass; however, the growth of the tumor may be very slow, particularly in pelvic tumors [49].

Chondrosarcomas can be classified based on their osseous location (intramedullary, peripheral, or periosteal) or by histological subtypes, with different grades of differentiation associated with varying prognoses and surgical treatments [47]. The most common subtype is conventional chondrosarcoma, which typically presents as a large calcified intramedullary lesion with a mixed lytic and sclerotic appearance.

Plain radiography of low-grade subtypes typically reveals a lobular, ill-defined osteolytic lesion with intralesional rings-and-arcs calcifications and endosteal scalloping. High-grade and dedifferentiated lesions, on the other hand, exhibit a

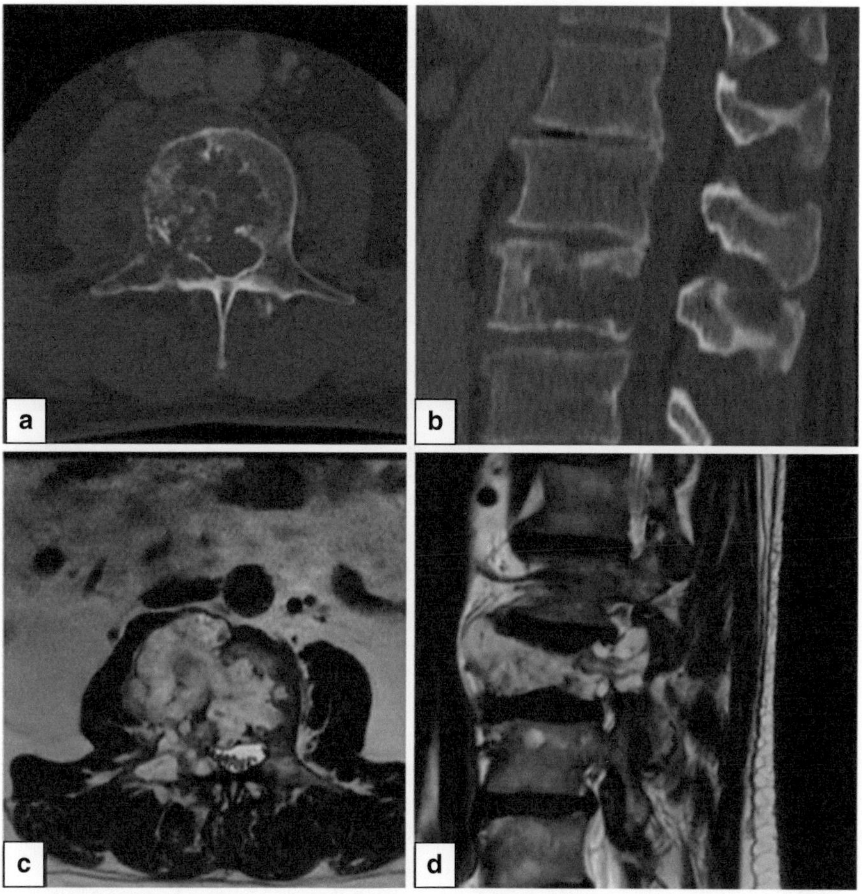

Fig. 1.5 Axial and sagittal CT (**a, b**) and T2 MRI (**c**) images show L3 vertebral body chordoma. Axial T2 image (**d**) better detects extraskeletal and epidural invasion

permeative or moth-eaten pattern, aggressive periosteal reactions, and fewer calcifications.

CT is better at detecting intra-tumoral calcifications, making it useful for categorizing lesions as chondroid. It is also more accurate in assessing endosteal scalloping, which is a key feature for differentiating low-grade chondrosarcoma from enchondroma. Other distinguishing features include periosteal reaction, soft tissue mass, cortical remodeling, size (larger than 5 cm), and pain.

On MRI, chondrosarcomas appear T1-hypointense and T2-hyperintense, with hypointense calcific foci and peripheral and septal contrast enhancement after contrast media injection (Fig. 1.6). Typically, they show no restricted diffusion on DWI, with high ADC values even in high-grade chondrosarcomas [50–56].

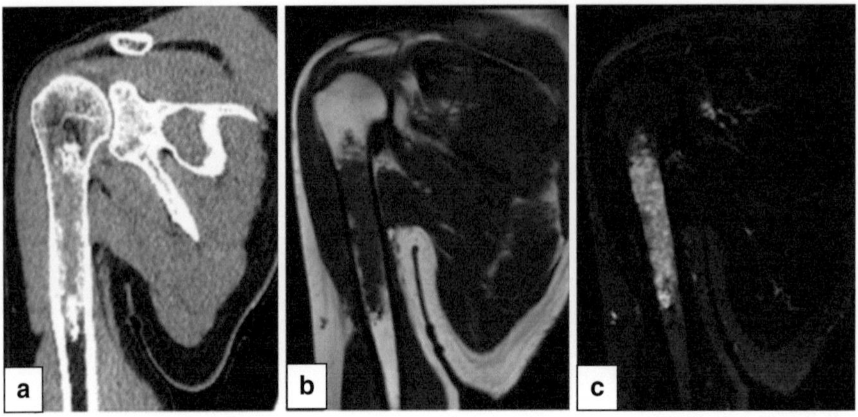

Fig. 1.6 Coronal CT (**a**), T1 (**b**), and STIR (**c**) MRI images show G1 chondrosarcoma of right humeral diaphysis

Chondrosarcomas are metabolically active, unlike enchondromas, and show increased uptake on bone scintigraphy. PET/CT reveals avid FDG uptake, which increases with higher grading of the cartilaginous tumor [57].

1.2.7 Multiple Myeloma

Multiple myeloma (MM) is the second most common hematologic malignancy, characterized by the clonal proliferation of plasma cells in bone marrow. This condition can lead to the production of excessive amounts of monoclonal immunoglobulins, which can be detected in serum and urine [58].

MM primarily affects patients in their seventh decade of life. Diagnosis is based on biological findings such as the so-called hypercalcemia, renal failure, anemia, and lytic bone lesions on imaging (CRAB) criteria and the pathological demonstration of bone marrow infiltration.

Plain radiography has low sensitivity for the detection of bone lytic lesions, with the most common sites of disease including the axial skeleton, ribs, skull, shoulders, pelvis, and long bones.

CT scans using a low-dose protocol enhance the detection of punched-out lytic lesions, diffuse osteopenia, fractures, and, in rare cases, osteosclerosis. However, CT cannot reliably differentiate between active and responsive lesions, as lytic foci often maintain a consistent appearance for months (Fig. 1.7). Therefore, it is not recommended for evaluating treatment response.

MRI provides improved detection of intra- and extraosseous lesions and the ability to differentiate between physiological and myeloma-infiltrated bone marrow. Typical lesions in MM are marrow-based and appear T1-hypointense and T2/STIR hyperintense, with contrast enhancement following the administration of contrast media.

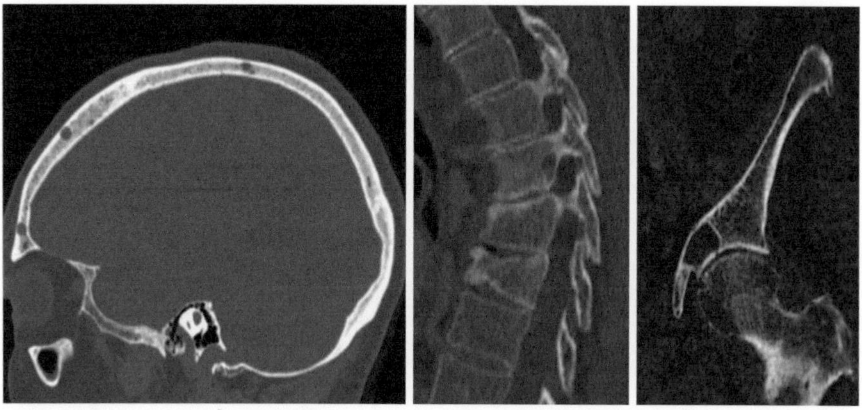

Fig. 1.7 CT low-dose protocol detects multiple punched-out lytic lesions typical of MM that involve widely skull, spine (with pathological fracture of D7 vertebral body) and pelvis

The bone marrow involvement in multiple myeloma can be classified into three different patterns: focal lesions, homogeneous diffuse bone marrow infiltration, and a mixed "salt-and-pepper" pattern with remaining islets of fatty bone marrow [35, 59].

Whole-body MRI (WB-MRI) and PET/CT play crucial roles in initial staging, response evaluation, and detection of minimal residual disease. WB-MRI has superior sensitivity for detecting diffuse bone marrow involvement, while 18F-FDG-PET/CT is more effective for identifying relevant residual abnormalities and extraosseous lesions [60].

1.3 Conclusion

Malignant bone tumors represent a diverse and complex group of neoplasms that require accurate diagnosis, staging, and follow-up to guide appropriate therapeutic strategies. Imaging plays a central role throughout the clinical course, from initial detection to posttreatment surveillance, with each modality contributing unique diagnostic value. Conventional radiography remains the first-line tool, while MRI and CT offer superior anatomical detail and lesion characterization. Nuclear medicine techniques, particularly PET/CT and WB-MRI, have revolutionized the evaluation of disease extent and treatment response.

Given the heterogeneity of malignant bone tumors—from aggressive lesions like osteosarcoma and Ewing sarcoma to more indolent entities like chordomas and chondrosarcomas—a multidisciplinary approach is essential. Collaboration between radiologists, oncologists, pathologists, surgeons, and interventional specialists is crucial to optimizing patient outcomes. Continuous advancements in imaging protocols and the integration of radiomics and AI hold promise for further improving diagnostic precision and personalized care in bone oncology.

References

1. ESMO/European Sarcoma Network Working Group. Bone sarcomas: ESMO clinical practice guidelines for diagnosis, treatment and follow-up. Annal Oncol. 2014;25:iii113–23. https://doi.org/10.1093/annonc/mdu256.
2. Green NM, Abas S, Sajid S, Cribb GL. Presentation of bone tumours: clinical findings and initial management of patients. Orthop Trauma. 2021;35:108–14. https://doi.org/10.1016/j.mporth.2021.03.001.
3. Debs P, Ahlawat S, Fayad LM. Bone tumors: state-of-the-art imaging. Skeletal Radiol. 2024;53:1783–98. https://doi.org/10.1007/s00256-024-04621-7.
4. Pozzi G, Albano D, Messina C, et al. Solid bone tumors of the spine: diagnostic performance of apparent diffusion coefficient measured using diffusion-weighted MRI using histology as a reference standard. J Magn Reson Imaging. 2018;47:1034–42. https://doi.org/10.1002/jmri.25826.
5. Bellelli A, Silvestri E, Barile A, et al. Position paper on magnetic resonance imaging protocols in the musculoskeletal system (excluding the spine) by the Italian College of Musculoskeletal Radiology. Radiol Med. 2019;124:522–38. https://doi.org/10.1007/s11547-019-00992-3.
6. Albano D, Messina C, Gitto S, et al. Differential diagnosis of spine tumors: my favorite mistake. Semin Musculoskelet Radiol. 2019;23:026–35. https://doi.org/10.1055/s-0038-1675551.
7. Messina C, Bignone R, Bruno A, et al. Diffusion-weighted imaging in oncology: an update. Cancers (Basel). 2020;12:1493. https://doi.org/10.3390/cancers12061493.
8. Behzadi AH, Raza SI, Carrino JA, et al. Applications of PET/CT and PET/MR imaging in primary bone malignancies. PET Clin. 2018;13:623–34. https://doi.org/10.1016/j.cpet.2018.05.012.
9. Costelloe CM, Chuang HH, Madewell JE. FDG PET/CT of primary bone tumors. Am J Roentgenol. 2014;202:W521–31. https://doi.org/10.2214/AJR.13.11833.
10. O'Sullivan GJ. Imaging of bone metastasis: an update. World J Radiol. 2015;7:202. https://doi.org/10.4329/wjr.v7.i8.202.
11. Isaac A, Dalili D, Dalili D, Weber M-A. State-of-the-art imaging for diagnosis of metastatic bone disease. Radiologe. 2020;60:1–16. https://doi.org/10.1007/s00117-020-00666-6.
12. Coleman RE. Metastatic bone disease: clinical features, pathophysiology and treatment strategies. Cancer Treat Rev. 2001;27:165–76. https://doi.org/10.1053/ctrv.2000.0210.
13. Vassiliou V, Andreopoulos D, Frangos S, et al. Bone metastases: assessment of therapeutic response through radiological and nuclear medicine imaging modalities. Clin Oncol. 2011;23:632–45. https://doi.org/10.1016/j.clon.2011.03.010.
14. Yang H-L, Liu T, Wang X-M, et al. Diagnosis of bone metastases: a meta-analysis comparing 18FDG PET, CT, MRI and bone scintigraphy. Eur Radiol. 2011;21:2604–17. https://doi.org/10.1007/s00330-011-2221-4.
15. Albano D, Stecco A, Micci G, et al. Whole-body magnetic resonance imaging (WB-MRI) in oncology: an Italian survey. Radiol Med. 2021;126:299–305. https://doi.org/10.1007/s11547-020-01242-7.
16. Shie P, Cardarelli R, Brandon D, et al. Meta-analysis: comparison of F-18 Fluorodeoxyglucose-positron emission tomography and bone scintigraphy in the detection of bone metastases in patients with breast cancer. Clin Nucl Med. 2008;33:97–101. https://doi.org/10.1097/RLU.0b013e31815f23b7.
17. Scoccianti G, Rigacci L, Puccini B, et al. Primary lymphoma of bone: outcome and role of surgery. Int Orthop. 2013;37:2437–42. https://doi.org/10.1007/s00264-013-2055-6.
18. Krishnan A, Shirkhoda A, Tehranzadeh J, et al. Primary bone lymphoma: radiographic–MR imaging correlation. Radiographics. 2003;23:1371–83. https://doi.org/10.1148/rg.236025056.
19. Stefanini FS, Gois FWC, de TCSB A, et al. Primary bone lymphoma: pictorial essay. Radiol Bras. 2020;53:419–23. https://doi.org/10.1590/0100-3984.2019.0137.
20. Albano D, La Grutta L, Grassedonio E, et al. Pitfalls in whole body MRI with diffusion weighted imaging performed on patients with lymphoma: what radiologists should know. Magn Reson Imaging. 2016;34:922–31. https://doi.org/10.1016/j.mri.2016.04.023.

21. Albano D, Patti C, Matranga D, et al. Whole-body diffusion-weighted MR and FDG-PET/CT in Hodgkin lymphoma: predictive role before treatment and early assessment after two courses of ABVD. Eur J Radiol. 2018;103:90–8. https://doi.org/10.1016/j.ejrad.2018.04.014.
22. Galia M, Albano D, Tarella C, et al. Whole body magnetic resonance in indolent lymphomas under watchful waiting: the time is now. Eur Radiol. 2018;28:1187–93. https://doi.org/10.1007/s00330-017-5071-x.
23. Albano D, Patti C, La Grutta L, et al. Comparison between whole-body MRI with diffusion-weighted imaging and PET/CT in staging newly diagnosed FDG-avid lymphomas. Eur J Radiol. 2016;85:313–8. https://doi.org/10.1016/j.ejrad.2015.12.006.
24. Kanavos T, Birbas E, Papoudou-Bai A, et al. Primary bone lymphoma: a review of the literature with emphasis on histopathology and Histogenesis. Diseases. 2023;11:42. https://doi.org/10.3390/diseases11010042.
25. Yarmish G, Klein MJ, Landa J, et al. Imaging characteristics of primary osteosarcoma: nonconventional subtypes. Radiographics. 2010;30:1653–72. https://doi.org/10.1148/rg.306105524.
26. Murphey MD, Robbin MR, McRae GA, et al. The many faces of osteosarcoma. Radiographics. 1997;17:1205–31. https://doi.org/10.1148/radiographics.17.5.9308111.
27. Ta HT, Dass CR, Choong PFM, Dunstan DE. Osteosarcoma treatment: state of the art. Cancer Metastasis Rev. 2009;28:247–63. https://doi.org/10.1007/s10555-009-9186-7.
28. Crombé A, Simonetti M, Longhi A, et al. Imaging of osteosarcoma: presenting findings, metastatic patterns, and features related to prognosis. J Clin Med. 2024;13:5710. https://doi.org/10.3390/jcm13195710.
29. Chianca V, Cuocolo R, Gitto S, et al. Radiomic machine learning classifiers in spine bone tumors: a multi-software. Multi-Scanner Study Eur J Radiol. 2021;137:109586. https://doi.org/10.1016/j.ejrad.2021.109586.
30. Ilaslan H, Sundaram M, Unni KK, Shives TC. Primary vertebral osteosarcoma: imaging findings. Radiology. 2004;230:697–702. https://doi.org/10.1148/radiol.2303030226.
31. Lee SY, Cho WH, Song WS, Park JH. Different radiological findings with the same pathologic diagnosis due to different age in primary osteosarcoma. Acta Radiol. 2006;47:841–4. https://doi.org/10.1080/02841850600812736.
32. deSantos L, Bernardino M, Murray J. Computed tomography in the evaluation of osteosarcoma: experience with 25 cases. Am J Roentgenol. 1979;132:535–40. https://doi.org/10.2214/ajr.132.4.535.
33. Cannavò L, Albano D, Messina C, et al. Accuracy of CT and MRI to assess resection margins in primary malignant bone tumours having histology as the reference standard. Clin Radiol. 2019;74:736.e13–21. https://doi.org/10.1016/j.crad.2019.05.022.
34. Inarejos Clemente EJ, Navarro OM, Navallas M, et al. Multiparametric MRI evaluation of bone sarcomas in children. Insights Imaging. 2022;13:33. https://doi.org/10.1186/s13244-022-01177-9.
35. Liu F, Zhang Q, Zhou D, Dong J. Effectiveness of 18F-FDG PET/CT in the diagnosis and staging of osteosarcoma: a meta-analysis of 26 studies. BMC Cancer. 2019;19:323. https://doi.org/10.1186/s12885-019-5488-5.
36. Lee I, Byun BH, Lim I, et al. Comparison of 99mTc-methyl diphosphonate bone scintigraphy and 18F-fluorodeoxyglucose positron emission tomography/computed tomography to predict histologic response to neoadjuvant chemotherapy in patients with osteosarcoma. Medicine. 2018;97:e12318. https://doi.org/10.1097/MD.0000000000012318.
37. Murphey MD, Senchak LT, Mambalam PK, et al. From the radiologic pathology archives: Ewing sarcoma family of tumors: radiologic-pathologic correlation. Radiographics. 2013;33:803–31. https://doi.org/10.1148/rg.333135005.
38. Coppola A, Albano D, Messina C, et al. Imaging of bone tumors of the spine: radiologic-pathologic correlation. J Radiol Rev. 2019;6 https://doi.org/10.23736/S2283-8376.19.00187-6.
39. Mar WA, Taljanovic MS, Bagatell R, et al. Update on imaging and treatment of Ewing sarcoma family tumors. J Comput Assist Tomogr. 2008;32:108–18. https://doi.org/10.1097/RCT.0b013e31805c030f.

40. Gitto S, Corino VDA, Annovazzi A, et al. 3D vs. 2D MRI radiomics in skeletal Ewing sarcoma: feature reproducibility and preliminary machine learning analysis on neoadjuvant chemotherapy response prediction. Front Oncol 12. 2022; https://doi.org/10.3389/fonc.2022.1016123.
41. Sobic Saranovic DP, Nikitovic M, Saponjski J, et al. Post-treatment FDG PET/CT predicts progression-free survival in young patients with small round blue cell tumors: Ewing sarcoma and PNET. Eur J Radiol. 2020;129:109076. https://doi.org/10.1016/j.ejrad.2020.109076.
42. Santegoeds RGC, Temel Y, Beckervordersandforth JC, et al. State-of-the-art imaging in human Chordoma of the Skull Base. Curr Radiol Rep. 2018;6:16. https://doi.org/10.1007/s40134-018-0275-7.
43. Farsad K, Kattapuram SV, Sacknoff R, et al. Sacral Chordoma. Radiographics. 2009;29:1525–30. https://doi.org/10.1148/rg.295085215.
44. Sciubba DM, Chi JH, Rhines LD, Gokaslan ZL. Chordoma of the spinal column. Neurosurg Clin N Am. 2008;19:5–15. https://doi.org/10.1016/j.nec.2007.09.006.
45. Santos P, Peck KK, Arevalo-Perez J, et al. T1-weighted dynamic contrast-enhanced MR perfusion imaging characterizes tumor response to radiation therapy in Chordoma. Am J Neuroradiol. 2017;38:2210–6. https://doi.org/10.3174/ajnr.A5383.
46. Park S-A, Kim HS. F-18 FDG PET/CT evaluation of Sacrococcygeal Chordoma. Clin Nucl Med. 2008;33:906–8. https://doi.org/10.1097/RLU.0b013e31818c4e88.
47. Kim J-H, Lee SK. Classification of chondrosarcoma: from characteristic to challenging imaging findings. Cancers (Basel). 2023;15:1703. https://doi.org/10.3390/cancers15061703.
48. Lloret I, Server A, Bjerkehagen B. Primary spinal chondrosarcoma: radiologic findings with pathologic correlation. Acta Radiol. 2006;47:77–84. https://doi.org/10.1080/02841850500406852.
49. Ollivier L. Imaging of chondrosarcomas. Cancer Imaging. 2003;4:36–8. https://doi.org/10.1102/1470-7330.2003.0022.
50. Murphey MD, Walker EA, Wilson AJ, et al. From the archives of the AFIP. Radiographics. 2003;23:1245–78. https://doi.org/10.1148/rg.235035134.
51. Sharif B, Lindsay D, Saifuddin A. The role of imaging in differentiating low-grade and high-grade central chondral tumours. Eur J Radiol. 2021;137:109579. https://doi.org/10.1016/j.ejrad.2021.109579.
52. Gitto S, Cuocolo R, Emili I, et al. Effects of Interobserver variability on 2D and 3D CT- and MRI-based texture feature reproducibility of cartilaginous bone tumors. J Digit Imaging. 2021;34:820–32. https://doi.org/10.1007/s10278-021-00498-3.
53. Gitto S, Annovazzi A, Nulle K, et al. X-rays radiomics-based machine learning classification of atypical cartilaginous tumour and high-grade chondrosarcoma of long bones. EBioMedicine. 2024;101:105018. https://doi.org/10.1016/j.ebiom.2024.105018.
54. Gitto S, Cuocolo R, Albano D, et al. MRI radiomics-based machine-learning classification of bone chondrosarcoma. Eur J Radiol. 2020;128:109043. https://doi.org/10.1016/j.ejrad.2020.109043.
55. Gitto S, Cuocolo R, Annovazzi A, et al. CT radiomics-based machine learning classification of atypical cartilaginous tumours and appendicular chondrosarcomas. EBioMedicine. 2021;68:103407. https://doi.org/10.1016/j.ebiom.2021.103407.
56. Fanciullo C, Gitto S, Carlicchi E, et al. Radiomics of musculoskeletal sarcomas: a narrative review. J Imaging. 2022;8:45. https://doi.org/10.3390/jimaging8020045.
57. Annovazzi A, Anelli V, Zoccali C, et al. 18F-FDG PET/CT in the evaluation of cartilaginous bone neoplasms: the added value of tumor grading. Ann Nucl Med. 2019;33:813–21. https://doi.org/10.1007/s12149-019-01392-3.
58. Derlin T. Imaging of multiple myeloma: current concepts. World J Orthop. 2014;5:272. https://doi.org/10.5312/wjo.v5.i3.272.
59. Albano D, Benenati M, Bruno A, et al. Imaging side effects and complications of chemotherapy and radiation therapy: a pictorial review from head to toe. Insights Imaging. 2021;12:76. https://doi.org/10.1186/s13244-021-01017-2.
60. Lecouvet FE, Vekemans M-C, Van Den Berghe T, et al. Imaging of treatment response and minimal residual disease in multiple myeloma: state of the art WB-MRI and PET/CT. Skeletal Radiol. 2022;51:59–80. https://doi.org/10.1007/s00256-021-03841-5.

Extra-Spinal Cementation and Screw Fixation

2

Federico Torre, Antonella Castrignano, Sylvain Guinebert, Giuseppe Guzzardi, Edouard Herin, and Mathieu Liberatore

2.1 Introduction

Percutaneous screw fixation has emerged as a pivotal technique in interventional radiology, offering a minimally invasive approach to stabilizing skeletal structures compromised by fractures, metastatic lesions, or degenerative conditions [1–4]. As imaging technology [5, 6] and procedural precision have advanced [7–9] this technique has become an essential tool for radiologists involved in musculoskeletal interventions.

This chapter provides an in-depth analysis of the biomechanical principles underlying percutaneous screw fixation [10–12], particularly in relation to the pelvis and axial skeleton. The distribution of gravitational and mechanical forces plays a crucial role in determining fixation strategies [13–15], ensuring optimal stability, and mitigating risks of hardware failure. Understanding the interplay between compressive, tensile, and shear forces is fundamental for achieving effective structural reinforcement in vulnerable skeletal regions.

A detailed discussion is presented on anatomical considerations, procedural planning, and technical execution. Key topics include imaging guidance for precise screw placement, selection of screw type and trajectory, and the integration of

Supplementary Information The online version contains supplementary material available at https://doi.org/10.1007/978-3-032-00018-7_2.

F. Torre (✉) · A. Castrignano · G. Guzzardi · E. Herin · M. Liberatore
Radiology and Interventional Radiology Department, Princess Grace Hospital Center, Monaco, Monaco
e-mail: federico.torre@chpg.mc; antonella.castrignano@chpg.mc; giuseppe.guzzardi@chpg.mc; herin.e@chu-nice.fr; ; mathieu.liberatore@chpg.mc

S. Guinebert
Musculoskeletal Biology, Bioengineering and Bioimaging (B3OA), UMR7052 U1271, Paris, France

C. Pusceddu, S. Marsico (eds.), *Malignant Bone Lesions and Beyond*,
https://doi.org/10.1007/978-3-032-00018-7_2

adjunct techniques such as cement augmentation [16, 17]. The role of percutaneous screw fixation in managing pathological fractures, particularly in oncological cases, is also explored, emphasizing its impact on patient mobility, pain relief, and overall prognosis [18–21].

By addressing both theoretical and practical aspects, this chapter aims to equip radiology specialists with the knowledge required to perform percutaneous screw fixation safely and effectively. The integration of biomechanical principles with cutting-edge imaging modalities underscores the importance of a multidisciplinary approach in optimizing patient outcomes in interventional musculoskeletal radiology [22–24].

2.2 Biomechanical Load Transfer in the Skeleton and Pelvis

The distribution of gravitational forces on the skeleton and pelvic ring is fundamental to human biomechanics. Below are described the key principles of gravitational load transmission through the skeleton and pelvis: [25, 26].

Gravitational Forces on Skeleton

Gravity acts along the body's longitudinal axis, generating compressive loads on the bone structures. The distribution of forces varies depending on posture and movement:

- In an upright position, body weight is distributed along the spine and transferred through the pelvis to the lower limbs.
- While walking or running, the load changes dynamically, with oscillations in ground reaction forces and joint torsions.
- While sitting, the force is redistributed through the ischium and spine, increasing pressure on the intervertebral discs.

Distribution of Forces on the Pelvic Ring

The pelvic ring, composed of the ilium, ischium, pubis, and sacroiliac joints, is essential for force transmission between the trunk and lower limbs.

Ascending and Descending Forces

- The weight of the upper body is transmitted through the spine and unloaded onto the sacroiliac joints.
- Ground reaction forces rise from the lower limbs and are absorbed by the pelvis before being transferred to the spine.
- Stabilizing Effect of Joints and Muscles: The sacroiliac joints play a key role in dissipating shear and torsional forces; muscles such as the gluteus medius and piriformis stabilize the hip, while the pelvic floor provides support and resistance to internal loads (such as abdominal pressure).

Distribution in Different Postures:

- Standing: The pelvic ring balances the weight between the right and left sides.
- Walking: Compression and torsion alternate with hip movement.
- Sitting: The load is concentrated on the ischial tuberosities, reducing stress on the sacroiliac joints.

In summary, gravity influences the biomechanics of the skeleton and pelvic ring, which function as support and force transmission structures between the trunk and lower limbs, ensuring stability and efficient movement.

The biomechanical analysis of the pelvic ring involves studying the forces, bony structures, joints, and soft tissues that contribute to the stability and functionality of the pelvis.

2.3 Structure of Pelvic Ring

The pelvic ring comprises:

- Bones: Ilium, ischium, pubis (collectively forming the hip bones), sacrum, and coccyx.
- Joints: Sacroiliac joints, pubic symphysis, and lumbosacral joints.
- Ligaments: Anterior and posterior sacroiliac ligaments, sacrotuberous and sacrospinous ligaments, pubic ligaments, and iliolumbar ligaments.
- Muscles: Stabilizing muscles such as the pelvic floor muscles (levator ani and coccygeus), core muscles (transversus abdominis, obliques), and gluteal muscles.

2.4 Pathologies and Clinical Implications

- Pelvic Fractures: Can compromise the stability of the pelvic ring and may require surgical fixation.
- Sacroiliac Joint Dysfunctions: Cause lumbopelvic pain and postural alterations.
- Pelvic Floor Weakness: Can lead to urinary incontinence or prolapse.

Understanding the biomechanical aspects of the pelvic ring is essential for rehabilitation, injury prevention, and the design of orthopedic prostheses or supports.

2.5 Histology of Bone Metastases

Bone metastases result from the spread of tumor cells from a primary cancer to bone tissue, altering normal bone architecture through processes of osteolysis, osteogenesis, or a combination of both [27].

Histologically, bone metastases exhibit different characteristics depending on the origin of the tumor and the type of bone alteration they cause:

(a) Osteolytic Metastases (Bone Destruction).
  - Typical Examples: Breast, lung, kidney, and thyroid cancers.
  - Mechanism: Tumor cells secrete factors that activate osteoclasts, leading to bone resorption.
  - Histological Features: Increased number of activated osteoclasts, enlarged Howship's lacunae (due to high osteoclastic activity), loss of normal bone matrix, and tumor cells infiltrating between bone trabeculae.

(b) Osteoblastic Metastases (Abnormal Bone Formation).
  - Typical Examples: Prostate cancer, some breast and gastrointestinal cancers.
  - Mechanism: Tumor cells stimulate osteoblasts, leading to excessive but disorganized bone formation.
  - Histological Features: Thickened but disorganized trabecular bone, presence of hyperactive osteoblasts, and deposits of immature (osteoid) bone.

(c) Mixed Metastases (Osteolytic and Osteoblastic).
  - Typical Examples: Breast cancer and some sarcomas.
  - Mechanism: Coexistence of bone destruction and new bone formation.
  - Histological Features: Areas of bone resorption adjacent to irregular bone formation, simultaneous presence of active osteoclasts and osteoblasts, and altered trabecular architecture.

2.6 Structural Changes in Bone Tissue

Bone metastases profoundly alter bone tissue structure, affecting its strength and biomechanical function [28].

(a) Changes in Osteolytic Metastases.
  - Loss of bone density, with reduced mineral content.
  - Mechanical weakening, increasing the risk of pathological fractures.
  - Disorganization of bone trabeculae, with marrow spaces filled by tumor cells.

(b) Changes in Osteoblastic Metastases.
  - Trabecular thickening, but with a disorganized and less resistant structure.
  - Increased bone stiffness, leading to paradoxical fragility and risk of microfractures.
  - Decreased bone matrix quality, with irregular mineralization.

(c) Changes in Mixed Metastases.
  - Alternating areas of osteolysis and osteosclerosis, creating a highly heterogeneous bone structure.
  - Increased bone fragility, with a high risk of complex fractures.
  - Modification of bone marrow composition, often replaced by tumor cells and fibrotic tissue.

The histology of bone metastases varies depending on the type of tumor and its interaction with the bone microenvironment. Changes in bone tissue structure compromise its mechanical strength, increasing the risk of fractures and pain, with significant implications for patient treatment and prognosis [28].

Bone metastases are a common complication in cancer patients, significantly impacting both quality of life and healthcare costs. In the United States, the economic burden associated with managing bone metastases is particularly significant.

According to the American Cancer Society, approximately 1.6 million new cases of malignant tumors were diagnosed in the United States in 2013, with about half having a predisposition to develop bone metastases. Additionally, cases of myeloma and bone lymphoma contribute to a total of approximately 174,000 patients with skeletal involvement.

A study estimated that the economic burden for managing patients with bone metastases in the United States amounts to approximately $12.6 billion per year. This highlights that patients experiencing skeletal-related events (SREs) incur significantly higher medical costs than those without such complications [11, 13].

Bone metastases represent a major challenge for the US healthcare system, both clinically and economically. The high costs associated with their management underscore the need for effective preventive strategies and targeted therapeutic interventions to reduce the incidence of skeletal-related events and improve patients' quality of life.

2.7 Literature Review

Cementoplasty is a minimally invasive procedure that involves injecting an acrylic cement Polymethylmethacrylate (PMMA) into weakened bone to provide stabilization and pain control. This technique is commonly used to treat lytic bone lesions, such as bone metastases, which can cause significant pain and increase the risk of pathological fractures. However, cementoplasty alone may not provide adequate stabilization in areas subjected to torsional or shear forces, such as the pelvis and femoral neck. In these cases, the combination of cementoplasty with percutaneous screw fixation, known as cement-augmented osteosynthesis, represents an innovative and effective approach. This combination improves the resistance of the cement to mechanical stress, offering greater structural stability.

Deschamps et al. [29–31] have shown that percutaneous cement-augmented osteosynthesis is a safe and effective technique for stabilizing lytic sacral lesions, with significant clinical improvement in terms of pain relief and functionality after one month of treatment. Moreover, the combination of percutaneous screw fixation and cement injection, guided by imaging, has been recognized as an innovative, effective, safe, and minimally invasive approach for fragile patients with lytic bone metastases.

In the literature, numerous studies describe the combined technique of cementoplasty and screw fixation for the treatment of pathological fractures. There is a fairly widespread consensus regarding the indications for this procedure. The patient's clinical condition is crucial, particularly the presence of pain, reduced mobility, impaired ambulation, or prolonged bed rest. The latter can lead to numerous complications, such as thromboembolic diseases and infections, which can have devastating consequences for extremely fragile patients. Therefore, not only a significant reduction in quality of life but also an increased risk of mortality constitute the primary indications for performing an interventional radiology procedure.

Of course, the clinical assessment must be supported by radiological findings at multiple levels. Every pain and symptom must be justified by the presence of a metastasis capable of causing such pain, with radiological semeiotics as clear as possible in favor of a secondary localization. As previously mentioned, metastases can appear as lytic, sclerotic, or mixed lesions. Purely sclerotic lesions rarely lead to pathological fractures, whereas this is far more common in the presence of lytic or mixed lesions (Deschamps et al. [31]).

Regarding force distribution, biomechanics plays a crucial role in the decision to perform combined osteoplasty and screw fixation. If the compressive forces acting on the pelvic bone are accompanied by torsional forces and shear stress, cement alone proves ineffective and must be combined with screws.

Thus, beyond the clinical assessment and the radiological evaluation of metastasis nature and extension, understanding the biomechanics of force distribution is essential for tailoring the optimal treatment for each anatomical site. For instance, the vertebral body of S1 cannot be considered biomechanically or therapeutically equivalent to the posteroinferior portion of the sacral wings [32].

The outcome of a treatment adapted to the type of lesion is described in the literature as a reduction in pain, an improvement in quality of life, and a return to as normal mobility as possible [33].

This study therefore demonstrated a statistically significant reduction in postprocedure pain, with a decreasing trend in the consumption of morphine-based medications. Additionally, patients were able to resume daily activities or at least maintain an adequate weight-bearing position approximately 48 h after the procedure. Dien et al. [34] even reported that nearly all patients in their study (a multicenter study on 138 patients) were able to walk within 24 h.

The benefit to the patient is therefore significant, particularly in terms of quality of life. The complication rate reported in the literature is relatively low. The use of CT guidance, the ability to plan and monitor screw placement, and the proper distribution of cement help prevent technical failures and complications related to the injury of sensitive anatomical structures near the surgical site.

However, some complications have been described, including disease progression around the implanted material, postoperative infection requiring material removal, and subcutaneous or muscular hematomas [35].

A key advantage, given the low complication rate and minimal invasiveness, is the ability to continue chemotherapy, radiotherapy, or hormone therapy without delay after the procedure [36].

2.8 Approach to the Percutaneous Consolidation of a Pelvic Lesion

Every patient undergoing treatment, whether a simple cementoplasty or one combined with screw fixation, must be discussed in a dedicated multidisciplinary meeting for the assessment of bone lesions. This meeting involves interventional radiologists, radiation oncologists, oncologists, orthopedic surgeons, rehabilitation specialists, palliative care professionals, and a nursing representative.

During the multidisciplinary meeting, several aspects are evaluated, including the type of pain, the characteristics of the bone lesion in relation to the primary tumor, the contribution of various imaging modalities (such as PET-CT, MRI, and CT), and the available therapeutic options, all supported by solid scientific literature.

Once an interventional radiology treatment is collectively indicated, the patient undergoes a specialist consultation to receive a detailed explanation of the surgical technique, its advantages, potential complications, and postoperative management after hospital discharge. It is crucial to perform the procedure within the first few weeks following the multidisciplinary discussion, particularly in the presence of lytic lesions at risk of fracture and highly aggressive histological patterns.

In general, a combined and integrated approach involving interventional radiology, chemotherapy, and radiotherapy is always preferable. While surgery remains the best option for structural and biomechanical integrity, it carries a significant perioperative burden, especially for frail patients. Radiotherapy is excellent for pain control but has limited efficacy in ensuring stability.

In this context, interventional radiology plays a crucial role [37, 38], as it can effectively address both biomechanical and pain-related aspects while remaining a well-tolerated procedure for patients.

2.8.1 Technique

The procedure is performed under general anesthesia or spinal anesthesia for the pelvis and lower limbs in a dedicated interventional suite equipped with CT or cone-beam CT combined with fluoroscopy. A preprocedure scan is acquired to further assess the lesion and optimize the procedural planning. It is essential to determine the entry point of the material on the skin, at the bone level, and the screw trajectory, ensuring that sensitive anatomical structures such as nerves and blood vessels are preserved.

Once the surgical landmarks are established, they are marked on the patient's skin under complete aseptic conditions. A Chiba needle is positioned in contact with the periosteum. An 8G, 15 cm trocar is then inserted using the Chiba needle as a guide and advanced into the bone under combined CT and fluoroscopic guidance.

In patients undergoing corticosteroid treatment and presenting with lytic lesions, the trocar is advanced manually. However, in cases of mixed lesions with a sclerotic component, a surgical hammer may be necessary to facilitate its progression.

Once the trocar is fully inserted, in order to reach the distal part of the lesion, the inner cannula is removed, and a Kirschner-type guidewire is placed inside the working cannula. The guidewire is then advanced with light hammer taps until it reaches the predetermined point. At this stage, after a volumetric CT check, it is possible to select the exact screw size down to the millimeter.

In addition to the size, the type of screw must be determined:

- Fully Threaded Screw: It is used when the screw serves only as a core around which the cement can diffuse, and there is no fracture.
- Partially Threaded Screw: It is chosen when the goal is to join the two ends of a fracture, creating a metallic bridge.

The selected screw is then slid over the guidewire with the help of a cannulated screwdriver, after removing the outer part of the trocar. If necessary, a second screw can be inserted afterward.

Regarding cementoplasty, the procedure involves inserting a 13- Gauge trocar into the lesion, following a parallel or perpendicular approach to the screw under combined CT and fluoroscopic guidance. Once positioned, cement (PMMA) is injected until optimal filling of the lesion is achieved, ensuring distribution to the adjacent healthy bone for better anchorage.

In the following examples, the various treatment possibilities and combinations will be described based on anatomical localization and the forces acting on them.

2.9 Adapted Technique According to Biomechanical Features

2.9.1 Vertebra S1

The vertebral body of S1 is crucial in transmitting loads from the spine to the sacroiliac joints. The totality of forces acting on the sacral promontory are compressive forces. Secondary tumor lesions located at this level can therefore benefit from a simple cementoplasty via a transpedicular or trans-iliac approach, as explained in Figs. 2.1a, b, 2.2a, b, 2.3a–d, and 2.4a, b.

2.9.2 SI Joints and Sacral Ala

The sacroiliac joints and sacral wings are essential in transmitting forces to the pelvis. There are two biomechanically important areas:

- The anterior and middle parts of the sacroiliac joints are primarily subjected to compressive forces, so a simple sacroplasty is sufficient to restore integrity and stability.
- The dorsal and cranial parts, however, are subjected to tensile and shear stresses, meaning that cementoplasty alone would not be sufficient. Therefore, adding screws is mandatory to enhance stability.

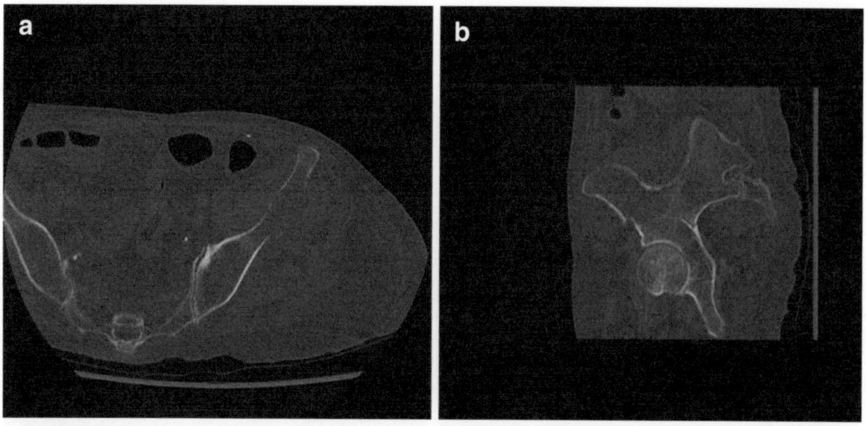

Fig. 2.1 Preoperative CT evaluation of an osteolytic lesion of the left iliac bone. (**a**) Axial CT section showing a well-defined osteolytic lesion characterized by significant cortical thinning and disruption of normal trabecular bone structure. (**b**) Sagittal CT reconstruction illustrating lesion localization, size, and relationship to adjacent anatomical structures, supporting the indication for percutaneous screw fixation combined with cementoplasty

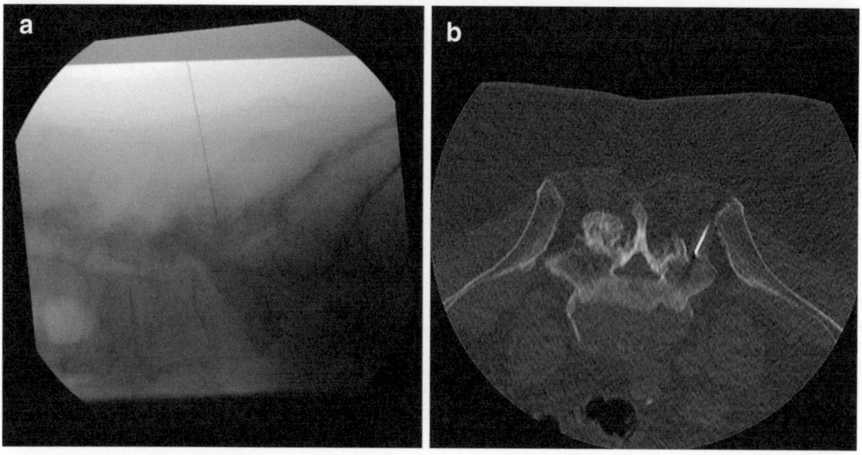

Fig. 2.2 Intraprocedural fluoroscopic and axial CT-guided placement of a break-away tip Chiba needle into the posteromedial facet of the interapophyseal joint at S1. (**a**) Fluoroscopic views demonstrating stepwise progression of a 20-gauge, 15 cm Chiba needle (break-away tip) toward the posteromedial facet, serving simultaneously for step-by-step local anesthesia and accurate guidance of the trocar through the Chiba needle. (**b**) Corresponding axial CT images confirming controlled and precise advancement of the Chiba needle tip into the targeted cortical region of the posteromedial facet, ensuring proper positioning for subsequent guidewire function after detachment of the needle head

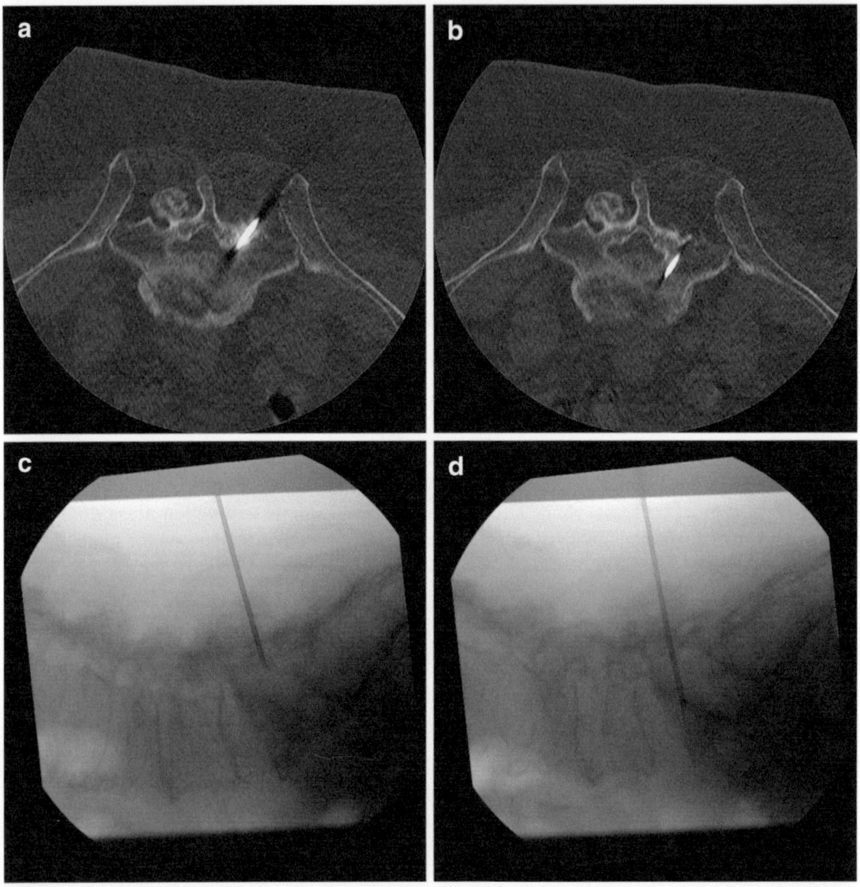

Fig. 2.3 Intraprocedural axial CT and fluoroscopic imaging demonstrating insertion and placement of the trocar. (**a**, **b**) Axial CT images illustrating controlled progression of an 11-gauge, 15 cm t'am trocar (Thiebaud Biomedical Devices, Margencel, France) through the previously positioned Chiba needle guide, and precise trajectory into the lesion under the S1 endplate, verifying optimal placement prior to cement injection. (**c**, **d**) Sequential lateral fluoroscopic images confirm the accurate final positioning of the trocar tip centrally within the osteolytic lesion

Cadaveric studies show that placing two parallel trans-sacroiliac screws in S1 and S2, combined with sacroplasty, provides the strongest mechanical resistance. The advantage of sacroplasty is to improve stability and prevent potential screw loosening (Figs. 2.5a, b, 2.6a–d, 2.7a, b).

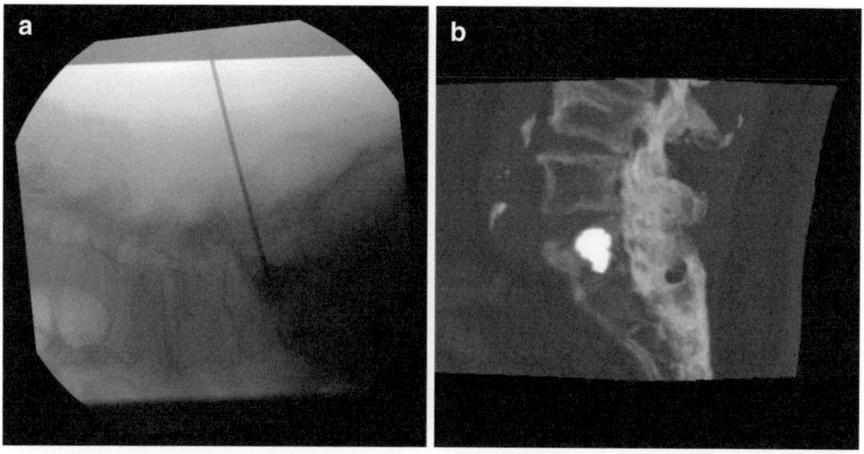

Fig. 2.4 Intraprocedural fluoroscopic control and postprocedural CT imaging confirming successful cementoplasty of the S1 osteolytic lesion. (**a**) Real-time lateral fluoroscopic control image during cement injection, demonstrating progressive and homogeneous filling of the lesion without cement leakage or extravasation. (**b**) Postprocedural lateral Maximum Intensity Projection (MIP) CT reconstruction confirming complete and correct filling of the lesion, with no evidence of procedural complications

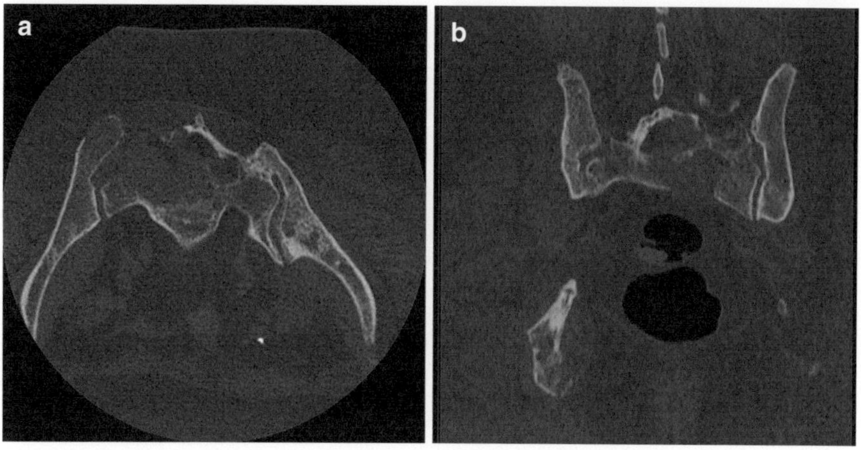

Fig. 2.5 Preprocedural CT evaluation showing an extensive osteolytic lesion of the left sacral ala associated with pelvic ring instability. (**a**) Axial CT image demonstrating a large osteolytic lesion involving the left sacral wing, which is characterized by extensive posterior cortical disruption and direct extension into the S1 and S2 sacral neural foramina. (**b**) Coronal CT reconstruction highlighting the full extent of the lesion, illustrating the inferior cortical breaches, and confirming neural foramina involvement, responsible for structural weakening, pelvic instability, and clinical symptoms of pain

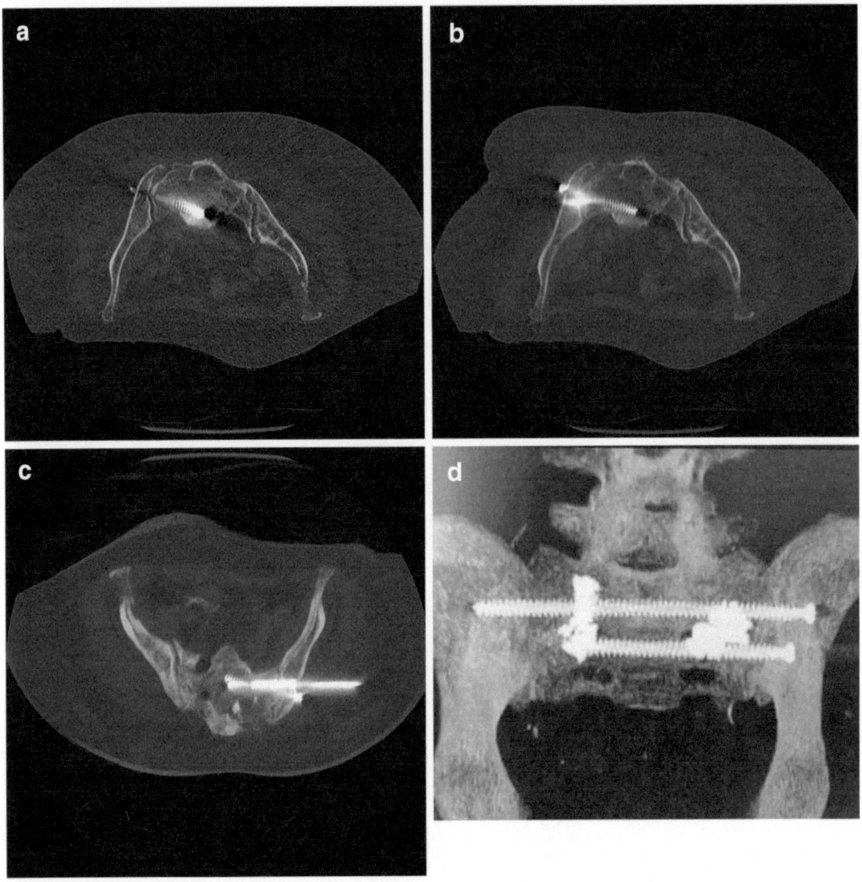

Fig. 2.6 Intraprocedural axial CT guidance demonstrating trans-sacral screw placement for stabilization of the left sacral osteolytic lesion. (**a, b**) Axial CT images illustrating controlled progression of a trans-sacroiliac screw inserted from the left iliac bone, crossing through the osteolytic lesion, with the screw tip securely anchored in healthy trabecular bone of the contralateral right sacral ala. This strategic positioning creates a bridging construct through the lesion, restoring biomechanical stability and force transmission across the compromised pelvic ring. (**c, d**) Axial and coronal MIP CT reconstructions confirm the accurate and stable placement of screws at the S1 and S2 levels, ensuring optimal mechanical reinforcement and correction of pelvic instability

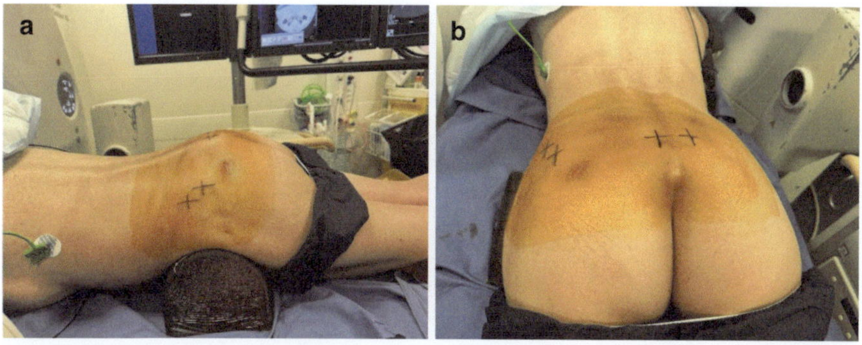

Fig. 2.7 Patient positioning for sacral percutaneous procedures. (**a**) Lateral view showing the patient in the prone (ventral decubitus) position with proper alignment. (**b**) Close-up view of pelvic support placement to elevate the pelvis and optimize exposure of the sacrum, ensuring a favorable trajectory for fluoroscopic or CT-guided sacral access

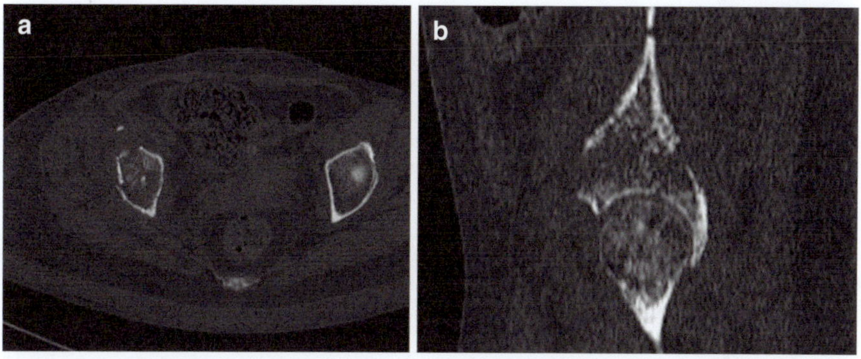

Fig. 2.8 Preoperative CT evaluation of Harrington grade I lytic lesion of the acetabular roof with non-displaced fracture. (**a**) Axial CT image (bone window) demonstrating a lytic lesion affecting the acetabular roof with a subtle, non-displaced fracture line. (**b**) Sagittal CT reconstruction confirming the lesion's extent and the fracture orientation within the acetabular roof

2.9.3 Acetabulum

The acetabulum plays a crucial role in transmitting forces to the lower limbs, especially the supra-acetabular area, also known as the acetabular roof, which corresponds to the superior and lateral portion of the acetabulum.

Compressive forces are primarily concentrated on the lateral side, while tensile forces act on the medial side. For this reason, any lytic lesion located in this key area for force distribution must always be reinforced, as the risk of fracture is extremely high.

The literature extensively describes the use of cementoplasty, which provides good biomechanical stabilization. Additionally, an increasing number of studies report combining screw fixation with cementoplasty, anchoring the screws into healthy bone. However, no clear superiority of this combined approach over cement alone has been demonstrated.

If the lytic lesion erodes both cortices of the acetabular roof, surgery is the only viable option (Figs. 2.8a, b, 2.9a, b, 2.10a–d, and 2.11).

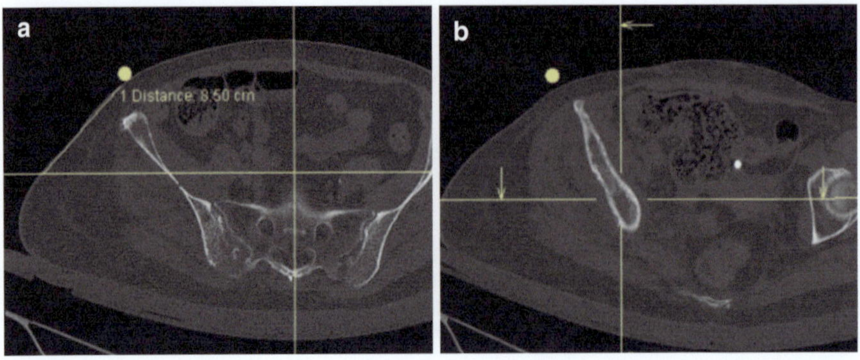

Fig. 2.9 Axial CT identification of trocar entry point. (**a**) Axial CT image showing the anatomical landmarks used to localize the anterosuperior iliac crest. (**b**) Axial CT image illustrating the planned downward trajectory from the iliac crest toward the acetabular roof and ensuring safe and targeted trocar access to the lesion

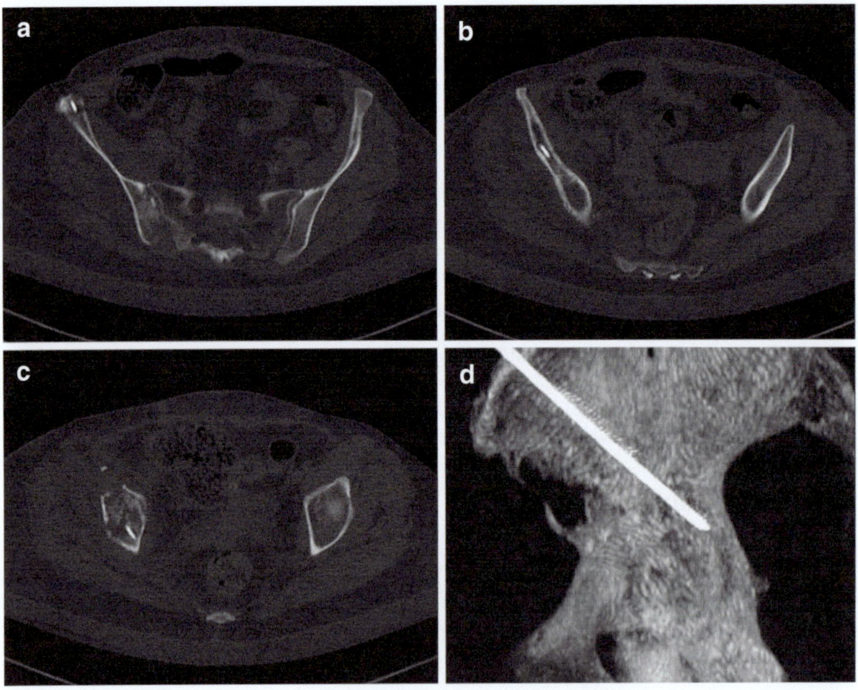

Fig. 2.10 CT-guided progression and positioning of the trocar toward the acetabular roof. (**a, b**) Axial CT image showing the initial advancement of the trocar along the planned downward trajectory, guided by the iliac cortical walls. (**c**) Axial CT image demonstrating the trocar tip reaching healthy trabecular bone beneath the acetabular roof, ensuring optimal anchorage for screw placement. (**d**) Sagittal MIP CT reconstruction confirming the overall trajectory and depth of the trocar, aligned with the axis of the acetabular roof for precise stabilization

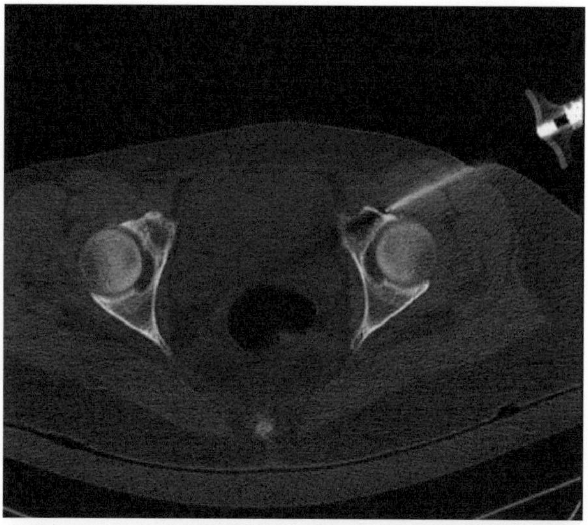

Fig. 2.11 Axial CT image demonstrating direct acetabular positioning of a second trocar for targeted cementoplasty. This image shows the precise placement of a second t'am trocar (Thiebaud Biomedical Devices) into the distal osteolytic lesion, positioned to allow cement injection around the tip of the screw that will be inserted through the primary access route

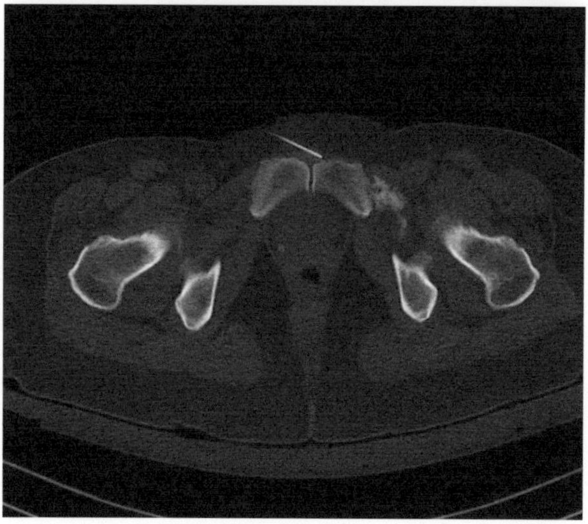

Fig. 2.12 CT-guided Chiba placement. This image demonstrates the advancement of a 20-gauge, 15 cm break-away tip Chiba needle (Thiebaud Biomedical Devices) along the preplanned trajectory, serving both for sequential local anesthesia and as a guidewire for subsequent trocar placement

2.9.4 Iliopubic Ramus

The iliopubic branch and, to a lesser extent, the ischiopubic branch can be sites of pathological fractures, as they provide support for the insertion of numerous muscle groups.

In a healthy patient, an iliopubic fracture heals and consolidates without specific treatment. However, in the case of a pathological fracture, the insertion of a screw, possibly combined with distal cementoplasty, can be proposed to relieve pain and enable ambulation (Figs. 2.12, 2.13a–c, 2.14a–c, and 2.15a–d, Video 2.1 (Pelvis–Screw 1)).

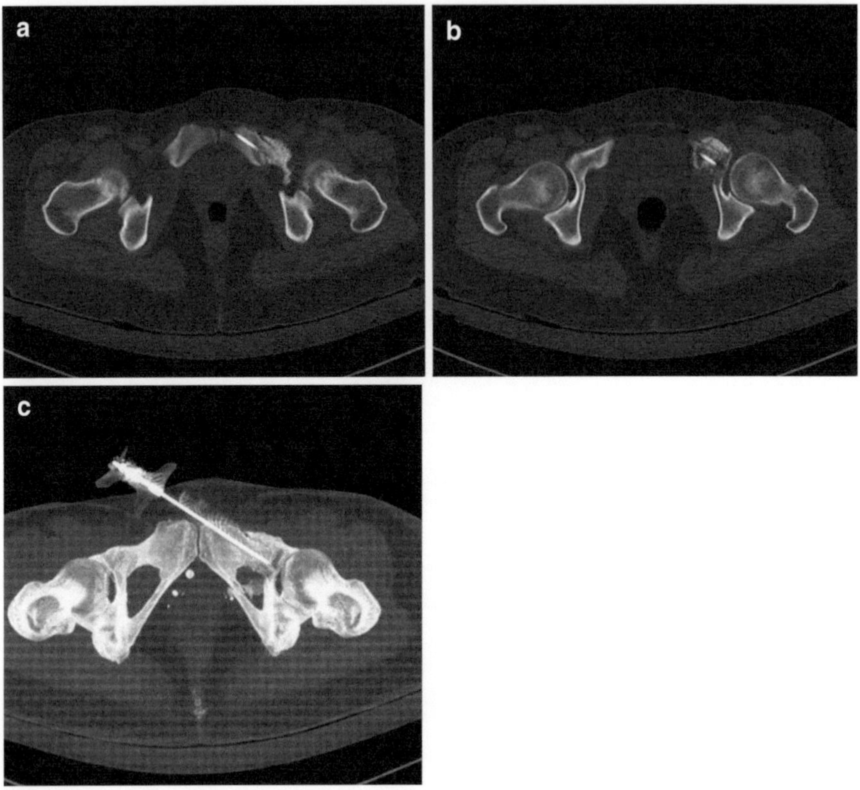

Fig. 2.13 CT-guided trocar insertion in left pubic branch lesion. (**a, b**) Axial CT images showing progressive advancement of the t'am trocar (Thiebaud Biomedical Devices) transfixing the osteolytic lesion and reaching healthy trabecular bone. (**c**) Axial MIP CT reconstruction illustrating the complete trajectory and confirming the correct final positioning of the trocar for effective stabilization

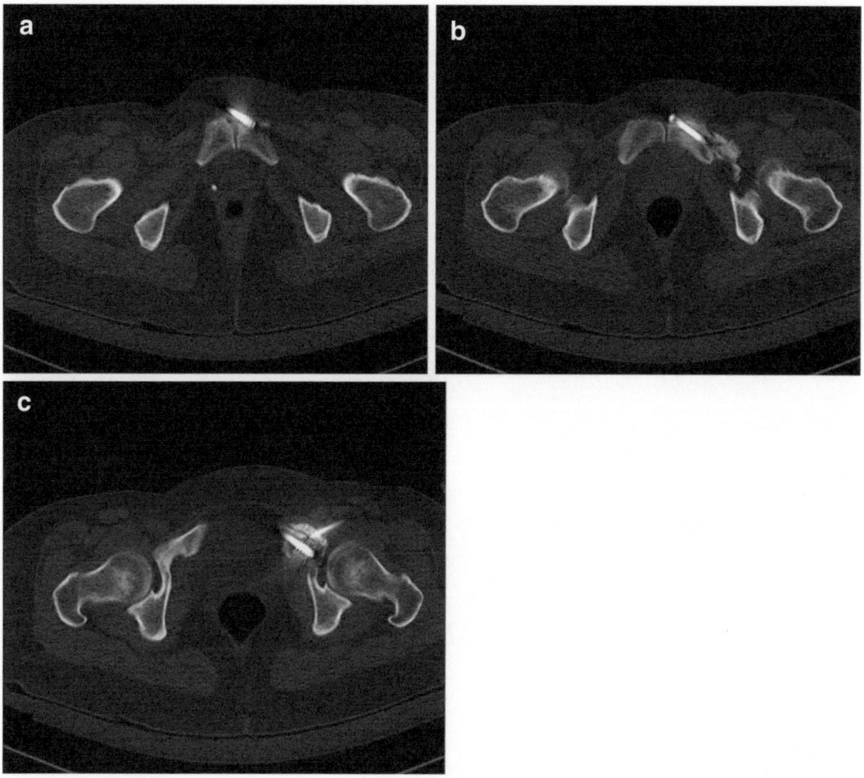

Fig. 2.14 Axial CT images demonstrating sequential progression of the screw along the fractured left pubic branch. (**a**) Initial axial CT image showing the screw's entry at the proximal aspect of the fractured pubic branch. (**b**) Intermediate axial CT image illustrating further advancement of the screw along the fracture line within the osteolytic lesion. (**c**) Final axial CT image confirming the screw's optimal positioning, effectively stabilizing the fracture and providing internal support

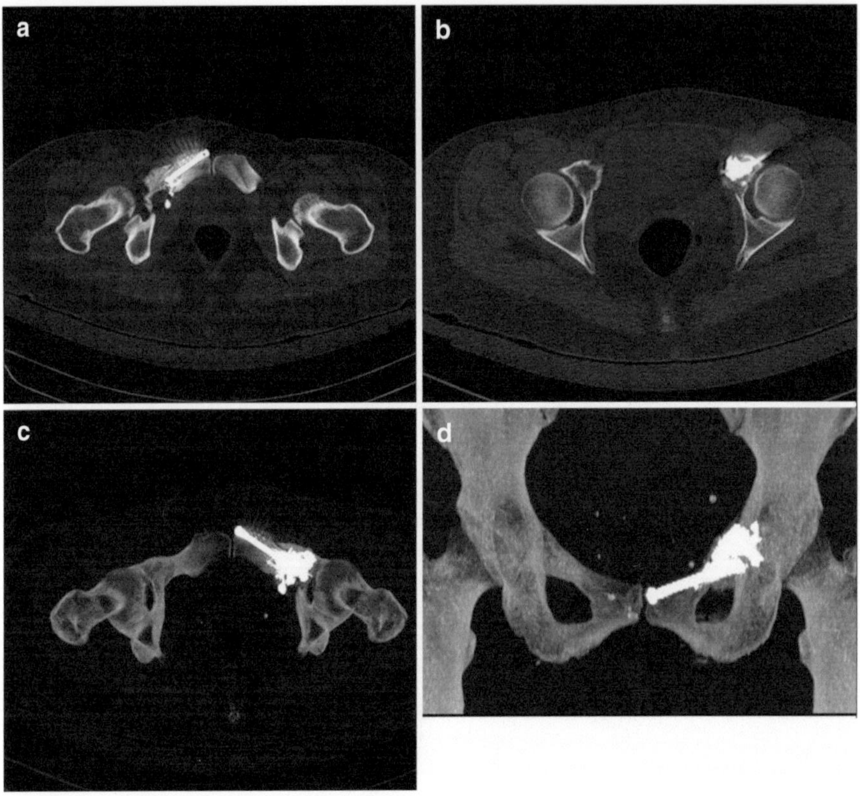

Fig. 2.15 Postprocedural CT evaluation of screw and cement placement in the left pubic branch. (**a, b**) Axial CT images demonstrating correct placement of the screw and cement, with a minimal, asymptomatic leak of cement into the obturator foramen. (**c, d**) Axial and coronal MIP reconstructions illustrating the overall stabilization, with effective cement distribution reinforcing the fracture and minimizing the risk of further osteolytic progression

2.9.5 Iliac Wing

The iliac wing, despite its marginal role in load transmission, can be the site of painful pathological fractures, as it serves as an insertion point for numerous muscle groups.

These fractures are usually associated with large lytic lesions extending to the cortices, making them difficult to treat with simple cementoplasty. The combined use of screws and cement enhances the stability of the iliac wing and any resulting pathological fractures (Figs. 2.16a, b, 2.17a–d, 2.18a–c, and 2.19a–c). Video 2.2 (Pelvis–Screw 3 and pelvis–screw detail).

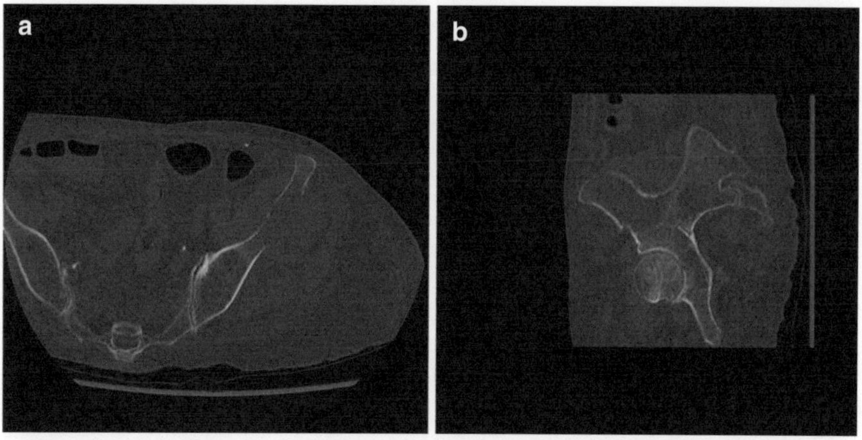

Fig. 2.16 Preoperative CT evaluation of an osteolytic lesion of the left iliac bone. (**a**) Axial CT section showing a well-defined osteolytic lesion characterized by significant cortical thinning and disruption of normal trabecular bone structure. (**b**) Sagittal CT reconstruction illustrating lesion localization, size, and relationship to adjacent anatomical structures, supporting the indication for percutaneous screw fixation combined with cementoplasty

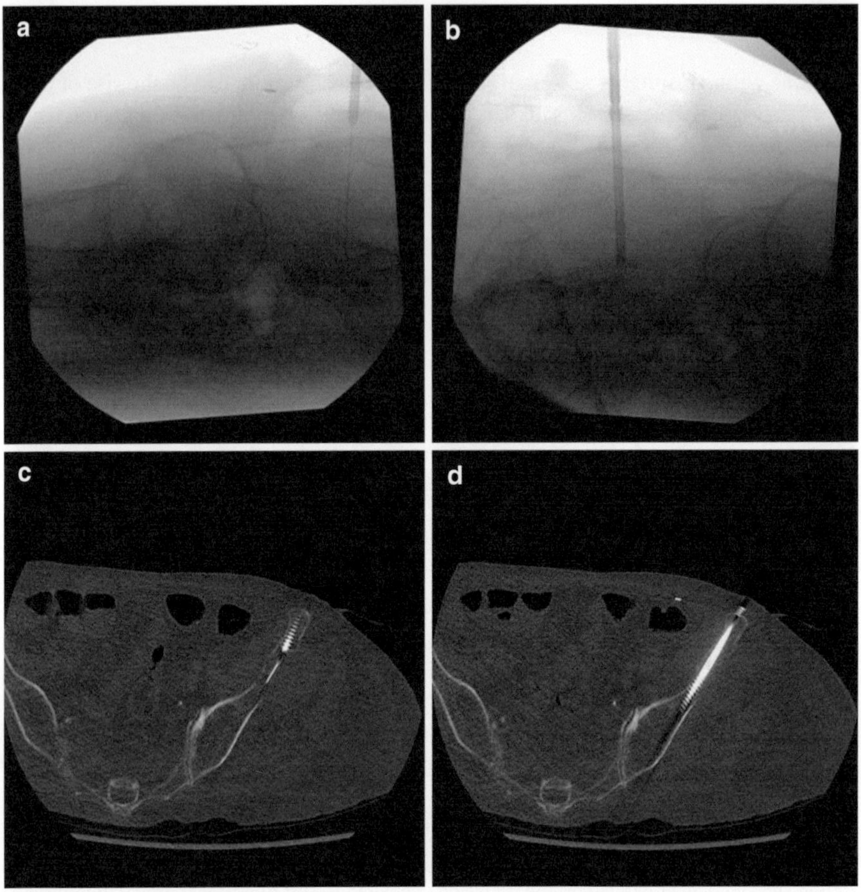

Fig. 2.17 Intraprocedural fluoroscopic and CT guidance illustrating percutaneous insertion of a Synthes bone screw into the osteolytic lesion using a Chiba needle as a guidewire. (**a, b**) Sequential lateral fluoroscopic images demonstrating the progression and placement of a 20-gauge, 15 cm Chiba needle (break-away tip), acting as a Kirschner-type guidewire, followed by advancement of a cannulated, self-drilling, self-tapping bone screw (Synthes Gesellschaft mit beschränkter Haftung (GmbH), Oberdorf, Switzerland, 6.5 mm diameter, 60 mm length) into the lesion. (**c, d**) Corresponding axial CT images confirming precise co-axial positioning of both the Chiba needle and the bone screw, verifying proper screw trajectory and placement within the iliac osteolytic lesion

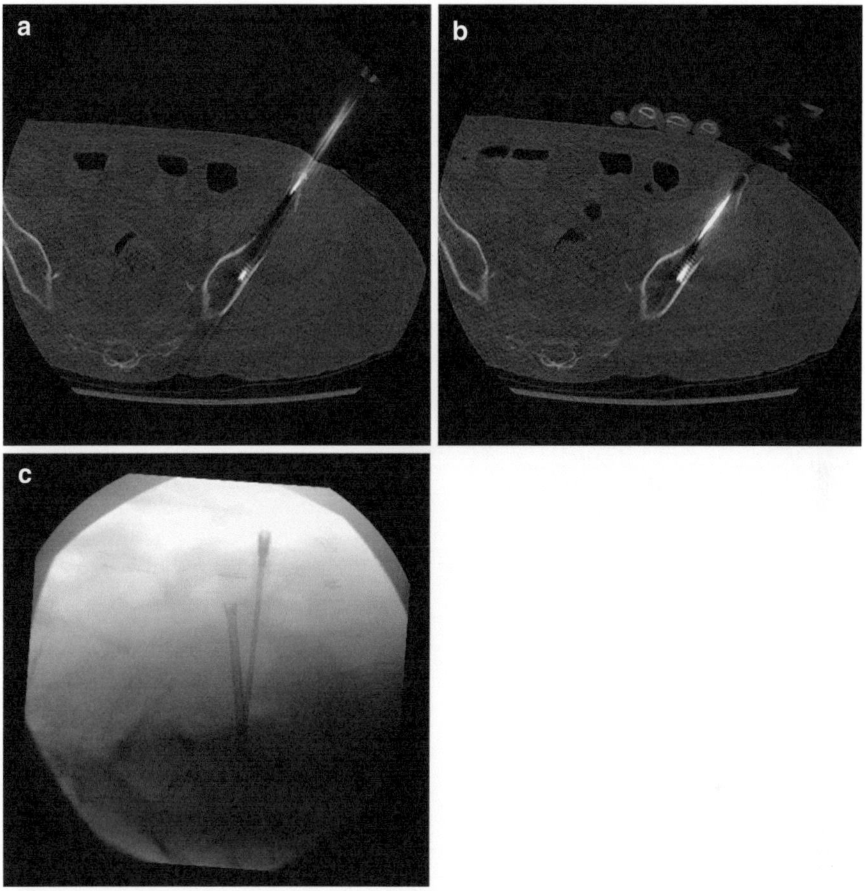

Fig. 2.18 Intraprocedural axial CT and fluoroscopic imaging illustrating trocar placement for cementoplasty within the osteolytic lesion of the left iliac bone. (**a, b**) Axial CT images demonstrating insertion and precise positioning of the 11-gauge-15 cm t'am trocar (Thiebaud Biomedical Devices, Margencel, France) within the lesion, verifying accurate trajectory prior to cement injection. (**c**) Lateral fluoroscopic image confirming the trocar position adjacent and parallel to the previously inserted bone screw, ensuring optimal cement consolidation and mechanical reinforcement of the fixation

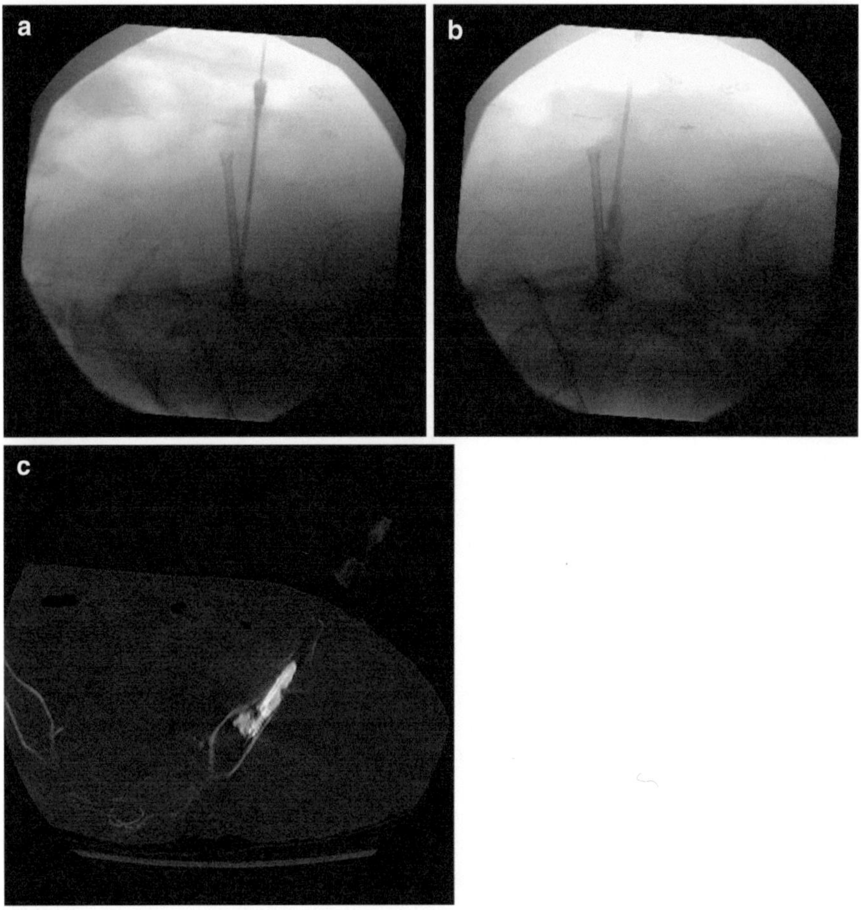

Fig. 2.19 Intraprocedural fluoroscopic and postprocedural CT imaging demonstrating cementoplasty of the left iliac osteolytic lesion. (**a**) Initial lateral fluoroscopic view showing injection of polymethylmethacrylate cement via the previously positioned trocar. (**b**) Subsequent fluoroscopic image demonstrating progressive cement injection during controlled withdrawal of the trocar, ensuring homogeneous filling and mechanical reinforcement around the inserted bone screw. (**c**) Postprocedural axial CT control confirming satisfactory cement distribution within the lesion, optimal integration around the screw fixation, and absence of procedural complications such as cement leak

2.9.6 Clinical Case

A lytic lesion of the femoral neck cannot be considered an intended fracture of the pelvic ring. However, the femur is the first step—the site where all forces from the pelvis are discharged. A high-risk lesion at the femoral neck represents a challenge for the interventional radiologist if the patient cannot undergo surgery.

The femoral neck is subjected to compressive forces and shear stress, making the ideal treatment a combination of screws and cement. Special metal rods can also be used to create a structure—a metallic core—around which cement is injected to restore functional integrity.

It is preferable to introduce two screws and anchor them into healthy bone using a lateral approach through the greater trochanter (Figs. 2.20a–c, 2.21a–b, 2.22, and 2.23a–c).

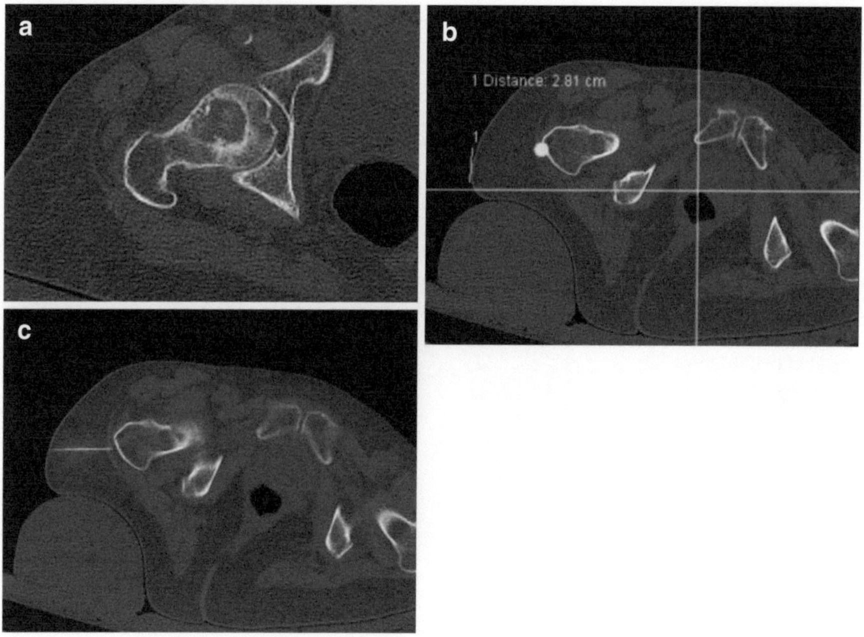

Fig. 2.20 Preprocedural CT evaluation of an osteolytic lesion of the femoral head and neck at high risk of pathological fracture. (**a**) Axial CT image showing a well-defined osteolytic lesion involving the femoral neck and extending into the femoral head, with cortical thinning and structural compromise. (**b**) Axial CT image used for preprocedural planning, demonstrating the optimal trajectory for trocar insertion into the femoral neck and head. The pathway is carefully aligned to cross the osteolytic lesion while avoiding neurovascular structures, ensuring safe and effective access for screw placement and cementoplasty. (**c**) Insertion of a 20-gauge, 15 cm Chiba needle under image guidance. The needle is advanced to perform sequential local anesthesia down to the femoral bone. Once at the cortical surface, the Chiba serves as a guidewire for subsequent trocar placement, ensuring a safe and accurate trajectory toward the osteolytic lesion

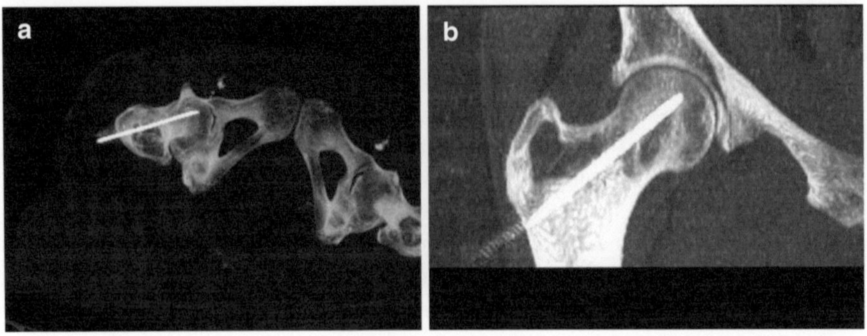

Fig. 2.21 MIP CT reconstructions confirming accurate trocar placement through the femoral osteolytic lesion. (**a**) Axial MIP CT image demonstrating correct alignment of the trocar traversing the osteolytic lesion within the femoral neck and reaching subchondral intact trabecular bone of the femoral head. (**b**) Coronal MIP reconstruction confirming appropriate depth and orientation of the trocar, ensuring optimal positioning for subsequent cement injection while avoiding articular cartilage breach

Fig. 2.22 Axial CT images showing final hardware positioning within the femoral head and neck. Axial CT image showing a second trocar (t'am Thiebaud Biomedical Devices, Margencel, France) positioned adjacent to the screw, providing access for cementoplasty to reinforce the surrounding bone and enhance mechanical stability

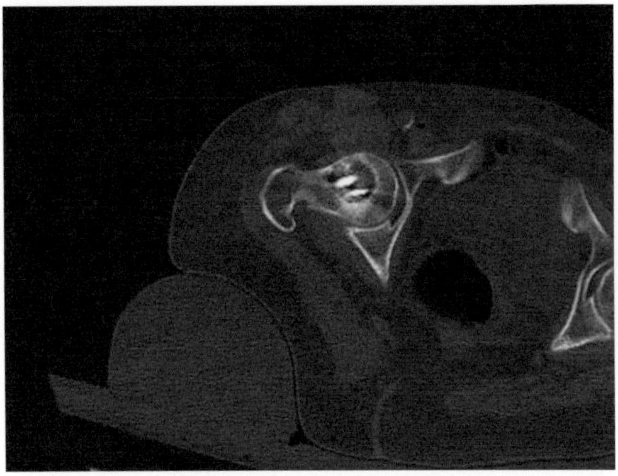

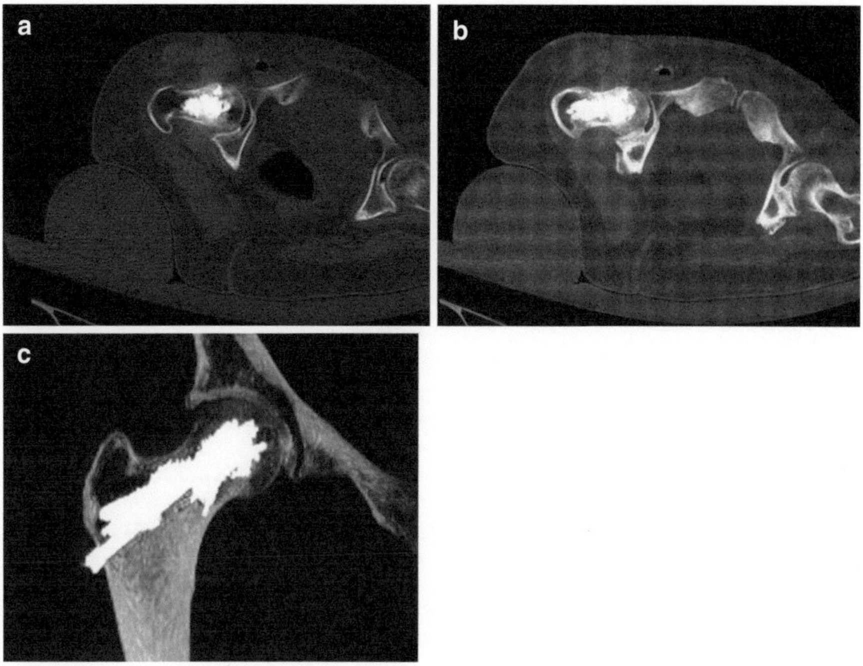

Fig. 2.23 Postprocedural CT control confirming successful cementoplasty of the femoral head and neck lesion. (**a, b**) Axial CT images showing homogeneous filling of the osteolytic lesion with polymethylmethacrylate (PMMA) cement, fully encompassing the screw and providing robust reinforcement of the surrounding trabecular bone. (**c**) Coronal MIP CT reconstruction confirming appropriate cement distribution around the pin and within the lesion, with no evidence of cement leakage or procedural complication, and optimal implant positioning for biomechanical support

2.10 Conclusion

Percutaneous screw fixation, particularly when combined with cementoplasty, represents a pivotal advancement in the management of skeletal fragility due to metastatic disease and pathological fractures. This technique offers a tailored biomechanical solution that effectively balances structural stabilization with the imperative to minimize procedural morbidity, especially critical in frail and oncologic patients.

By integrating biomechanical principles, histopathological understanding of bone metastases, and advanced imaging guidance, interventional radiologists can optimize screw placement, select the most appropriate fixation strategies, and enhance the distribution of mechanical forces through compromised skeletal regions. The adaptability of percutaneous screw fixation across diverse anatomical sites—such as the sacrum, acetabulum, iliac wing, and femoral neck—underscores its versatility and clinical utility.

Furthermore, the low complication rate, rapid postprocedural recovery, and the potential to maintain continuity of systemic oncologic therapies position this technique as an essential tool in multidisciplinary cancer care. Its role is not limited to structural support but extends to improving patient quality of life, reducing pain, restoring mobility, and preventing skeletal-related events.

Ultimately, successful outcomes depend on accurate biomechanical assessment, meticulous preprocedural planning, and precise technical execution. As interventional radiology continues to evolve, percutaneous screw fixation—especially when guided by robust anatomical, biomechanical, and pathological understanding—will remain at the forefront of minimally invasive musculoskeletal oncology.

References

1. Pusceddu C, Fancellu A, Ballicu N, et al. CT-guided percutaneous screw fixation plus cementoplasty in the treatment of painful bone metastases with fractures or a high risk of pathological fracture. Skeletal Radiol. 2017;46:539–45 .
2. Kurup AN, Callstrom MR. Expanding role of percutaneous ablative and consolidative treatments for musculoskeletal tumors. Clin Radiol. 2017;72:645–56.
3. Buy X, Cazzato RL, Catena V, Roubaud G, Kind M, Palussiere J. Techniques de consolidation osseuse guidée par imagerie en oncologie: cimentoplastie et vissage. Bull Cancer. 2017;104(5):423–32.
4. Hesler M-C, Buy X, Catena V, et al. Assessment of risk factors for occurrence or worsening of acetabular fracture following percutaneous cementoplasty of acetabulum malignancies. Eur J Radiol. 2019;120:108694.
5. Amoretti N, Thariat J, Nouri Y, et al. Imaging of bone metastases. Bull Cancer. 2013;100:1109–14.
6. Morse AS, Gonzalez MR, Kang HP, et al. Comparison of percutaneous techniques for stabilization of osteolytic lesions of the periacetabular region due to metastatic bone disease. Ann Surg Oncol. 2025;32:1529–40.
7. Iannessi A, Amoretti N, Marcy P-Y, Sedat J. Percutaneous cementoplasty for the treatment of extraspinal painful bone lesions, a prospective study. Diagn Interv Imaging. 2012;93:859–70.
8. Assouline J, Tselikas L, Roux C, et al. Prophylactic percutaneous consolidation of large osteolytic tumors of the pelvic ring using fixation by internal cemented screws. Radiol Imaging Cancer. 2021;3:e200137.
9. Cazzato RL, Dalili D, De Marini P, et al. Bone consolidation: a practical guide for the interventional radiologist. Cardiovasc Intervent Radiol. 2023;46:1458–68.
10. Enneking WF. The anatomic considerations in turner surgery: pelvis. Musculoskelet Turner Surg. 1983;2:483–529.
11. Dindo D, Demartines N, Clavien P-A. Classification of surgical complications: a new proposal with evaluation in a cohort of 6336 patients and results of a survey. Ann Surg. 2004;240:205–13.
12. Garnon J, Jennings J, Meylheuc L, et al. Biomechanics of the osseous pelvis and its implication for consolidative treatments in interventional oncology. Cardiovasc Intervent Radiol. 2020;43:1589–99.
13. Jawad MU, Scully SP. In Brief. Classifications in brief. Mirels' classification: metastatic disease in long bones and impending pathologic fracture. Clin Orthop. 2010;468:2825–7.
14. Damron TA, Mann KA. Fracture risk assessment and clinical decision making for patients with metastatic bone disease. J Orthop Res. 2020;38:1175–90.
15. Le Corroller T, Arrigoni F. ESR essentials: percutaneous bone consolidation – practice recommendations by the European Society of Musculoskeletal Radiology. Eur Radiol. 2025.
16. Moulin B, Tselikas L, De Baere T, et al. CT guidance assisted by electromagnetic navigation system for percutaneous fixation by internal cemented screws (FICS). Eur Radiol. 2020;30:943–9.

17. Amoretti N, Hovorka I, Marcy P-Y, et al. Computed axial tomography-guided fixation of sacroiliac joint disruptions: safety, outcomes, and results at 3-year follow-up. Cardiovasc Intervent Radiol. 2009;32:1227–34.
18. Deschamps F, Farouil G, Hakime A, et al. Cementoplasty of metastases of the proximal femur: is it a safe palliative option? J Vase Interv Radiol. 2012;23:1311–6.
19. Rosenthal D, Callstrom MR. Critical review and state of the art in interventional oncology: benign andv metastatic disease involving bone. Radiology. 2012;262:765–80.
20. Wood TJ, Racano A, Yeung H, et al. Surgical management of bone metastases: quality of evidence and systematic review. Ann Surg Oncol. 2014;21:4081–9.
21. Hindiskere S, Kim H-S, Han I. Postoperative delirium in patients undergoing surgery for bone metastases. Medicine (Baltimore). 2020;99:e20159.
22. Yevich S, Tselikas L, Kelekis A, et al. Percutaneous management of metastatic osseous disease. Chin Clin Oncol. 2019;8:62.
23. Dassa M, Roux C, Tselikas L, et al. Image-guided percutaneous fixation with internal cemented screws of impending femoral neck pathologic fractures in patients with metastatic cancer. Safety, efficacy, and durability. Radiology. 2020;297:721–9.
24. Cornelis FH, Petitpierre F, Fabre T, et al. Percutaneous low-pressure bone stenting to control cement deposition in extensive lytic lesions. Eur Radiol. 2017;27:3942–6.
25. Tsuzuki S, Park SH, Eber MR, et al. Skeletal complications in cancer patients with bone metastases. Int J Urol. 2016;23:825–32.
26. Randall RL. Metastatic bone disease: an integrated approach to patient care. New York: Springer; 2016.
27. Li S, Peng Y, Weinhandl ED, et al. Estimated number of prevalent cases of metastatic bone disease in the US adult population. Clin Epidemiol. 2012;4:87–93.
28. Saad F, Lipton A, Cook R, et al. Pathologic fractures correlate with reduced survival in patients with malignant bone disease. Cancer. 2007;110:1860–7.
29. Deschamps F, de Baere T, Hakime A, et al. Percutaneous osteosynthesis in the pelvis in cancer patients. Eur Radiol. 2016;26:1631–9.
30. Bennard E, Foti P, Kastler A, Amoreni N. Percutaneous vertebroplasty under local anaesthesia: feasibility regarding patients' experience. Eur Radiol. 2017;27:1512–6.
31. Deschamps F, Yevich S, Gravel G, et al. Percutaneous fixation by internal cemented screw for the treatment of unstable osseous disease in cancer patients. Semin Interv Radiol. 2018;35:238–47.
32. Garnon J, Jennings JW. Percutaneous consolidation for extraspinal osteolytic lesions: to cementoplasty and beyond. J Vase Interv Radiol. 2020;31:659–60.
33. Letty Q, Grange R, Bertholon S, et al. Percutaneous fixation with internal cemented screws for iliac lytic bone metastases: assessment of pain and quality of life on long term follow-up. Cardiovasc Intervent Radiol. 2024;47:980–90.
34. Dien E, Stacoffe N, Pavan LJ, et al. Restoring mobility: roles of percutaneous consolidation for pelvic ring bone lesions – a multicenter study. Eur Radiol. 2024.
35. Roux C, Tselikas L, Yevich S, et al. Fluoroscopy and cone-beam CT-guided fixation by internal cemented screw for pathologic pelvic fractures. Radiology. 2019;290:418–25.
36. Dien E, Stacoffe N, Pavan LJ, et al. Restoring mobility: roles of percutaneous consolidation for pelvic ring bone lesions – a multicenter study. Eur Radiol. 2024
37. Dekimpe C, Andreani O, De Dompsure RB, et al. CT-guided fixation of pelvic fractures after high-energy trauma, by interventional radiologists: technical and clinical outcome. Eur Radiol. 2020;30:961–70.
38. Bertholon S, Grange R, Thomas T, et al. Combination of percutaneous screw fixation and cementoplasty for lytic bone metastases: feasibility, safety and clinical outcomes. Cardiovasc Intervent Radiol. 2022;45:1129–33.

3 Spinal Procedures: Vertebroplasty, Kyphoplasty, and Vertebral Implants

Salvatore Marsico and Claudio Pusceddu

3.1 Introduction

The vertebral column is the most common site of skeletal metastases, involved in up to 70% of patients with systemic malignancy and in as many as 90% of patients at autopsy with advanced cancer [1, 2]. Among these, thoracic vertebrae are most frequently affected (60–80%), followed by lumbar and cervical regions [2]. Vertebral metastases commonly arise from breast, prostate, lung, renal, and thyroid cancers, while hematologic malignancies such as multiple myeloma and lymphoma frequently involve the spine with diffuse osteolysis and risk of collapse [1, 3].

Pathological fractures occur in approximately 20–40% of patients with spinal metastases and may result in severe pain, kyphotic deformity, and sometimes neurologic deficits due to spinal canal encroachment [3]. These events are associated with reduced mobility, opioid dependency, and may delay or prevent continuation of systemic oncologic therapies [1]. Standard treatments include analgesia, corticosteroids, and radiotherapy [2]. However, these approaches may be inadequate for patients with mechanical instability, rapid disease progression, or poor tolerance to medication [3].

S. Marsico (✉)
Department of Radiology, Hospital del Mar, Barcelona, Spain

Interventional Oncology Institute, Barcelona, Spain

C. Pusceddu
Department of Radiology, Mater Olbia Hospital, Olbia, Cagliari, Italy

Interventional Oncology Institute, Barcelona, Spain

C. Pusceddu, S. Marsico (eds.), *Malignant Bone Lesions and Beyond*,
https://doi.org/10.1007/978-3-032-00018-7_3

3.1.1 The Role of Percutaneous Image-Guided Interventions

Percutaneous image-guided procedures, including vertebroplasty and kyphoplasty, have become established techniques for the treatment of painful vertebral compression fractures in cancer patients [3–5]. They provide rapid pain relief, improve quality of life, and are associated with low complication rates when performed in experienced centers. Vertebroplasty consists of the injection of polymethylmethacrylate (PMMA) cement into the vertebral body, exerting its effect through mechanical stabilization and thermal/chemical denervation [6]. Kyphoplasty adds a balloon tampering step to create an intravertebral cavity, restore height, and possibly reduce cement leakage [7]. More recently, vertebral implants such as SpineJack®, KIVA® Vertebral Compression Fracture (VCF) Implant System (KIVA), and Vertebral Body Stent (VBS®) have demonstrated efficacy in height restoration and load distribution with encouraging outcomes [8]. The 2017 and 2022 CIRSE Standards of Practice support vertebral augmentation for vertebral metastases and myeloma-related fractures in patients with pain refractory to conservative management or radiation therapy. They also endorse cementoplasty combined with ablation in patients with radioresistant or oligometastatic disease [9, 10]. The 2020 ESMO Clinical Practice Guidelines for bone health in cancer patients recommend vertebroplasty and kyphoplasty as safe and effective interventions for painful vertebral fractures [11]. According to international Myeloma Treatment Pathways, vertebral augmentation is a first-line option even in the absence of collapse, aimed at preserving mobility and limiting opioid use [12].

3.1.2 Identifying Candidates: The Spinal Instability Neoplastic Score (SINS)

The Spinal Instability Neoplastic Score (SINS) was developed to assess instability in patients with spinal neoplastic disease [13]. It evaluates six categories:

1. Location of the lesion
2. Pain characteristics (mechanical vs. nonmechanical)
3. Bone lesion quality (lytic, blastic, and mixed)
4. Radiographic spinal alignment
5. Vertebral body collapse
6. Posterolateral involvement

The total score ranges from 0 to 18:

- 0–6: Stable
- 7–12: Indeterminate (potentially unstable)
- 13–18: Unstable

SINS correlates well with treatment decisions, especially in defining the need for percutaneous versus surgical intervention. It has been validated in multicenter studies and shows high interobserver reliability [13].

3.2 Indications and Patient Selection (Fig. 3.1)

Proper patient selection is essential to ensure the clinical success and safety of percutaneous vertebral interventions. Indications for vertebroplasty, kyphoplasty, and vertebral implant placement must be grounded in a combination of clinical, imaging, and oncologic criteria. These procedures are primarily indicated for:

- Painful vertebral compression fractures secondary to malignant disease (metastasis, myeloma).
- Mechanical instability, particularly when the SINS score exceeds 6 [6].
- Inadequate response to conservative management or radiation therapy.
- Urgent need to restore mobility and functional autonomy to enable continuation of systemic cancer treatment.

CIRSE guidelines [9, 10] define the key indications for percutaneous cementoplasty as:

- Intractable mechanical pain from vertebral body lesions.
- High risk of fracture progression due to osteolytic destruction.
- Pathologic fractures compromising biomechanics, even in the absence of neurological symptoms.
- Adjunctive use in conjunction with ablative therapies in oligometastatic or radioresistant tumors.

Inclusion Criteria
- Localized vertebral pain with mechanical features.
- Imaging-confirmed lytic or mixed vertebral lesions with or without fracture.
- Intact posterior vertebral wall or limited cortical disruption.
- ECOG performance status 0–3.
- Platelet count $>50 \times 10^9$/L and INR <1.5 if not corrected.

Exclusion Criteria
- Complete vertebral body collapse with loss of height >80%.
- Extensive posterior wall destruction with epidural mass or spinal cord compression.
- Active systemic infection or uncorrected coagulopathy.
- Severe neurologic symptoms requiring urgent decompression.

	Indication	Description	Supporting Literature
1	Painful vertebral compression fractures	Fractures due to metastases or myeloma with mechanical pain refractory to medical/radiation therapy	Anselmetti et al. 2005; CIRSE 2017; ESMO 2020
2	Mechanical instability (SINS >6)	Segmental instability identified via SINS score indicating need for stabilization	Fourney et al. 2011; CIRSE 2022
3	Oligometastatic/radioresistant tumors	Tumors less responsive to radiotherapy may benefit from cementoplasty and adjunctive ablation	CIRSE 2022; Pusceddu et al. 2023
4	Multiple vertebral lesions in myeloma	Diffuse or focal osteolytic lesions in plasma cell disorders with high risk of collapse	McDonald et al. 2008; Hirsch et al. 2022
5	Failure of conservative or radiation therapy	Persistent pain or loss of mobility after adequate non-invasive treatment	ESMO 2020; Myeloma UK Pathway 2020
6	Prevention of collapse in osteolytic metastases	Lesions from renal, breast, thyroid tumors with impending collapse or instability	Noriega et al. 2021; Marcia et al. 2022
7	Benign vertebral pathology (select cases)	Cases of hemangiomas or refractory osteoporotic fractures unresponsive to other therapy	Filippiadis et al. 2017

Fig. 3.1 Indications for vertebral augmentation in oncologic patients
This table summarizes the primary clinical indications for vertebroplasty, kyphoplasty, and vertebral implant placement in patients with malignant spinal involvement. Indications are supported by major guidelines and clinical studies and include mechanical instability, painful compression fractures, failure of conservative therapy, and disease-specific considerations such as multiple myeloma and radioresistant metastases. The integration of literature sources provides an evidence-based framework for appropriate patient selection

3.3 Preprocedural Planning and Imaging (Fig. 3.2)

- Accurate preprocedural planning is a cornerstone of successful intervention. It involves a comprehensive clinical evaluation and a multimodality imaging assessment.
- Imaging Modalities
  - MRI: Gold standard for evaluating soft tissue involvement, vertebral edema, and spinal canal status. It is essential for identifying cord compression, epidural extension, and bone marrow infiltration [14–16].
  - CT scan: Ideal for assessing cortical integrity, degree of lysis, fracture morphology, and for precise planning of needle trajectory [17].
  - PET-CT: Useful for staging, especially in cases of unknown primary, and identifying metabolically active lesions in multimetastatic disease [18].

	Category	Component	Description
1	Imaging Modality	MRI	Evaluation of spinal canal, epidural extension, bone marrow edema, and soft tissue involvement
2	Imaging Modality	CT	Assessment of cortical integrity, lytic destruction, fracture morphology, and needle path planning
3	Imaging Modality	PET-CT	Identification of metabolically active lesions and staging in patients with unknown or disseminated disease
4	Planning Element	Pain-to-lesion correlation	Confirm lesion responsible for symptoms and match with imaging findings
5	Planning Element	SINS score calculation	Evaluate mechanical stability and determine need for augmentation
6	Planning Element	Vertebral morphology	Assess vertebral height loss, kyphosis, cortical breach, and alignment
7	Planning Element	Approach planning	Select transpedicular, parapedicular, or extrapedicular access based on anatomy
8	Planning Element	Multilevel evaluation	Check adjacent vertebrae for potential treatment during the same session
9	Planning Element	Need for biopsy	Plan image-guided biopsy if lesion is atypical or ablation is considered
10	Procedural Setup	Anesthesia choice	Use local anesthesia with conscious sedation; general anesthesia for multilevel or complex cases
11	Procedural Setup	Imaging guidance	Fluoroscopy (biplanar) or CT navigation mandatory for accuracy and safety
12	Procedural Setup	Equipment preparation	Confirm availability of cement system, ablation device if needed, and backup tools
13	Risk Management	Informed consent	Explain risks: cement leakage, embolism, neural damage, adjacent fractures

Fig. 3.2 Procedural planning and setup overview for vertebral augmentation
This table provides a comprehensive breakdown of the key components involved in preprocedural evaluation and intraoperative setup for vertebroplasty, kyphoplasty, and vertebral implant procedures. It is structured into four thematic sections:

Imaging modalities: Describes the role of MRI, CT, and PET-CT in evaluating lesion characteristics, structural integrity, and metastatic disease burden

Planning elements: Outlines the essential steps for determining lesion relevance, spinal instability (via SINS score), vertebral morphology, and the need for multilevel or biopsy planning

Procedural setup: Summarizes anesthetic strategies, image-guided navigation requirements, and equipment preparation

Risk management: Highlights the importance of informed consent, infection prophylaxis, and preprocedural coagulation assessment

This framework supports clinical decision-making and ensures procedural safety, consistency, and efficacy across oncologic vertebral interventions

- Planning Elements
  - Verify lesion site corresponds with pain location and SINS evaluation.
  - Assess vertebral height, degree of kyphosis, cortical breach, and spinal alignment.
  - Measure pedicle width and choose approach (transpedicular, extrapedicular).
  - Evaluate adjacent levels for potential multilevel treatment.
  - Consider biopsy if lesion etiology is unclear or if ablation is planned.

Integration of SINS
SINS score remains essential to determine eligibility and guide the interventional strategy. Lesions scoring 7–12 should be carefully discussed in a multidisciplinary team to assess the risk of progression. Scores >12 justify vertebral augmentation or hybrid approaches combining stabilization and decompression [13].

Anesthesia and Procedural Environment
Most procedures are performed under local anesthesia with conscious sedation. In high-risk patients or multilevel cases, general anesthesia may be preferred. Image guidance is mandatory—preferably fluoroscopy in two planes and/or CT navigation systems in complex lesions.

Informed Consent and Risk Stratification
Patients should be informed of potential complications, including:

- Cement leakage (up to 30%, mostly asymptomatic).
- Neural injury.
- Pulmonary embolism (rare).
- Adjacent-level fracture due to altered biomechanics.

Prophylactic antibiotics are recommended, and coagulation parameters should be reviewed within 48 hours preprocedure.

3.4 Techniques

3.4.1 Vertebroplasty

Vertebroplasty is a percutaneous interventional procedure in which bone cement (typically polymethylmethacrylate, PMMA) is injected into the vertebral body to stabilize pathologic fractures and provide immediate pain relief. Initially described in the late 1980s for aggressive vertebral hemangiomas, its application rapidly expanded to osteoporotic, metastatic, and myeloma-related fractures [19].

Objectives
- Achieve rapid analgesia through mechanical stabilization.
- Prevent further vertebral collapse.
- Reduce the risk of spinal deformity and instability.

Step-by-Step Technique

1. Patient Positioning: The patient is positioned prone on a radiolucent table. Proper support under the chest and pelvis helps maintain lumbar lordosis.
2. Imaging Setup: Biplanar fluoroscopy is most commonly used. Alternatively, CT or cone-beam CT guidance provides superior anatomical detail and is particularly useful in complex or previously treated vertebrae.
3. Approach Selection [20]:
   - Transpedicular: Standard approach in lumbar and lower thoracic vertebrae.
   - Parapedicular/Paravertebral: Preferred for upper thoracic vertebrae where pedicles are small or distorted.
   - Costovertebral or Extrapedicular: Used in cases of altered anatomy or tumor-related destruction of conventional access routes.
4. Local Anesthesia: Infiltration is performed at the skin and along the needle tract. Conscious sedation is used in most cases, though general anesthesia may be required in complex or multilevel procedures.
5. Needle Advancement: Under real-time fluoroscopic guidance, a bone access needle is advanced into the anterior third of the vertebral body, ideally avoiding cortical breach or posterior wall involvement.
6. Cement Preparation and Injection [21]:
   - PMMA is mixed to achieve a toothpaste-like consistency. Viscosity should be adapted based on lesion size and risk of leakage.
   - Cement types may include standard PMMA, radiopaque variants (barium/zirconium), antibiotic-loaded cement, or high-viscosity cements for controlled injections.
   - Cement is injected under continuous fluoroscopy to monitor spread and detect early signs of leakage. Injection should be halted if cement approaches the posterior wall or venous channels.
7. Postprocedural Care: The patient is monitored for 1–2 h, then mobilized. Most patients experience significant pain relief within 24–72 h.

Cement Types and Properties

PMMA remains the gold standard due to its mechanical strength, ease of handling, and long track record. Newer formulations vary in:

- Viscosity: Low viscosity allows longer working time; high viscosity reduces leakage.
- Radiopacity: Barium or zirconium additives improve visualization.
- Antibiotic loading: Useful in patients at high infection risk.
- Bioactive fillers: Calcium phosphate-based cements are under investigation for biologic remodeling.

Choice of cement depends on lesion characteristics, operator preference, and risk profile [21].

3.4.2 Kyphoplasty

Kyphoplasty is a vertebral augmentation procedure that evolved from vertebroplasty to address two key limitations: lack of vertebral height restoration and increased risk of cement leakage. First introduced in the late 1990s, kyphoplasty incorporates the use of inflatable bone tamps (balloons) to create a cavity within the collapsed vertebral body, enabling partial height restoration and more controlled cement injection. This innovation was particularly driven by the need to correct kyphotic deformity and improve spinal alignment, especially in patients with significant vertebral collapse due to osteolytic tumors or myeloma-related fractures [7].

In oncologic contexts, kyphoplasty plays a critical role in restoring stability and anatomy while also minimizing risks associated with cement extravasation. This is particularly relevant when treating patients with painful vertebral compression fractures that impact daily functioning and quality of life.

Objectives

- Reduce pain through vertebral stabilization.
- Restore lost vertebral body height and correct deformity.
- Reduce risk of cement leakage via cavity creation.

Step-by-Step Technique

1. Patient Positioning: Similar to vertebroplasty, the patient is placed in a prone position with attention to spinal alignment and support.
2. Imaging Setup: Biplanar fluoroscopy is standard, though CT guidance or hybrid imaging (CT + C-arm) can enhance accuracy, especially postablation.
3. Needle Access: Access is gained via a transpedicular or parapedicular route, depending on vertebral level and anatomy. In upper thoracic levels, a paravertebral or extrapedicular approach may be required.
4. Balloon Placement and Inflation:
   - A working cannula is inserted into the vertebral body.
   - An inflatable bone tamp (balloon) is advanced and inflated under fluoroscopic guidance.
   - Inflation compresses cancellous bone and creates a cavity, displacing tumor or necrotic debris.
   - The balloon is then deflated and removed, leaving a void.
5. Cement Injection:
   - PMMA is injected into the cavity at high viscosity, reducing the risk of venous extravasation.
   - The cavity limits lateral or posterior migration, enhancing control.
6. Postprocedural Care: Patients are monitored and mobilized similarly to vertebroplasty.

Advanced Balloon Technologies

- Curved Balloons: Allow bilateral cavity creation from a single unipedicular approach. These are especially useful in narrow pedicles, altered anatomy, or when reducing procedural time and access-related risks is critical.
- Directional Tamps: Newer systems enable height restoration in targeted segments, potentially improving segmental alignment [22–24].

Imaging Considerations

- Cavity creation is monitored in real-time via fluoroscopy or CT.
- Preablation CT helps assess vertebral anatomy and guides safe balloon expansion.
- In cases involving tumor ablation, cavity creation after ablation enables cement injection into the necrotic zone with reduced risk of leakage.

Clinical Outcomes

Kyphoplasty provides pain relief and functional improvement in over 85% of treated patients. In contrast to vertebroplasty, it offers measurable restoration of vertebral body height and correction of kyphosis, especially in fractures with moderate collapse. Its role is particularly significant in vertebral compression fractures from myeloma or metastatic disease with preserved posterior wall integrity [25].

Complications

- Balloon Rupture: Rare, mitigated by using pressure-controlled inflation systems.
- Cement Leakage: Less frequent than in vertebroplasty due to cavity formation and higher cement viscosity.
- Neurological or Embolic Events: Very rare when using proper technique and imaging.

Kyphoplasty expands the therapeutic scope of vertebral augmentation, offering biomechanical and clinical advantages in appropriately selected oncologic patients. The technique is especially advantageous when vertebral height restoration is desirable and cement control is essential [25].

3.4.3 Vertebral Implants

Vertebral implant systems were developed as an evolution of kyphoplasty, aiming to provide not only vertebral height restoration but also long-term internal support through permanent implantable devices. These systems allow cavity formation and mechanical stabilization without the use of inflatable balloons, thus minimizing the trauma associated with balloon inflation and providing a stable structure within the vertebral body prior to cement injection.

The concept was first introduced with mechanical expandable implants that restore height by exerting outward pressure. Unlike kyphoplasty, the cavity is created through the implant itself, which remains in place and supports the vertebral body even before cement injection. These systems have gained popularity due to their biomechanical reliability and reduced risk of height loss postprocedure [26].

Common Systems and Technologies

- SpineJack® (Stryker): Titanium implants inserted bilaterally via transpedicular access. Once deployed, they expand vertically to restore vertebral height and generate a central cavity. Their symmetrical expansion enables balanced load distribution. Cement is injected after mechanical expansion, stabilizing the construct [26].
- VBS® (Vertebral Body Stent, DePuy Synthes): A mesh-like metallic expandable stent inserted bilaterally through a cannula. When deployed, it expands radially to provide circumferential internal support. PMMA is then injected within and around the stent to reinforce the vertebral body, making this ideal for circumferential cortical compromise [27].
- KIVA® System: A coil-shaped PEEK implant inserted percutaneously in a helical fashion via a single unipedicular approach. As the coil is advanced, it displaces cancellous bone laterally, creating a central channel for cement. Its design allows directional control of cement delivery with minimal extrusion [8].
- Stent-Screw-Assisted Internal Fixation (SAIF): Combines bilateral expandable stents with percutaneous pedicle screws, followed by PMMA injection. The technique offers internal vertebral support and segmental fixation, particularly suitable for high-risk vertebral collapse due to severe neoplastic or osteoporotic damage. The screws are inserted directly through the pedicles into the stent-reinforced vertebral body, and cement secures the entire construct [28].

According to CIRSE and recent literature [9, 10], the indications for vertebral implant placement largely mirror those of kyphoplasty:

- Painful vertebral compression fractures from metastases or myeloma.
- Fractures with partial collapse and significant height loss.
- Cases where kyphotic correction is desirable.
- Patients at high risk of recurrent collapse or biomechanical instability.

Technical Approach

- Access: Transpedicular or extrapedicular approach under fluoroscopic or CT guidance.
- Deployment: The implant is delivered in a collapsed configuration and expanded within the vertebral body to restore height and generate a cavity.
- Cement Injection: PMMA or high-viscosity cement is injected around the implant, locking it into place and filling the residual cavity.

Advantages
- Mechanical height restoration without balloon inflation.
- Permanent internal scaffold supports long-term stability.
- Controlled cement distribution with reduced leakage risk.
- Higher compressive resistance and potential reduction in adjacent-level fractures.

Limitations
- Technically more demanding with a steeper learning curve.
- Higher procedural cost.
- Requires careful preprocedural planning to ensure appropriate access and sizing.

3.5 Complications and Management

Despite being minimally invasive and generally well tolerated, spinal augmentation procedures are not devoid of risks. A thorough understanding of potential complications is essential for appropriate patient counseling, procedural planning, and timely intervention.

Cement-Related Complications
- Cement Leakage: Most common complication. This can occur through venous channels, cortical defects, or into intervertebral discs. Though often asymptomatic, leakage into the spinal canal or foramina may cause neurological symptoms.
- Pulmonary Cement Embolism: Rare but potentially life-threatening. Risk increases with low-viscosity cement or rapid injection.
- Embolization into Epidural Veins: May result in spinal cord or nerve root compression [25].

Mechanical Complications
- Adjacent-Level Fractures: Biomechanical stress transfer to adjacent vertebrae can result in new fractures, especially in osteoporotic bone. Incidence ranges from 10% to 20%.
- Vertebral Body Recollapse: Particularly relevant when posterior cortical integrity is compromised or insufficient cement volume is used.
- Implant Migration or Failure: Rare, more relevant in improperly sized or malpositioned vertebral implants.

Neurological Complications
- Spinal Cord or Nerve Root Injury: From cement extrusion or direct mechanical trauma during needle or implant placement.
- Radiculopathy: Can result from foraminal leakage or compression.

Infectious Complications

- Infection or Abscess Formation: Rare (<1%), often related to breach in sterile technique. Prophylactic antibiotics are routinely administered.

Management Strategies

- Prevention: Includes meticulous imaging planning, use of high-viscosity cement, controlled injection under fluoroscopy or CT, and correct implant sizing.
- Early Detection: Real-time imaging allows for immediate response to signs of leakage or misplacement.
- Symptomatic Leakage: May require corticosteroids, surgical decompression, or evacuation.
- Fracture Recurrence: Treated with reintervention or bracing, depending on severity.

Complication rates are generally low in experienced hands, and most issues are preventable with appropriate technique and intraoperative vigilance. Awareness and preparedness are the best tools to minimize adverse outcomes in spinal augmentation [29–31].

3.6 Clinical Outcomes and Evidence Review

Percutaneous vertebral augmentation techniques have consistently demonstrated clinical efficacy in the oncologic setting, particularly in improving pain, function, and quality of life. Their role is central in the palliative management of spinal metastases and myeloma [9, 10].

Pain Control and Quality of Life

- Numerous studies show significant reductions in pain scores, particularly on the Visual Analog Scale (VAS), with mean reductions of 5–7 points within the first week postprocedure.
- Vertebroplasty and kyphoplasty have demonstrated comparable analgesic effects, though some studies suggest more rapid relief with kyphoplasty due to mechanical decompression.
- Pain relief is often sustained for months and may persist until the end of life in palliative cases [32, 33].

Functional Outcomes

- Improvements in Oswestry Disability Index (ODI) and Karnofsky Performance Status are consistently observed.
- Patients experience early mobilization (typically within 24–48 h), reduction in analgesic requirements, and restoration of ambulation.
- These gains are critical in maintaining independence and allowing continuation of systemic oncologic therapies [32, 33].

Long-Term Stability and Vertebral Integrity

- Kyphoplasty and implant-based techniques (e.g., SpineJack®, VBS®) offer superior restoration of vertebral height and kyphosis correction, reducing progressive collapse.
- Cemented vertebrae exhibit high mechanical strength, especially with circumferential or stent-assisted constructs, minimizing the risk of recollapse.
- Implant systems provide added load redistribution, which may reduce the incidence of adjacent-level fractures compared to vertebroplasty alone.

Comparative Effectiveness

- Kyphoplasty vs. Vertebroplasty: Similar pain outcomes. Kyphoplasty is superior in vertebral height restoration and lower cement leakage rates [34].
- Implants vs. Balloon Techniques: Implant-based techniques demonstrate equivalent or improved mechanical outcomes and allow for controlled cement delivery. However, they require more experience and planning [27].

3.7 Special Considerations in Oncology

Vertebral Augmentation Without Ablation: Evidence and Outcomes

Numerous studies have consistently confirmed the clinical effectiveness of vertebral augmentation techniques, including percutaneous vertebroplasty (PVP) and kyphoplasty (PKP), in the treatment of vertebral compression fractures [35, 36]. The first documented application of vertebral augmentation for spinal tumors was reported by Galibert and Deramond in 1987 for vertebral hemangiomas. Since then, growing evidence has highlighted its significant role in alleviating pain caused by spinal metastases. PKP, in particular, aims to reduce pain and reinforce vertebral structural integrity. Several earlier investigations have demonstrated its notable analgesic benefits in patients with metastatic spinal disease. Although the precise mechanisms underlying its pain-relieving effects remain under debate, two main theories have been proposed: (1) Mechanically, PKP increases vertebral stability and (2) chemically, the polymethylmethacrylate (PMMA) cement may exert cytotoxic effects on tumor cells either through toxic monomers or the heat released during polymerization. In patients with lung cancer and bone metastases, osteolytic lesions are most common, leading to destruction of trabecular bone and localized vertebral collapse. These pathological fractures frequently result in kyphotic deformities. Compared to PVP, PKP is considered more effective in correcting kyphosis due to the balloon's capacity to restore vertebral height prior to cement injection [37–40].

Steerable Devices, Curved Balloons, and Cavity Creation

Recent advancements in vertebral tumor treatment include the adoption of steerable ablative technologies and curved balloon catheters to optimize local tumor control, reduce intravertebral pressure, and enhance the distribution of high-viscosity cement.

A 2023 study by Pusceddu et al. evaluated a combined protocol employing a steerable radiofrequency (RFA) probe (STAR™), directional cavity creation (Arcadia™ steerable balloon), and cement delivery (StabiliT® MX system) in 16 patients with painful thoracolumbar spinal metastases. All procedures achieved technical success with no major complications. Median VAS dropped from 8 to 2 after 1 week, and to 0.5 after 1 month, with functional mobility significantly improved (FMS $p = 0.002$) [24].

Vertebral Implants

Noriega et al. (2021) compared SpineJack implants to balloon kyphoplasty in patients with vertebral fractures, demonstrating superior vertebral height restoration, less cement use, and a lower incidence of adjacent-level fractures (3–5% vs. 15–20%) [27].

Pusceddu et al. retrospectively analyzed 39 multiple myeloma patients with 49 vertebral compression fractures treated by vertebroplasty using SpineJack implants. The procedure achieved 100% technical success, with VAS scores dropping from 5.4 to 0.2 and no major complications. Results support SpineJack as a safe, effective option for pain relief and vertebral stabilization [41].

Pusceddu et al. retrospectively evaluated 28 cancer patients with 36 painful vertebral compression fractures treated using a combined approach of microwave ablation, bilateral expandable SpineJack implants, and vertebroplasty. The procedure achieved 100% technical success, restored vertebral height in 58% of cases, and reduced VAS scores from 6.3 to 0.4 at 6 months. No major complications, implant displacement, or local recurrence were observed, confirming the technique's safety, efficacy, and tumor control benefit [42].

Cornelis et al. (2022) employed cone-beam CT to guide SpineJack placement in patients with tumor-infiltrated vertebrae, reporting technical success and enhanced cement control [43]. Cianfoni et al. (2023) introduced the SAIF (Stent-Assisted Internal Fixation) technique, combining expandable stents, percutaneous pedicle screws, and cement in patients with unstable vertebral fractures from metastatic disease, with excellent outcomes in terms of pain control and biomechanical stabilization [28].

3.7.1 Integration with Tumor Ablation

The combination of thermal ablation with vertebral augmentation has become an advanced and targeted approach in the treatment of spinal metastases, offering both tumor debulking and mechanical stabilization. Different modalities offer distinct advantages and have been evaluated in a growing number of clinical studies.

Radiofrequency Ablation (RFA)

Radiofrequency ablation (RFA) is a percutaneous technique that uses alternating high-frequency electric current to generate heat, inducing coagulative necrosis of tumor tissue. Under CT or fluoroscopic guidance, a specialized electrode is positioned within the bone lesion, achieving temperatures between 60 °C and 90 °C for

4–8 min depending on tumor size. Monopolar or bipolar configurations can be used, and thermocouples are employed to monitor temperatures during treatment.

RFA is particularly suited for contained osteolytic spinal metastases, offering precise tumor control with minimal risk of damage to surrounding tissues.

A multicenter study by Goetz et al. treated 43 patients with painful bone metastases refractory to conventional therapies using percutaneous image-guided RFA. The results demonstrated a significant reduction in pain, with the mean worst pain score decreasing from 7.9 to 1.4 within 24 weeks posttreatment. Moreover, 95% of patients reported clinically significant pain relief and a reduction in opioid use [44].

Anchala et al. evaluated the effectiveness of a bipolar navigational RFA system in a multicenter retrospective study including 92 patients with 128 spinal metastatic lesions. Significant pain reduction was observed at 1 week, 1 month, and 6 months postprocedure, with 54% of patients reducing their analgesic consumption [45].

RFA provides the advantage of precise tumor debulking with minimal spread, making it particularly useful for treating osteolytic lesions with preserved posterior vertebral elements. It is often combined with cementoplasty to enhance vertebral stability and provide durable pain relief [46].

Cryoablation

Cryoablation uses argon gas-based cryoprobes to produce extremely low temperatures (−40 °C to −100 °C) and generate an ice ball that leads to tissue necrosis via freezing-thawing cycles. The ice ball is directly visible under CT, allowing precise ablation zone monitoring. Dual-cycle freezing is commonly applied (e.g., 10 min freeze, 5 min thaw, repeat). Cryoablation is especially beneficial when treating lesions near sensitive structures such as the spinal cord, due to a more favorable thermal gradient compared to RFA [47].

The multicenter study of cryoablation for palliation of painful bone metastases (MOTION) study, a pivotal prospective multicenter trial, evaluated cryoablation for painful bone metastases and demonstrated a median pain reduction of 4 points on the Visual Analog Scale (VAS) at 1 month, with sustained improvement at 6 months and minimal complications [48].

Microwave Ablation (MWA)

Microwave ablation relies on dielectric heating, whereby electromagnetic waves (typically 2.45 GHz) agitate water molecules within tissue, rapidly raising the temperature to cytotoxic levels (>60 °C). Unlike RFA, MWA is not dependent on electrical conductivity and is more effective in sclerotic or heterogeneous bone environments. MWA achieves larger ablation volumes in less time, with reduced heat sink effect near vasculature.

Pusceddu et al. (2013) evaluated MWA in 21 spinal metastases across 18 sessions, achieving >90% pain reduction on BPI scores within 4 weeks [49].

Sagoo et al. (2021) confirmed these results in a systematic review showing that MWA, combined with vertebroplasty, is effective in managing spinal metastases with low recurrence and improved cement distribution [50].

Combined Strategies

Recent developments combine thermal ablation, vertebral augmentation, and mechanical realignment.

These procedures are typically performed under CT-fluoroscopy guidance with curved balloon catheters or directional implants, allowing tailored therapy even in complex vertebral anatomy. Combined strategies are particularly relevant in lesions involving the anterior and middle columns with cortical compromise, or when local tumor control is critical to avoid recurrence. Furthermore, Mohme et al. (2021) suggested that augmentation alone may increase circulating tumor cells (CTCs), reinforcing the rationale for cytoreductive ablation prior to cement injection [51].

Overall, mounting evidence supports the use of thermal ablation—especially RFA, cryoablation, and MWA—in conjunction with vertebral augmentation as an effective, durable, and safe intervention for spinal metastases, with the added benefit of tumor control and prevention of further collapse.

- Radiosensitive tumors (myeloma, lymphoma) may be managed with augmentation alone.
- Radioresistant tumors (renal cell, sarcoma) often require combined ablation and cementoplasty to ensure durable pain control and stabilization.

3.8 Future Perspective and Emerging Technologies

The field of interventional spine oncology is rapidly evolving, driven by technological innovation, expanding indications, and the growing need for personalized, minimally invasive therapies. Several promising avenues are poised to reshape vertebral interventions in the coming decade.

Augmented Reality (AR) and Robotic Assistance

Augmented reality, which overlays digital imaging data in real-time onto the surgical field, is being integrated into preoperative planning and intraoperative navigation. AR platforms allow enhanced visualization of critical structures and needle trajectories, reducing operator dependence and exposure to radiation. Early pilot studies have demonstrated increased accuracy in vertebral targeting and cement delivery when using AR guidance, particularly in complex or multilevel lesions.

Robotic systems offer submillimetric precision in needle placement and trajectory control. Spine-specific robotic platforms now integrate with CT and cone-beam CT to plan and execute bipedicular and extrapedicular access with reproducible outcomes. The use of robotics also allows for remote operation, enabling specialists to perform high-risk procedures in underserved regions or pandemic situations. As these systems become more cost-effective and user-friendly, their adoption is likely to expand [52].

Advanced Navigation Systems

The fusion of imaging datasets—such as CT/MRI and fluoroscopy—enables dynamic real-time guidance during vertebral procedures. Hybrid operating suites now support seamless switching between modalities and advanced 3D reconstruction, reducing misplacement risk and procedural time. In particular, navigation systems linked with software-assisted lesion targeting are crucial in the integration of ablation and cementoplasty in anatomically challenging segments.

The advent of electromagnetic navigation further enhances the ability to treat posteriorly located lesions and navigate around epidural components, with minimal disruption of surrounding tissue. These systems have shown high accuracy in experimental and early clinical settings, especially when combined with steerable devices or directional tools [53].

Personalized and 3D-Printed Implants

The application of patient-specific implants, designed from preoperative imaging and produced via additive manufacturing, allows for the replacement of large or deformed vertebral segments in oncologic and postablative settings. These implants can be matched to the patient's spinal curvature and bone density profile, improving biomechanical distribution and reducing the risk of subsidence.

In addition, novel expandable implants with integrated anchoring mechanisms (e.g., antirotational flanges or trabecular mimicry) are under development for use in cases of severe vertebral destruction or deformity. These may complement or replace standard vertebral body stents in high-risk cases.

3.9 Conclusion

Minimally invasive image-guided interventions have become a cornerstone in the treatment of painful and unstable vertebral lesions in oncology. Techniques such as vertebroplasty, kyphoplasty, and vertebral implant placement—whether performed alone or in conjunction with thermal ablation—have demonstrated consistent efficacy in pain control, mobility restoration, and structural stabilization.

Key Takeaways Include:

Careful patient selection and multidisciplinary coordination are critical for procedural success.

Image-guided interventions are effective even in complex or fragile patients, with rapid recovery and low complication rates.

Integration with ablation and advanced implant systems allows tailored treatment in radioresistant tumors or severe fractures.

Evidence-based criteria such as the SINS score and functional metrics (VAS, FMS) should guide clinical decision-making.

Looking ahead, the integration of robotics, AR, advanced navigation, and biologically active materials promises to further expand the possibilities of vertebral oncology care. Personalization and technological precision will continue to improve safety, efficacy, and long-term outcomes. Ultimately, these techniques embody the principles of modern interventional oncology: targeted, patient-centric, and minimally disruptive, offering high-value care even in the most challenging clinical contexts.

3.10 Clinical Cases (Figs. 3.3, 3.4, 3.5, 3.6, 3.7, 3.8, and 3.9)

Case 1

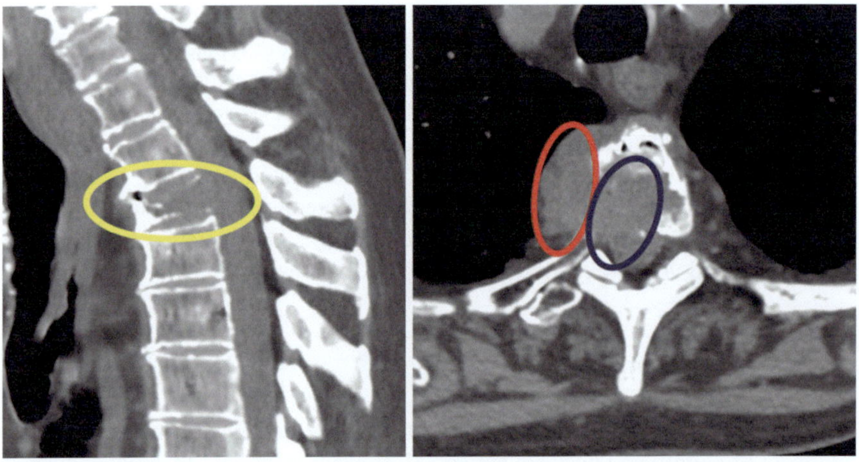

Fig. 3.3 Sagittal (left) and axial (right) contrast-enhanced CT images of the thoracic spine in an 83-year-old patient with known pulmonary carcinoma (cT3 cM1), previously treated with radiotherapy. *Left image (yellow circle):* Metastatic osteolytic fracture of the T2 vertebral body, with cortical destruction and partial collapse. *Right image:* Presence of a right paravertebral soft tissue mass (red circle), consistent with an associated tumor component extending from the vertebral lesion; mild effacement of the spinal canal is noted (blue circle), without evidence of spinal cord compression

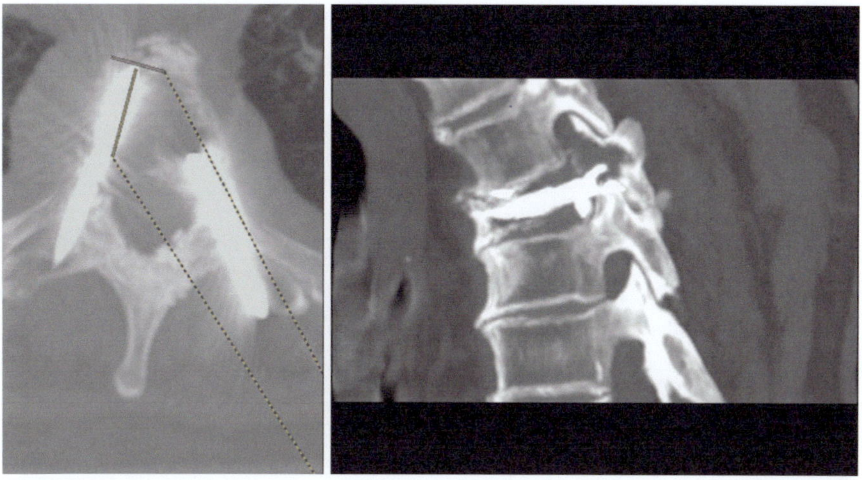

Fig. 3.4 Axial (left) and sagittal (right) CT images during and after treatment of a vertebral metastasis. *Left image:* Axial intraprocedural CT showing bilateral percutaneous access for *microwave ablation* targeting a right-sided vertebral metastasis. *Right image:* Sagittal postprocedural CT demonstrating vertebroplasty with optimal cement filling of the T2 vertebral body, without evidence of leakage or complications

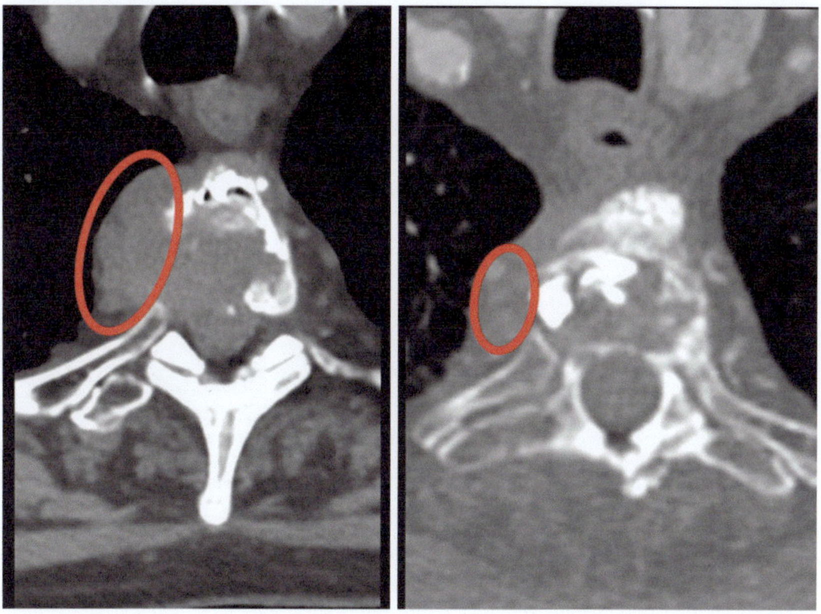

Fig. 3.5 Axial contrast-enhanced CT images before (left) and 4 months after (right) microwave ablation and vertebroplasty of a T2 vertebral metastasis. *Left image:* Preprocedural scan showing a right paravertebral soft tissue tumor component (red circle). *Right image:* Follow-up scan at 4 months demonstrating marked reduction in the paravertebral lesion (red circle) and stable cement filling of the treated vertebral body, with no evidence of complications

Case 2

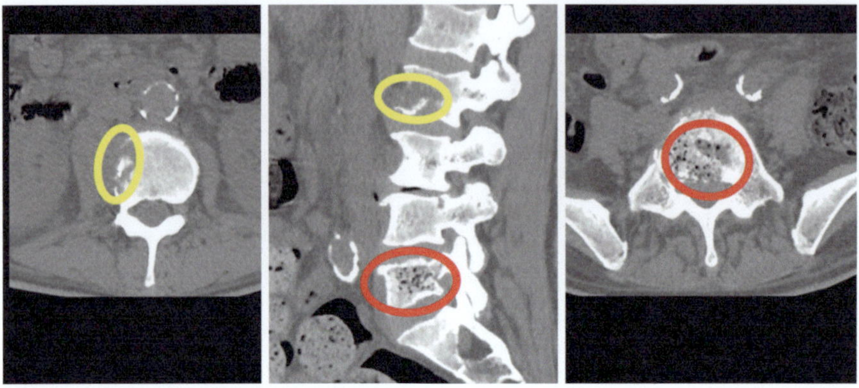

Fig. 3.6 Axial and sagittal CT images of the lumbar spine in a 43-year-old patient with stage IV (cM1) lung cancer presenting with lumbar pain. The sagittal reconstruction (center) reveals a *right hemivertebral lytic lesion at L2* (yellow circle), consistent with metastatic involvement. Additionally, a *pathological fracture of the L5 vertebral body* is seen (red circles), secondary to a destructive osteolytic metastasis, clearly visible on both sagittal and axial images

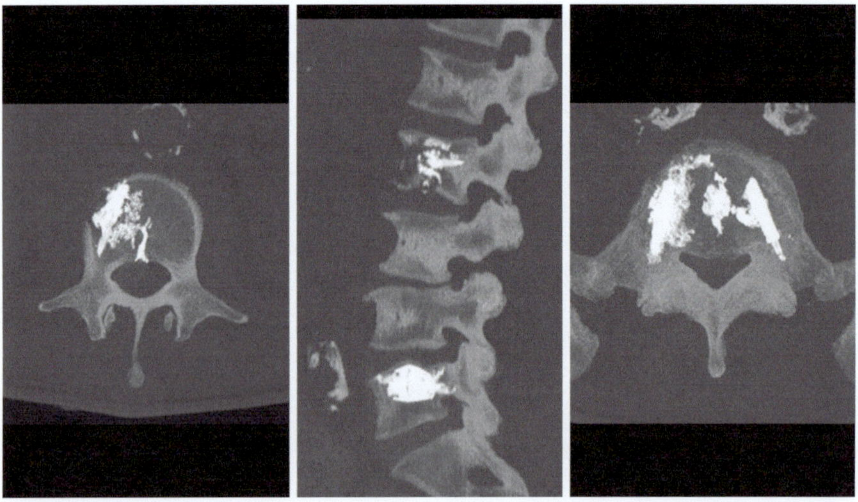

Fig. 3.7 Postprocedural CT images following combined percutaneous treatment of vertebral metastases. *Left image:* Axial CT view after microwave ablation and cementoplasty of the L2 vertebral body, showing adequate cement distribution without leakage. *Right image:* Axial CT scan demonstrating postablation vertebral stabilization with *SpineJack® implant* and cementoplasty at the L5 level. *Center image:* Sagittal CT reconstruction confirming correct positioning of the cement and implants at both treated levels (L2 and L5), with restoration of vertebral body height at L5

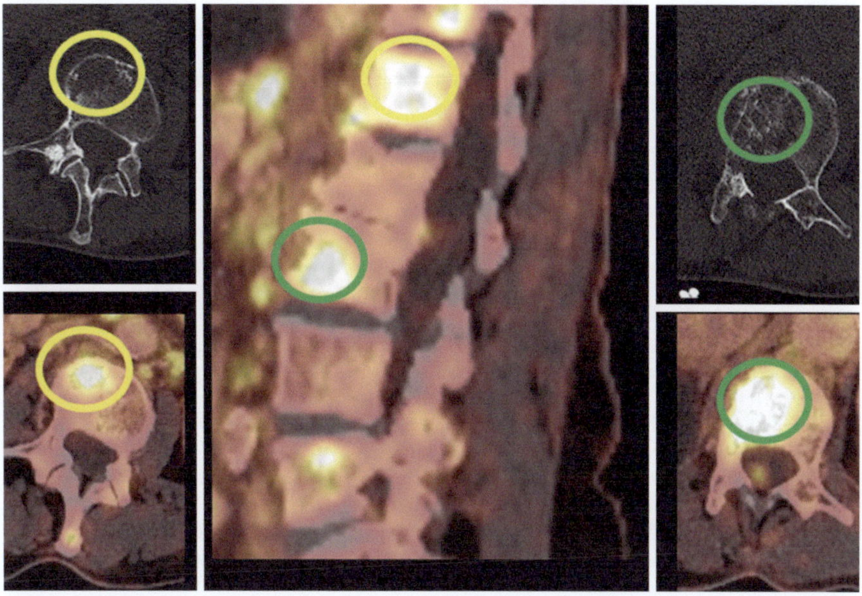

Fig. 3.8 PET/CT and CT images in a 69-year-old female patient with metastatic breast cancer and dorsal-lumbar pain. *Center image:* Sagittal PET/CT fusion showing multiple FDG-avid osteolytic vertebral metastases. The most significant hypermetabolic foci, correlating with clinical pain, are located at *L1 (yellow circle)* and *L3 (green circle)*. *Top left and right images:* Axial CT scans at L1 and L3 levels, respectively, showing osteolytic changes corresponding to PET-avid lesions. *Bottom left and right images:* Axial PET/CT fusion images confirming intense metabolic activity at L1 (yellow circle) and L3 (green circle)

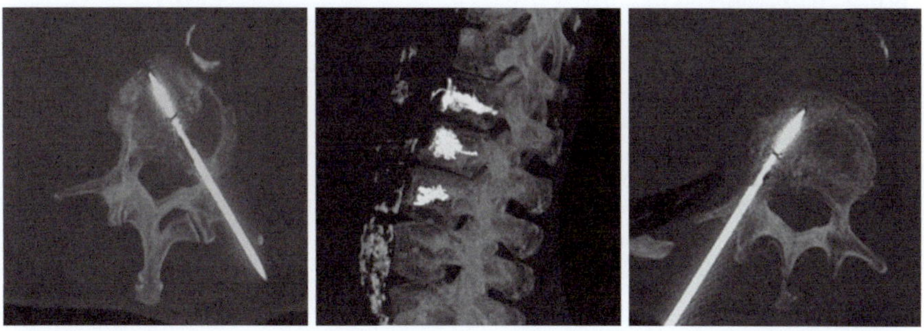

Fig. 3.9 Axial and sagittal CT images demonstrating percutaneous treatment of FDG-avid spinal metastases in a patient with metastatic breast cancer. *Left image:* Axial CT during *percutaneous image-guided microwave ablation* of the hypermetabolic L1 vertebral lesion. *Right image:* Axial CT showing *microwave ablation* of the FDG-avid lesion at the L3 level. *Center image:* Sagittal CT reconstruction showing the *final outcome with vertebroplasty at L1, L2, and L3*, demonstrating good cement distribution and no evidence of complications

References

1. Cole JS, Patchell RA. Metastatic epidural spinal cord compression. Lancet Neurol. 2008;7(5):459–66. https://doi.org/10.1016/S1474-4422(08)70120-7.
2. Sciubba DM, Petteys RJ, Dekutoski MB, Fisher CG, Fehlings MG, Ondra SL, et al. Diagnosis and management of metastatic spine disease. J Neurosurg Spine. 2010;13(1):94–108. https://doi.org/10.3171/2010.3.SPINE09202.
3. Fourney DR, Gokaslan ZL. Spinal instability and deformity secondary to neoplastic conditions. Neurosurg Clin N Am. 2004;15(4):499–509. https://doi.org/10.1016/j.nec.2004.03.001.
4. Wallace AN, Tomasian A, Chang RO, Jennings JW. Radiologic percutaneous treatment of spinal metastases. Semin Intervent Radiol. 2020;37(2):163–73. https://doi.org/10.1055/s-0040-1709364.
5. Tsou IY, Goh PY, Peh WC, Goh LA, Chee TS. Percutaneous vertebroplasty in the management of osteoporotic vertebral compression fractures: initial experience. Ann Acad Med Singap. 2002;31(1):15–20.
6. Deramond H, Wright NT, Belkoff SM. Temperature elevation caused by bone cement polymerization during vertebroplasty. Bone. 1999;25(2 Suppl):17S–21S.
7. Garfin SR, Yuan HA, Reiley MA. New technologies in spine: kyphoplasty and vertebroplasty for the treatment of painful osteoporotic compression fractures. Spine (Phila Pa 1976). 2001;26(14):1511–5. https://doi.org/10.1097/00007632-200107150-00020.
8. Tutton SM, Pflugmacher R, Davidian M, Beall DP, Facchini FR, Garfin SR. KAST study: the KIVA system as a vertebral augmentation treatment-a safety and effectiveness trial: a randomized, noninferiority trial comparing the KIVA system with balloon kyphoplasty in treatment of osteoporotic vertebral compression fractures. Spine (Phila Pa 1976). 2015;40(12):865–75. https://doi.org/10.1097/BRS.0000000000000906.
9. Tsoumakidou G, Too CW, Koch G, Caudrelier J, Cazzato RL, Garnon J, Gangi A. CIRSE guidelines on percutaneous vertebral augmentation. Cardiovasc Intervent Radiol. 2017;40(3):331–42. https://doi.org/10.1007/s00270-017-1574-8. Epub 2017 Jan 19.
10. Ryan A, Byrne C, Pusceddu C, Buy X, Tsoumakidou G, Filippiadis D. CIRSE standards of practice on thermal ablation of bone tumours. Cardiovasc Intervent Radiol. 2022;45(5):591–605. https://doi.org/10.1007/s00270-022-03126-x. Epub 2022 Mar 29. PMID: 35348870; PMCID: PMC9018647.
11. Body JJ, Bone HG, de Boer RH, et al. Bone health in cancer patients: ESMO clinical practice guidelines. Ann Oncol. 2020;31(12):1650–63. https://doi.org/10.1016/j.annonc.2020.09.006.
12. Terpos E, Zamagni E, Lentzsch S, Drake MT, García-Sanz R, Abildgaard N, Ntanasis-Stathopoulos I, Schjesvold F, de la Rubia J, Kyriakou C, Hillengass J, Zweegman S, Cavo M, Moreau P, San-Miguel J, Dimopoulos MA, Munshi N, Durie BGM, Raje N, Bone Working Group of the International Myeloma Working Group. Treatment of multiple myeloma-related bone disease: recommendations from the bone Working Group of the International Myeloma Working Group. Lancet Oncol. 2021;22(3):e119–30. https://doi.org/10.1016/S1470-2045(20)30559-3. Epub 2021 Feb 2.
13. Fisher CG, DiPaola CP, Ryken TC, et al. A novel classification system for spinal instability in neoplastic disease: an evidence-based approach and expert consensus from the spine oncology study group. Spine (Phila Pa 1976). 2010;35(22):E1221–9. https://doi.org/10.1097/BRS.0b013e3181e16ae2.
14. Park C, Lee JW, Kim Y, Ahn S, Lee E, Kang Y, Kang HS. Diagnosis of spinal metastasis: are MR images without contrast medium application sufficient? Clin Imaging. 2019;55:165–73. https://doi.org/10.1016/j.clinimag.2019.03.003. Epub 2019 Mar 11.
15. Ghanem NA, Pache G, Lohrmann C, Brink I, Bley T, Kotter E, Kelly T, Langer M. MRI and (18)FDG-PET in the assessment of bone marrow infiltration of the spine in cancer patients. Eur Spine J. 2007;16(11):1907–12. https://doi.org/10.1007/s00586-007-0350-x. Epub 2007 Apr 3. PMID: 17404763; PMCID: PMC2223344.

16. State-of-the-art imaging techniques in metastatic spinal cord compression. Cureus. 2022;14(6):e25923. https://doi.org/10.7759/cureus.25923.
17. Supple S, Ahmad S, Gaddikeri S, Jhaveri MD. Treatment of metastatic spinal disease; what the radiologist needs to know. Br J Radiol. 2022;95(1135):20211300. https://doi.org/10.1259/bjr.20211300. Epub 2022 June 7. PMID: 35604660; PMCID: PMC10996317.
18. Kwee TC, Kwee RM. Combined FDG-PET/CT for the detection of unknown primary tumors: systematic review and meta-analysis. Eur Radiol. 2009;19(4):731–44. https://doi.org/10.1007/s00330-008-1194-4.
19. Galibert P, Deramond H, Rosat P, Le Gars D. Preliminary note on the treatment of vertebral angioma by percutaneous acrylic vertebroplasty. Neurochirurgie. 1987;33(2):166–8.
20. Boss S, Srivastava V, Anitescu M. Vertebroplasty and kyphoplasty. Phys Med Rehabil Clin N Am. 2022;33(2):425–53. https://doi.org/10.1016/j.pmr.2022.01.008.
21. Wang Q, Dong JF, Fang X, Chen Y. Application and modification of bone cement in vertebroplasty: a literature review. Jt Dis Relat Surg. 2022;33(2):467–78. https://doi.org/10.52312/jdrs.2022.628. Epub 2022 July 6. PMID: 35852210; PMCID: PMC9361106.
22. Wang X, Zhu YH, Zhu QS. Efficacy and safety of robot-assisted versus fluoroscopy-assisted PKP or PVP for osteoporotic vertebral compression fractures: a systematic review and meta-analysis. J Robot Surg. 2023;17(6):2597–610. https://doi.org/10.1007/s11701-023-01507-5.
23. Ortiz A O. Vertebral body reconstruction: Review and update on vertebroplasty and kyphoplasty. Appl Radiol. 2008;37(1):12–20.
24. Pusceddu C, Marsico S, Derudas D, et al. Clinical rationale of using steerable technologies for radiofrequency ablation followed by cavity creation and cement augmentation in the treatment of painful spinal metastases. Curr Oncol. 2023;30(5):4257–68. https://doi.org/10.3390/curroncol30050400.
25. Fourney DR, Schomer DF, Nader R, et al. Percutaneous vertebroplasty and kyphoplasty for painful vertebral body fractures in cancer patients. J Neurosurg Spine. 2003;98(1 Suppl):21–30. https://doi.org/10.3171/spi.2003.98.1.0021.
26. Noriega DC, Marcia S, Theumann N, et al. A prospective, international, randomized, noninferiority study comparing an implantable titanium vertebral augmentation device versus balloon kyphoplasty in the reduction of vertebral compression fractures (SAKOS study). Spine J. 2019;19(11):1782–95. https://doi.org/10.1016/j.spinee.2019.07.009.
27. Rotter R, Martin H, Fuerderer S, Gabl M, Roeder C, Heini P, Mittlmeier T. Vertebral body stenting: a new method for vertebral augmentation versus kyphoplasty. Eur Spine J. 2010;19(6):916–23. https://doi.org/10.1007/s00586-010-1342-4.
28. Cianfoni A, Distefano D, Isalberti M, Reinert M, Scarone P, Kuhlen D, Hirsch JA, Bonaldi G. Stent-screw-assisted internal fixation: the SAIF technique to augment severe osteoporotic and neoplastic vertebral body fractures. J Neurointerv Surg. 2019;11(6):603–9. https://doi.org/10.1136/neurintsurg-2018-014481. Epub 2018 Dec 14.
29. Zhang Y, Wang L, Liu J, et al. Incidence and risk factors of adjacent vertebral fracture after percutaneous vertebroplasty or kyphoplasty in postmenopausal women: a retrospective study. Sci Rep. 2024;14(1):12345. https://doi.org/10.1038/s41598-024-68835-4.
30. Lee SH, Kim TH, Lee SY, et al. Risk factors for vertebral re-collapse after percutaneous vertebroplasty in osteoporotic vertebral compression fractures. J Orthop Surg Res. 2021;16(1):123. https://doi.org/10.1186/s13018-021-02456-7.
31. Gao X, Du J, Gao L, et al. Risk factors for bone cement displacement after percutaneous vertebral augmentation for osteoporotic vertebral compression fractures. Front Surg. 2022;9:947212. https://doi.org/10.3389/fsurg.2022.947212.
32. Berenson J, Pflugmacher R, Jarzem P, Zonder J, Spalding J, Tschegg E, Tillman JB, Reese ER, Vrionis F. Balloon kyphoplasty versus non-surgical care for vertebral compression fractures in patients with cancer: a randomized controlled trial. Lancet Oncol. 2011;12(3):225–35. https://doi.org/10.1016/S1470-2045(11)70008-0.
33. Kaufmann TJ, Jensen ME, Schweickert PA, Marx WF, Kallmes DF. Age of fracture and clinical outcomes of percutaneous vertebroplasty. AJNR Am J Neuroradiol. 2001;22(10):1860–3.

34. McCall T, Cole C, Dailey A. Vertebroplasty and kyphoplasty: a comparative review of efficacy and adverse events. Curr Rev Musculoskelet Med. 2008;1(1):17–23. https://doi.org/10.1007/s12178-007-9013-0. PMID: 19468894; PMCID: PMC2684146.
35. Mattie R, Brar N, Tram JT, McCormick ZL, Beall DP, Fox A, Saltychev M. Vertebral augmentation of cancer-related spinal compression fractures: a systematic review and meta-analysis. Spine (Phila Pa 1976). 2021;46(24):1729–37. https://doi.org/10.1097/BRS.0000000000004093.
36. Anselmetti GC, Manca A, Montemurro F, Hirsch J, Chiara G, Grignani G, Carnevale Schianca F, Capaldi A, Rota Scalabrini D, Sardo E, Debernardi F, Iussich G, Regge D. Percutaneous vertebroplasty in multiple myeloma: prospective long-term follow-up in 106 consecutive patients. Cardiovasc Intervent Radiol. 2012;35(1):139–45. https://doi.org/10.1007/s00270-011-0111-4. Epub 2011 Feb 9.
37. Galibert P, Deramond H, Rosat P, Le Gars D. Preliminary note on the treatment of vertebral angioma by percutaneous acrylic vertebroplasty. Neurochirurgie. 1987;33:166–8.
38. Zhang JX, Song ZR, Zou J, Ge J, Yang HL. Balloon kyphoplasty as palliative care for painful pathological spinal fracture followed by lung cancer metastasis: a cohort study. Front Surg. 2023;9:1081823. https://doi.org/10.3389/fsurg.2022.1081823. PMID: 36733676; PMCID: PMC9887125.
39. Kassamali RH, Ganeshan A, Hoey ETD, Crowe PM, Douis H, Henderson J. Pain management in spinal metastases: the role of percutaneous vertebral augmentation. Ann Oncol. 2011;22:782–6. https://doi.org/10.1093/annonc/mdq605.
40. Chen F, Xia YH, Cao WZ, Shan W, Gao Y, Feng BO, Wang D. Percutaneous kyphoplasty for the treatment of spinal metastases. Oncol Lett. 2016;11(3):1799–806. https://doi.org/10.3892/ol.2016.4121. Epub 2016 Jan 18. PMID: 26998079; PMCID: PMC4774488.
41. Pusceddu C, Faiella E, Derudas D, Ballicu N, Melis L, Zedda S, Marsico S. Re-expansion of vertebral compression fractures in patients with multiple myeloma with percutaneous vertebroplasty using spinejack implants: a preliminary and retrospective study. Front Surg. 2023;10:1121981. https://doi.org/10.3389/fsurg.2023.1121981. PMID: 37288134; PMCID: PMC10242080.
42. Pusceddu C, Marsico S, Derudas D, Ballicu N, Melis L, Zedda S, de Felice C, Calabrese A, De Francesco D, Venturini M, Santucci D, Faiella E. Percutaneous vertebral reconstruction (PVR) technique of pathological compression fractures: an innovative combined treatment of microwave ablation, bilateral expandable titanium SpineJack implants followed by Vertebroplasty. J Clin Med. 2023;12(13):4178. https://doi.org/10.3390/jcm12134178. PMID: 37445213; PMCID: PMC10342544.
43. Cornelis FH, Razakamanantsoa L, Ben Ammar M, Najdawi M, Gardavaud F, El-Mouhadi S, Barral M. Expandable intravertebral implant in cancer-related vertebral compression fractures: a retrospective review of 36 implantations. J Vasc Interv Radiol. 2022;33(1):14–8. https://doi.org/10.1016/j.jvir.2021.10.002.
44. Goetz MP, Callstrom MR, Charboneau JW, et al. Percutaneous image-guided radiofrequency ablation of painful metastases involving bone: a multicenter study. J Clin Oncol. 2004;22(2):300–6. https://doi.org/10.1200/JCO.2004.05.181.
45. Anchala PR, Irving WD, Hillen TJ, et al. Treatment of metastatic spinal lesions with a navigational bipolar radiofrequency ablation device: a multicenter retrospective study. Pain Physician. 2014;17(4):317–27.
46. Yevich S, Chen S, Metwalli Z, et al. Radiofrequency ablation of spine metastases: a clinical and technical approach. Semin Musculoskelet Radiol. 2021;25(6):795–804. https://doi.org/10.1055/s-0041-1740351.
47. Callstrom MR, Dupuy DE, Solomon SB, Beres RA, Littrup PJ, Davis KW, Paz-Fumagalli R, Hoffman C, Atwell TD, Charboneau JW, Schmit GD, Goetz MP, Rubin J, Brown KJ, Novotny PJ, Sloan JA. Percutaneous image-guided cryoablation of painful metastases involving bone: multicenter trial. Cancer. 2013;119(5):1033–41. https://doi.org/10.1002/cncr.27793. Epub 2012 Oct 12. PMID: 23065947; PMCID: PMC5757505.

48. Jennings JW, Prologo JD, Garnon J, Gangi A, Buy X, Palussière J, Kurup AN, Callstrom M, Genshaft S, Abtin F, Huang AJ, Iannuccilli J, Pilleul F, Mastier C, Littrup PJ, de Baère T, Deschamps F. Cryoablation for palliation of painful bone metastases: the MOTION Multicenter study. Radiol Imaging Cancer. 2021;3(2):e200101. https://doi.org/10.1148/rycan.2021200101. PMID: 33817650; PMCID: PMC8011449.
49. Pusceddu C, Fele RM, Sotgia B, Melis L. Treatment of bone metastases with microwave thermal ablation. J Vasc Interv Radiol. 2013;24(2):229–33.
50. Sagoo NS, Haider AS, Rowe SE, Haider M, Sharma R, Neeley OJ, Dahdaleh NS, Adogwa O, Bagley CA, El Ahmadieh TY, Aoun SG. Microwave ablation as a treatment for spinal metastatic tumors: a systematic review. World Neurosurg. 2021;148:15–23. https://doi.org/10.1016/j.wneu.2020.12.162. Epub 2021 Jan 8.
51. Mohme M, Riethdorf S, Dreimann M, et al. Circulating tumour cell release after cement augmentation of vertebral metastases. Sci Rep. 2017;7:7196. https://doi.org/10.1038/s41598-017-07649-z.
52. Bhatt FR, Orosz LD, Tewari A, Boyd D, Roy R, Good CR, Schuler TC, Haines CM, Jazini E. Augmented reality-assisted spine surgery: an early experience demonstrating safety and accuracy with 218 screws. Glob Spine J. 2023;13(7):2047–52. https://doi.org/10.1177/21925682211069321. Epub 2022 Jan 10. PMID: 35000409; PMCID: PMC10556900.
53. Hahn P, Oezdemir S, Komp M, Giannakopoulos A, Heikenfeld R, Kasch R, Merk H, Godolias G, Ruetten S. A new electromagnetic navigation system for pedicle screws placement: a human cadaver study at the lumbar spine. PLoS One. 2015;10(7):e0133708. https://doi.org/10.1371/journal.pone.0133708. PMID: 26221733; PMCID: PMC4519101.

4 Radiofrequency Ablation and Steerable Devices

Marc Viles Garcia, Ana Rodríguez Troyano, José María Maiques Llácer, Salvatore Marsico, and Claudio Pusceddu

4.1 Introduction

Image-guided ablation techniques for treating bone and soft tissue tumors of the musculoskeletal system have become an established therapeutic option for both benign and malignant lesions, providing safe, effective, and minimally invasive alternatives to conventional treatments such as surgery, radiotherapy, or chemotherapy [1–3]. These techniques offer several advantages, including reduced morbidity, shorter hospital stays, faster recovery times, and the ability to target tumors in anatomically challenging locations.

Ablative therapies can be categorized based on the type of energy used, distinguishing between ionizing and nonionizing modalities [4]. The key difference between these two approaches lies in the use of ionizing radiation, which is absent in nonionizing therapies.

M. V. Garcia (✉) · A. R. Troyano · J. M. M. Llácer
Department of Radiology, Hospital del Mar, Barcelona, Spain
e-mail: marc.viles.garcia@hmar.cat; ana.rodriguez.troyano@hmar.cat; jmaiques@hmar.cat

S. Marsico
Department of Radiology, Hospital del Mar, Barcelona, Spain

Interventional Oncology Institute, Barcelona, Spain

C. Pusceddu
Department of Radiology, Mater Olbia Hospital, Olbia, Cagliari, Italy

Interventional Oncology Institute, Barcelona, Spain

C. Pusceddu, S. Marsico (eds.), *Malignant Bone Lesions and Beyond*,
https://doi.org/10.1007/978-3-032-00018-7_4

4.1.1 Classification of Ablative Techniques

Ablation techniques are broadly divided into thermal and nonthermal modalities, each employing distinct mechanisms to induce tumor destruction [5].

- Thermal ablation relies on sustained temperature alterations to achieve tumor necrosis. The primary techniques in this category include:
  - Radiofrequency ablation (RFA).
  - Microwave ablation (MWA).
  - Cryoablation.
- Nonthermal ablation, in contrast, induces cell death through alternative biological pathways that do not depend on temperature modifications. Historically, techniques such as photodynamic therapy and alcohol ablation were employed in oncologic treatments; however, their use has largely declined in favor of more advanced, targeted techniques [2–5].

4.1.2 Historical Evolution of Thermal Ablation in Oncology

The application of thermal energy for tissue destruction dates back to the mid-nineteenth century, when direct current was used to create controlled lesions in animal brains. The later discovery of high-frequency alternating current as a means to induce predictable lesions led to the development of what is now termed radiofrequency ablation (RFA). The name is derived from the 300 kHz to 500 kHz frequencies, which were initially employed in radio transmission [3–5].

One of the earliest documented observations of temperature increases in biological tissues due to radiofrequency wave application was made by d'Arsonval in 1891 [6]. Subsequently, in the 1920s, the development of the Bovie electrosurgical scalpel introduced the use of radiofrequency energy in the form of alternating current for cauterization and surgical dissection [7]. This innovation marked a significant milestone in the clinical application of thermal energy in medicine.

4.1.3 Radiofrequency Ablation (RFA): From Hepatic Tumors to Musculoskeletal Applications

The first reported use of radiofrequency energy for tumor destruction occurred in 1992, when Roosi and McGahan et al. described its application for the ablation of hepatic tumors. In the same year, Rosenthal et al. successfully applied RFA to treat osteoid osteoma, establishing its role in musculoskeletal tumor management [8].

The early 2000s marked a turning point in the use of RFA for bone tumors, particularly for the treatment of spinal metastases. In a landmark study, Dupuy et al. published the first cases of RFA applied to vertebral metastases, demonstrating its feasibility in palliative oncology and pain management [9].

Since then, RFA has become a cornerstone in the interventional treatment of bone tumors, offering local tumor control, pain relief, and biomechanical stabilization when combined with vertebroplasty or cementoplasty. Its role continues to expand as technological advancements enhance precision, safety, and therapeutic outcomes.

4.1.4 Focus of This Chapter

This chapter explores the advantages and clinical applications of radiofrequency ablation (RFA) for bone tumors, with a particular emphasis on vertebral metastases, given their high prevalence and significant clinical impact. The discussion will highlight:

1. The fundamental principles of RFA and its mechanism of action in tumor destruction.
2. Indications and contraindications for RFA in musculoskeletal oncology.
3. Technical considerations, including patient selection, imaging guidance, and procedural execution.
4. The role of combination therapies (RFA + vertebroplasty/SpineJack) in enhancing pain relief and structural reinforcement.
5. Future directions in ablative therapy, including novel energy sources and augmented reality-guided interventions.

As research continues to refine minimally invasive ablation techniques, RFA remains a pivotal tool in interventional oncology, offering patients a less invasive yet highly effective alternative for the treatment of bone tumors and spinal metastases.

4.2 Principles of Radiofrequency Ablation and Devices

4.2.1 Mechanism of Radiofrequency Ablation (RFA)

Radiofrequency ablation (RFA) is a thermal-based tumor ablation technique that generates heat through a high-frequency alternating current (450–600 kHz) applied via an electrode. The process relies on the Joule effect, where electrical current induces ionic agitation, generating localized thermal energy as it passes through the electrode [2, 10, 11]. The resulting temperature elevation (60–100 °C) leads to cellular death via coagulative necrosis. The electrical circuit is completed by placing grounding pads on the patient's skin, ensuring proper energy distribution and procedural safety [12].

While temperatures between 60 and 100 °C are optimal for achieving tumor necrosis, exceeding 100 °C may reduce efficacy. Excessive heating can cause tissue dehydration, increasing electrical impedance and limiting further heat conduction, a phenomenon that can compromise ablation uniformity [9, 10, 13].

4.2.2 Heat Distribution and the Heat-Sink Effect

RFA-induced thermal lesions can be divided into three distinct zones [2, 9, 10]:

1. Central Zone (Coagulative Necrosis, >50 °C): The innermost area of ablation, where direct exposure to elevated temperatures results in complete cellular destruction via coagulative necrosis.
2. Peripheral/Transitional Zone (41–45 °C): A region where cellular apoptosis occurs due to prolonged exposure to moderate hyperthermia, leading to progressive cell death over time.
3. Surrounding Zone (Heat Dissipation and the Heat-Sink Effect): A region influenced by heat dissipation via blood circulation, which can reduce treatment efficacy by removing thermal energy from the ablation site [11–13].

The Heat-Sink Effect is a significant limitation of RFA, particularly in tumors adjacent to blood vessels. As circulating blood absorbs and dissipates thermal energy, it prevents sufficient heating of tumor margins, potentially leaving viable tumor cells within the treatment zone [14, 15]. See Fig. 4.1 [2, 10–13].

This figure illustrates the three distinct zones formed around the applicator tip during hyperthermic ablation:

1. Central Zone (Coagulation Necrosis, ≥50 °C) (Panel a).

- The core region surrounding the applicator experiences the highest temperatures (≥50 °C), leading to coagulative necrosis.
  - Key cellular effects include:
    - Cell Membrane Collapse: Loss of structural integrity causes cellular lysis.
    - Protein Denaturation: Heat-induced structural damage in essential proteins results in enzymatic dysfunction.
    - Halt in Enzyme Function and DNA Polymerase Activity: Cellular repair mechanisms cease, preventing recovery.
    - Mitochondrial Dysfunction: Disruption of oxidative phosphorylation and ATP production leads to cell death.
- Tumor cells in this area undergo irreversible thermal damage, leading to immediate cell death.

2. Peripheral or Transitional Zone (41–45 °C, Sublethal Damage) (Panel b).
   - Surrounding the central necrotic core, the transitional zone exhibits a steep temperature gradient, with temperatures between 41 and 45 °C, inducing sublethal but biologically significant effects:
     - Halted Metabolism: Enzymatic activity slows down, impairing key cellular functions.
     - Impaired DNA Repair: Heat stress inhibits DNA polymerase and repair enzymes, making the cells more susceptible to additional damage (e.g., radiation or chemotherapy).

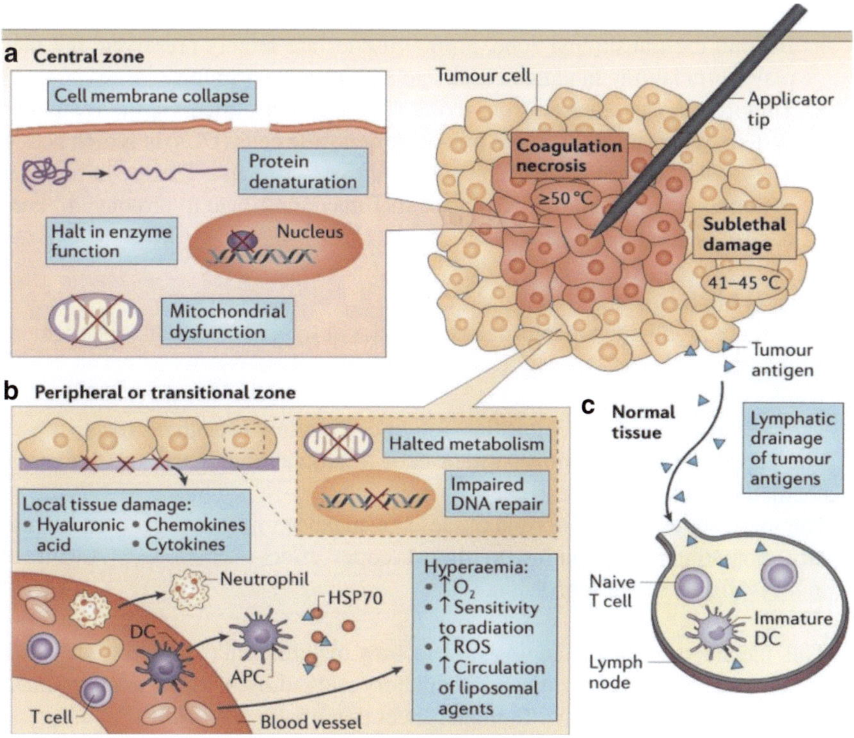

Fig. 4.1 Zones of hyperthermic ablation and their biological effects on tumor and surrounding tissues

- Local Tissue Damage: Release of hyaluronic acid, chemokines, and cytokines, promoting an inflammatory response.
- Hyperemia (Increased Blood Flow):
  - Increased oxygenation enhances radiosensitivity, making the region more vulnerable to radiation therapy.
  - Elevated levels of reactive oxygen species (ROS) cause oxidative stress, further weakening tumor cells.
  - Enhanced permeability of blood vessels facilitates drug delivery, improving chemotherapy efficacy.
- Immune Response Activation:
  - Heat shock protein 70 (HSP70) upregulation recruits antigen-presenting cells (APCs) and neutrophils.
  - Dendritic cell (DC) activation enhances antigen presentation, promoting an anti-tumor immune response.
  - Infiltration of T cells and macrophages contributes to tumor cell recognition and clearance.

3. Normal Tissue and Immune System Activation (Panel c).
   - Beyond the transitional zone, normal tissues are largely preserved, but they play a crucial role in antigen drainage and immune priming.
   - Tumor antigens released from dying cells are transported via the lymphatic system, where they encounter immature dendritic cells (DCs) in lymph nodes.
   - These DCs mature and present tumor antigens to naive T cells, initiating a systemic adaptive immune response that may contribute to prolonged tumor control beyond the ablation site.

Clinical Implications:

This figure highlights the multifaceted impact of hyperthermic ablation, demonstrating how:

- The central zone ensures immediate tumor destruction through necrosis.
- The peripheral zone sensitizes tumor cells to adjunct therapies (e.g., radiation, chemotherapy).
- The immune response in normal tissues can enhance systemic anti-tumor immunity, potentially contributing to the abscopal effect—where local treatment induces distant tumor regression.

This mechanistic understanding underscores hyperthermia's role not only as a cytotoxic tool but also as an immunomodulatory and radiosensitizing strategy, making it a powerful adjunct in multimodal cancer therapy [2, 10–13].

4.2.3 The Influence of Bone Composition on RFA Efficacy

Bone exhibits unique thermal properties that differentiate its response to radiofrequency ablation from that of soft tissues [16, 17]:

- Cortical Bone:
  - High thermal conductivity, acting as a heat barrier that prevents excessive energy dispersion.
  - However, the presence of numerous blood vessels can still facilitate heat dissipation, diminishing ablation efficiency [14, 15].
- Cancellous (Trabecular) Bone:
  - Low thermal conductivity, allowing greater heat retention and deeper tumor penetration.
  - In osteolytic lesions, this characteristic may enhance the efficacy of RFA, improving local tumor control [16, 17].

To counteract heat dissipation, various techniques have been developed, including:

- Bone Cement (Vertebroplasty): Polymethylmethacrylate (PMMA) cement has low thermal conductivity, preventing heat loss and prolonging the duration of tumor exposure to lethal temperatures [18].
- Increased Ablation Duration or Power: Extending energy application time or increasing RFA power output compensates for heat loss near vascularized regions.
- Pre-ablation Vascular Occlusion: Reducing blood flow via embolization before RFA helps mitigate the Heat-Sink Effect, maximizing tumor destruction [19].

4.2.4 Monopolar vs. Bipolar RFA Systems

RFA systems can be classified based on their electrode configuration, with two main types in clinical use:

Monopolar Radiofrequency Ablation (Fig. 4.2)

- Utilizes a single active electrode placed within the tumor.
- A grounding pad is positioned at a distant location (e.g., thigh or back) to complete the electrical circuit.
- Limited control over ablation size; energy dispersion may reduce treatment efficiency in larger tumors [19–22].

Bipolar Radiofrequency Ablation

- Features two active electrodes at the probe tip, both inserted within the tumor.
- Generates a localized electric field, enhancing tumor penetration and uniform energy distribution.
- More effective for large tumors, providing precise control over the ablation zone [22, 23].

Bipolar RFA is particularly advantageous for spinal metastases, as it allows greater energy deposition within confined vertebral spaces, minimizing thermal damage to surrounding structures [24].

4.2.5 Technological Advancements in RFA: Expandable and Steerable Systems

Initially, RFA procedures relied on straight, nonsteerable electrodes, which were effective for superficial or easily accessible lesions but were less suitable for complex anatomical locations [19, 22–24].

Expandable RFA Devices

- Feature extendable or articulated electrodes, increasing ablation coverage in large or irregularly shaped tumors.
- Enable greater lesion control, particularly in tumors near critical structures [13–15].

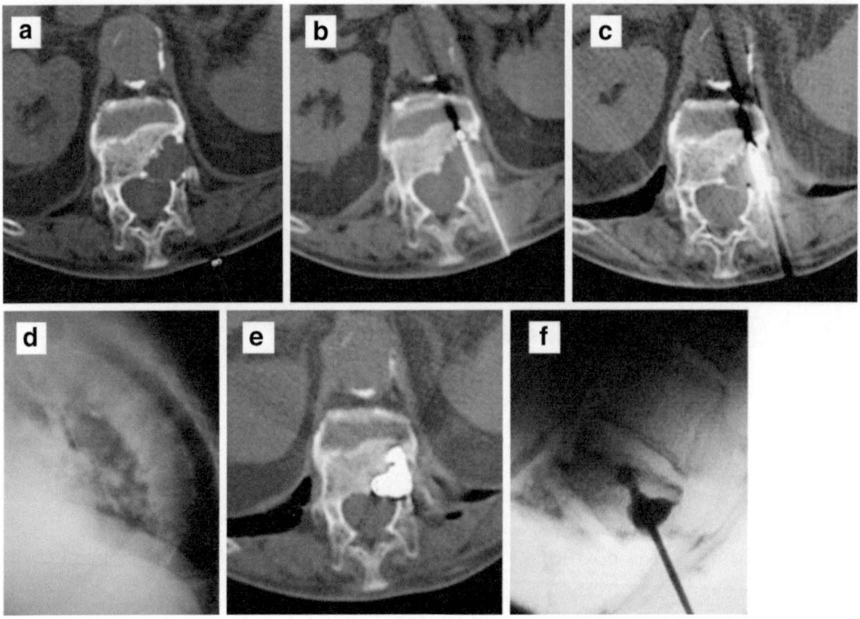

Fig. 4.2 Axial and fluoroscopic imaging of a metastatic D9 vertebral lesion from renal cell carcinoma in a 63-year-old male, treated with radiofrequency ablation (RFA) followed by vertebroplasty. Top row: (**a**) (Axial CT images). Preprocedural CT scan showing a lytic lesion in the left half of the D9 vertebral body, indicative of metastatic involvement from renal cell carcinoma. (**b**) (Axial CT images). Intraprocedural CT image demonstrating the insertion of the radiofrequency ablation (RFA) electrode into the lytic lesion within the D9 vertebral body. (**c**) (Axial CT images). Completion of the RFA procedure, with the electrode still in place, ensuring thermal ablation of the metastatic lesion while avoiding damage to adjacent critical structures. Bottom row: (**d**) (Fluoroscopic and CT images). Lateral fluoroscopic view confirming proper positioning of the vertebroplasty needle within the vertebral body. (**e**) (Fluoroscopic and CT images). Postprocedural axial CT showing polymethylmethacrylate (PMMA) cement filling the treated lytic area in the D9 vertebral body, providing structural reinforcement. (**f**) (Fluoroscopic and CT images). Intraprocedural fluoroscopic image capturing the controlled injection of PMMA cement, ensuring adequate vertebral stabilization without significant extravasation

Steerable RFA Systems [20, 22, 25]:

- Allow precise probe navigation via real-time image guidance (ultrasound, CT, magnetic resonance imaging (MRI)).
- Enable articulated distal segments, improving access to challenging anatomical regions.

For vertebral metastases, specialized bipolar RFA systems with integrated thermocouples allow for real-time temperature monitoring, enhancing both treatment precision and tissue protection [21, 22].

To see a summary of all available devices, see Table 4.1.

Table 4.1 Comparison of steerable devices in RFA

Device	Device type	Key features	Clinical applications	Advantages	Disadvantages
Straight, nonsteerable needles	Rigid needle	Fixed needle, no maneuverability	Superficial or fixed lesions	Simple and cost-effective, easy to use on accessible lesions	Limited precision, unsuitable for complex or deep lesions
Flexible RFA systems	Flexible radiofrequency probes	Increased flexibility, better access to deeper lesions	More complex lesions, organs, and surrounding structures	Greater precision, suitable for difficult-to-reach lesions	Requires greater skill, more expensive technology
Expandable RFA (extendable electrodes)	Probe with articulated or extendable electrode	Electrodes that extend or articulate to treat larger or complex areas	Large tumors or anatomically difficult locations	Improved access to difficult areas, more versatile	Requires more complex equipment, higher cost
Advanced articulated electrode RFA	Catheters with an advanced articulated electrode	Articulating electrodes for precise access to difficult sites	Larger tumors, complicated anatomical locations	High precision, controlled treatment area	Requires highly trained personnel, expensive

4.2.6 The Spinal Tumor Ablation with Radiofrequency (STAR™) System: Innovations in Spinal Tumor Ablation

One of the most advanced bipolar RFA technologies for bone tumors is the Spinal Tumor Ablation with Radiofrequency (STAR™) System, developed by Merit Medical.

SpineSTAR™ Ablation Instrument [20]:

- A bipolar, navigational, articulated device with an extendable, steerable tip that can curve up to 90°, enhancing tumor coverage (Figs. 4.3 and 4.4).
- Equipped with integrated thermocouples, providing real-time thermal monitoring of the ablation zone.

MetaSTAR™ Generator [20]:

- Displays simultaneous temperature readings from two thermocouples, allowing precise control over the ablation margins.
- Produces a 3:2 ablation zone ratio, with a maximum ablation area of 3 cm × 2 cm when the proximal thermocouple reaches 50 °C [25].

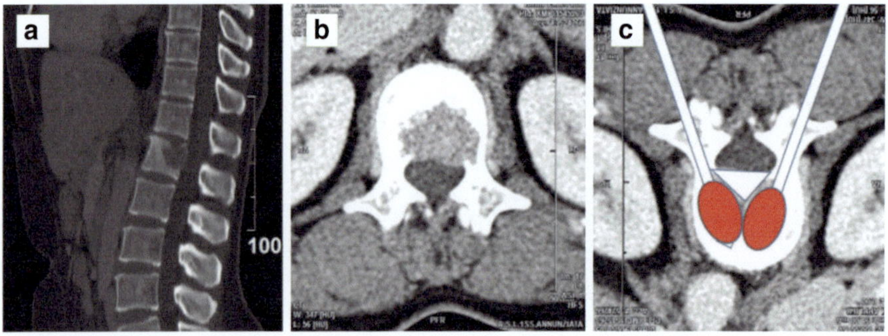

Fig. 4.3 CT imaging of a lytic metastatic lesion in the posterior portion of the L1 vertebral body from breast cancer in a 49-year-old female, highlighting the technical challenge of accessing the lesion using a straight needle approach. (**a**) (Sagittal CT): Preprocedural sagittal CT scan demonstrating a lytic metastatic lesion involving the posterior portion of the L1 vertebral body, compromising vertebral stability. The lesion originates from breast cancer metastasis, a common site for secondary spinal involvement. (**b**) (Axial CT): Axial CT image showing the posterior location of the lytic lesion at L1. The involvement of the posterior vertebral body makes standard vertebroplasty or biopsy more challenging due to the proximity of critical structures such as the spinal canal. (**c**) (Illustrative Diagram on CT): The schematic overlay illustrates the technical limitation of a straight needle approach (blue lines) in accessing the posterior and central portions of the lesion (red areas). Due to the specific anatomical configuration of the vertebral body and the challenging location of the lesion within it, a conventional transpedicular or extrapedicular approach using a straight needle may not allow sufficient access to the entire lesion. The linear trajectory of a rigid needle often limits the ability to reach posteriorly or eccentrically located tumor components, especially in anatomically complex or confined regions. As a result, standard straight-needle techniques may be inadequate for full lesion coverage, making it necessary to consider alternative access routes or the use of specialized, curved, or steerable needle systems that can navigate the anatomical constraints more effectively and ensure complete ablation

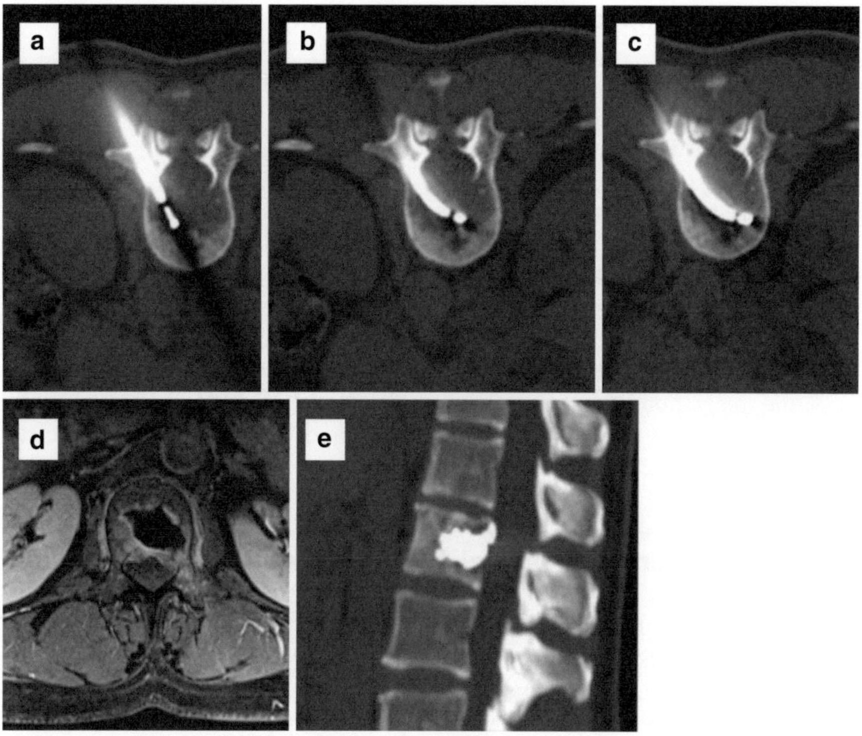

Fig. 4.4 (Case continued): (**a–c**) Top row (Axial CT images): Intraprocedural axial CT image demonstrating the insertion of the STAR™ curved ablation needle (Merit Medical, South Jordan, Utah, USA) into the metastatic lesion. The curved trajectory allows access to the posterior portion of the vertebral body, which would have been difficult to reach with a straight needle. (**d**, **e**) Bottom row: (**d**) Postprocedural axial MRI (T1-weighted postcontrast) demonstrating cement filling the ablated cavity with optimal distribution in the treated vertebral body, reinforcing structural integrity. No significant cement leakage is observed. (**e**) Postprocedural sagittal CT scan confirming successful cement augmentation following ablation. The polymethylmethacrylate (PMMA) cement is well distributed within the ablated tumor zone, providing structural reinforcement without significant leakage

The STAR™ system is particularly beneficial for treating [20, 25]:

- Spinal metastases adjacent to critical structures (e.g., spinal cord, nerve roots).
- Large, extravertebral metastases requiring extended ablation zones.
- Patients requiring vertebral augmentation (RFA + vertebroplasty in a single session).

Currently, an innovative radiofrequency device, the Cambridge Interventional System, has been developed with a power of up to 370 W. Using a single needle, it has achieved 6.5 × 5 cm ablations in just 15 min, providing greater control over the ablation area and effectively reducing the Heat-Sink Effect [26, 27].

4.2.7 Clinical Impact of Steerable Bipolar RFA

The selection of a steerable bipolar RFA probe is crucial for managing large, extravertebral, and anatomically challenging bone metastases. By allowing precise articulation of the distal probe segment, operators can:

- Maximize tumor coverage through a single bone access channel.
- Reduce the number of needle insertions, minimizing procedural morbidity.
- Enhance safety by selectively ablating tumor tissue while preserving adjacent structures [26].

As technological advancements continue to refine bipolar and steerable RFA systems, the integration of real-time imaging guidance (CT, MRI, fluoroscopy) will further enhance the accuracy, safety, and efficacy of spinal and musculoskeletal tumor ablation [20, 22, 23].

4.3 Indications and Clinical Applications

The initial success of radiofrequency ablation (RFA) in treating hepatic malignancies has expanded its role in musculoskeletal oncology, with growing applications in renal, breast, lung, and bone neoplasms [28]. The technique has proven particularly beneficial in bone metastases, which represent a frequent and debilitating complication of advanced cancer, occurring in 70–90% of patients with prostate or breast cancer and in 30–40% of those with thyroid, lung, or renal cancer [28]. Other malignancies, including melanoma, sarcoma, hepatocellular carcinoma, and uterine carcinoma, may also metastasize to bone, with vertebral involvement present in approximately 60–70% of patients [29, 30].

Up to 50% of patients with metastatic bone disease suffer from treatment-resistant pain, primarily due to tumor-induced periosteal stretching, osteoclast-mediated bone resorption, and the release of neurostimulating cytokines [28]. Although medical therapies (e.g., analgesics, bisphosphonates, and denosumab) and radiotherapy are widely used, pain remains inadequately controlled in 55–82% of cases [31].

Despite its role in palliation and local tumor control, radiotherapy (RT) has several limitations, including [32]:

- Ineffectiveness against radioresistant tumors (e.g., renal cell carcinoma, melanoma).
- Latency period of 1–2 weeks before significant pain relief [33].
- High recurrence rates, with pain returning in 50% of cases within 20–24 weeks posttreatment.

- Cumulative dose constraints that may prevent further treatment in previously irradiated sites.
- Lack of immediate structural reinforcement, failing to prevent pathological fractures.

Given these limitations, the European Society for Medical Oncology (ESMO) guidelines already incorporate RFA, cryoablation, and vertebroplasty (VP) as viable alternatives to radiotherapy, with comparable outcomes in terms of pain relief and even some advantages for vertebral metastases [34]. Specifically, the combination of RFA and vertebroplasty has been shown to reduce tumor burden, create an ablation cavity, and stabilize the vertebral body, making it an effective multimodal approach [34, 35].

4.3.1 Patient Selection [31]

Inclusion Criteria:

- Painful vertebral metastases, with or without pathological fracture.
- Poor tolerance or inadequate response to systemic analgesia.
- Moderate or better performance status.
- Life expectancy >3 months.
- Failure or ineligibility for external beam radiation therapy (EBRT).
- BMI <40, particularly in cases requiring prone positioning.

Relative Contraindications [31]

- BMI >40, especially in patients with osteoporosis or poor bone quality.
- Metastases with epidural extension, increasing the risk of spinal cord thermal injury due to a lack of cortical bone as a heat barrier.
- Poor baseline performance status, limiting procedural feasibility.
- Extensive soft-tissue metastatic disease, where RFA may not provide sufficient disease control.
- Life expectancy <3 months, as RFA is intended for patients expected to benefit from pain relief and functional improvement.
- Presence of a pacemaker or cardiac defibrillator, requiring cardiology consultation to assess interference risks.

Absolute Contraindications [31, 36]

- Spinal instability, requiring surgical fixation rather than percutaneous ablation.
- Neurological deficits, indicating nerve compression or spinal cord involvement.
- Systemic infection, increasing the risk of osteomyelitis or abscess formation.
- Irreversible coagulopathy, leading to uncontrolled bleeding risks.

4.3.2 Combined Applications: RFA with Vertebroplasty, SpineJack, and Extraspinal Metastases

The highest burden of metastatic bone disease occurs in the axial skeleton, leading to pathological fractures and severe pain [35, 37]. The resulting functional decline, loss of mobility, and deteriorated quality of life significantly affect survival outcomes and healthcare costs. In severe cases, vertebral collapse can lead to acute spinal cord compression [34, 35, 37].

Since RFA alone does not provide mechanical reinforcement, combining it with vertebral augmentation techniques is essential for restoring bone stability and reducing fracture risk (Figs. 4.5, 4.6, 4.7, and 4.8).

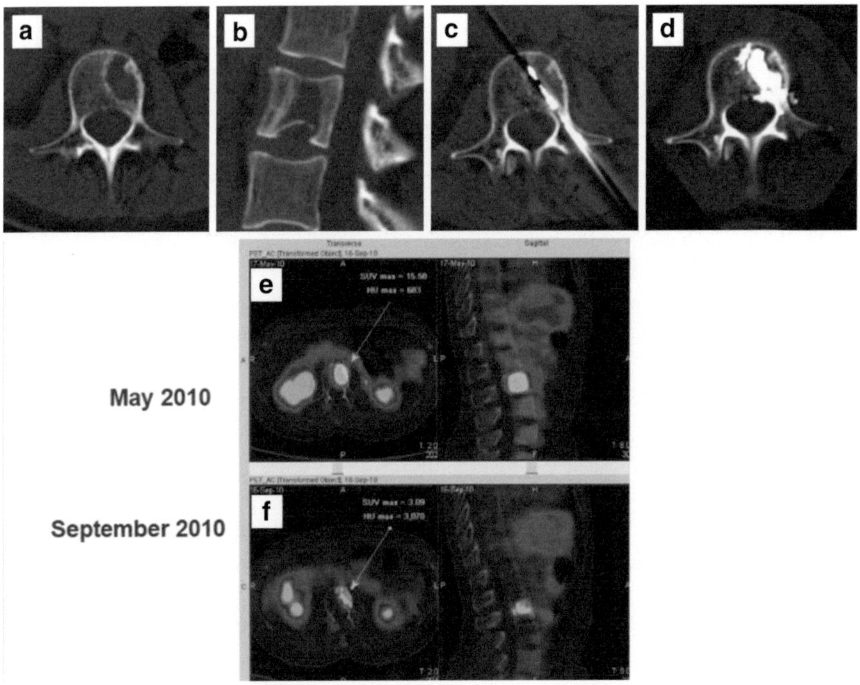

Fig. 4.5 Radiofrequency ablation (RFA) and vertebroplasty (VTP) for a lytic vertebral metastasis at L2 in a 50-year-old female with breast cancer. The patient presented in June 2010 with a lytic metastatic lesion at L2 vertebral body, measuring 2 × 1.5 cm, and a baseline Visual Analogue Scale (VAS) pain score of 7. Given her poor surgical candidacy, a minimally invasive approach combining radiofrequency ablation (RFA) and vertebroplasty (VTP) was chosen to achieve tumor control and vertebral stabilization. The top images (CT scans) illustrate the preprocedural axial (**a**) and sagittal (**b**) views of the L2 metastasis (arrow) and the intraprocedural steps, including RFA probe insertion (**c**) and postablation cement augmentation (**d**). The bottom images (PET-CT scans) show metabolic tumor activity before (**e**) and after (**f**) treatment. In May 2010 (preprocedure), the lesion exhibited high Fluorodeoxyglucose (FDG) uptake (SUVmax = 16.68), indicating active disease. In September 2010 (3 months postprocedure), follow-up PET-CT demonstrated a significant reduction in metabolic activity (SUVmax = 2.78), confirming successful tumor ablation and disease control

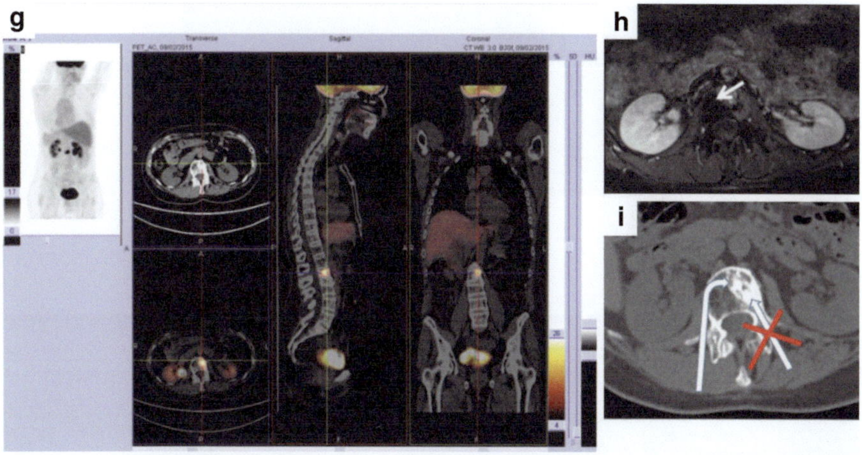

Fig. 4.6 Case continuation: After 55 months, the patient experienced a rise in tumor markers, prompting a PET-CT scan (G) that revealed increased FDG uptake in the previously ablated and cemented vertebral lesion, suggesting local recurrence. The MRI scan (H, axial view) confirmed this suspicion, showing contrast enhancement (white arrow) in the treated vertebra, consistent with active disease. Retreatment via a standard left pedicular approach was deemed unfeasible due to the presence of cement, which would obstruct needle placement (bottom right image). Instead, a contralateral transpedicular approach (I, blue trajectory) was proposed as an alternative, allowing safe access to the recurrent tumor while avoiding cement-related complications (I, red X marks the blocked access route)

Vertebroplasty (VP) and Cementoplasty

Percutaneous vertebroplasty (VP) is a minimally invasive procedure aimed at stabilizing symptomatic vertebral compression fractures using polymethylmethacrylate (PMMA) bone cement. It works by:

1. Enhancing spinal stability, reducing collapse progression.
2. Leveraging the thermal and chemical analgesic effects of cement on nociceptors.
3. Maximizing lesion filling, reducing the risk of secondary fractures [38, 39].

Pusceddu et al. analyzed RFA combined with cementoplasty for extraspinal metastases (e.g., pelvic and extremity tumors) and observed a significant pain reduction (VAS 7.75 → 0.5), with improved mobility in 6/7 previously wheelchair-bound patients within 1 month [40].

See Table 4.2. Results of local control and survival rate [67, 72–76].

Wang F. et al. analyzed RFA combined with cementoplasty for vertebral neoplastic lesions and observed a significant pain reduction (8.4–1.7) with a 6-month follow-up [41].

Similarly, Gazeloglu et al. studied 20 patients undergoing RFA + cementoplasty for pelvic and sacral metastases, reporting significant reductions in pain (VAS scores) and improvements in Karnofsky performance status [34].

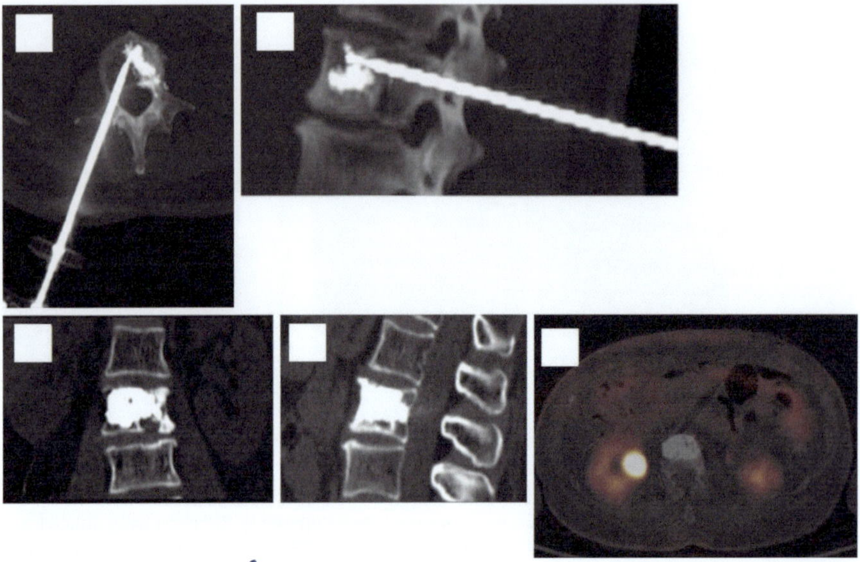

Fig. 4.7 (**a, b**) The top row (axial and sagittal CT images) demonstrates the intraprocedural phase of the retreatment, where a curved radiofrequency ablation (RFA) needle was used to precisely access and thermally ablate the recurrent lesion, overcoming the limitations posed by previous cement augmentation. Following ablation, vertebroplasty was performed, ensuring structural reinforcement of the treated vertebra. (**c, d**) The bottom row (left images, coronal and sagittal CT scans) shows the postprocedural appearance with successful cement augmentation in the previously treated vertebra. (**e**) The bottom right image (PET-CT at 6 months postprocedure) confirms the absence of FDG uptake, indicating effective local tumor control with no metabolic evidence of residual or recurrent disease

Fig. 4.8 In this case, we have an 83-year-old male diagnosed with lung adenocarcinoma (stage IV) due to bone, adrenals, retroperitoneal metastases, and possible retrocrural lymphadenopathy. The patient continues to have pain in the lumbar region despite analgesic treatment and antipain radiotherapy. A multidisciplinary committee was formed, and it was decided to perform radiofrequency ablation combined with vertebroplasty for pain treatment as palliative therapy. (**a**). This axial CT image, with bone filter, illustrates the left posterolateral level and with slight extension to the left pedicle, with a dense soft tissue component that breaks the cortex of the posterior wall, and with slight extension toward the central canal. No foraminal involvement is observed. (**b**). Placement, sedation, and percutaneous access: the patient was positioned in a prone position. Conscious sedation was performed. A posterior approach was performed at the L1 level, and a bilateral transpedicular approach was performed using CT and fluoroscopy. (**c, d**). Procedure. These axial CT images with a bone filter illustrate the sequence of the radiofrequency ablation technique performed. First, an 11-gauge bone trocar was introduced under CT and fluoroscopy guidance. Once the position was confirmed as satisfactory, the curved ablation probe was introduced through the coaxial trocar. (**e, f**). Vertebroplasty. These images identify the axial section (**e**) and sagittal section (**f**) with Maximum Intensity Projection (MIP). Following ablation, vertebroplasty was performed. Bilateral posterior vertebral cementation was performed with predominantly central and right lateral distribution. Minimal right posterolateral venous leak with no clinical significance. The final image shows well-distributed cement placement within the center of the ablation zone, ensuring structural reinforcement. Postprocedure: the procedure was well-tolerated and had no immediate complications. Bed rest was recommended. Sideways move was permitted, raising the head of the patient at 45° for meals. Control of the puncture site and vital signs to rule out bleeding and analgesia according to the guidelines (ablation may cause a slight increase in pain in the first few hours)

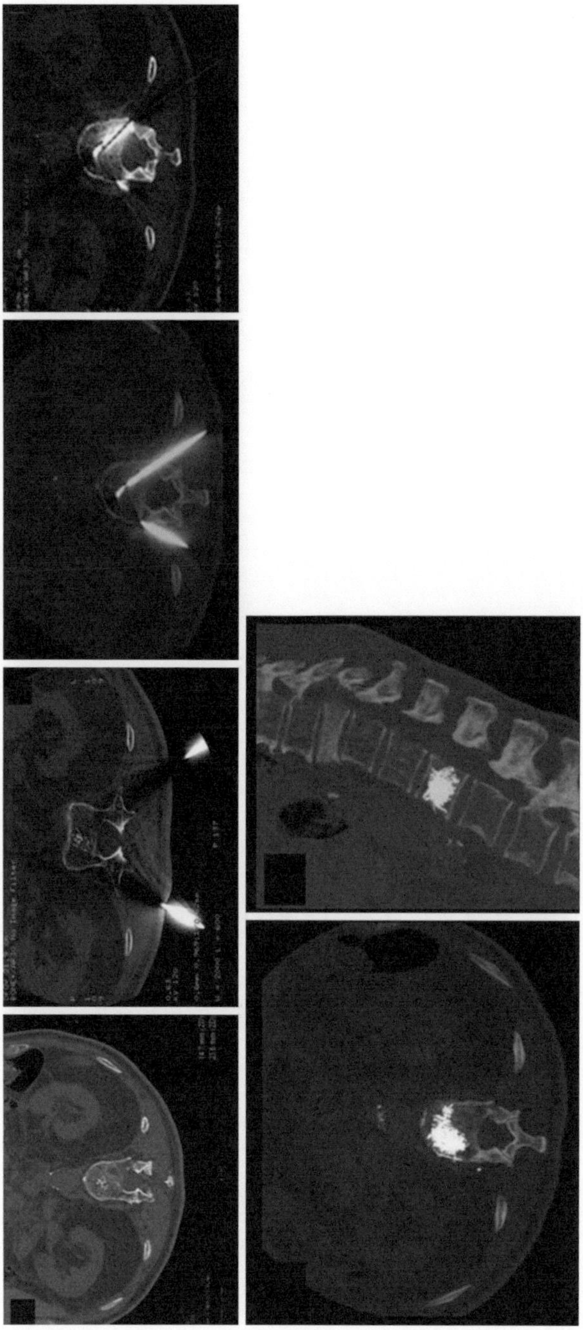

Table 4.2 Results of local control and survival rate [67, 72–76]

Author	Year	Title	N	% Local control	Survival rate	Follow-up (months)	% Complications
Koo et al. [72]	2021	The Efficacy of Radiofrequency Ablation for Bone Tumors Unsuitable for Radical Excision	43	85%			
Cazzato et al. [67]	2021	Percutaneous Thermal Ablation of Sacral Metastases: Assessment of Pain relief and Local Tumor Control	23	7 (30%)	NR	21	22
Luigi et al. [73]	2018	Percutaneous Image-Guided Ablation of Bone Metastases: Local Tumor Control in Oligometastatic Patients	46	71.7% 1 year	95.4% 2 years	34	10
Ma et al. [74]	2018	Percutaneous Image-Guided Ablation in the Treatment of Osseous Metastases from Non-small Cell Lung Cancer	45	68% 1 year	NR	NR	2,6
Wasmani et al. [75]	2018	Radiographic Local Tumor Control and Pain Palliation of Sarcoma Metastases within the Musculoskeletal System with Percutaneous Thermal Ablation	13	100% 1 year	NR	12	5
Erie et al. [76]	2017	Retrospective Review of Percutaneous Image-Guided Ablation of Oligometastatic Prostate Cancer: A Single-Institution Experience	16	83%	100% 2-year	27	0
Wallace et al. [50]	2016	Radiographic Local Control of Spinal Metastases with Percutaneous Radiofrequency Ablation and Vertebral Augmentation	NR [53]	70% 1 year	NR	7, 9	0

SpineJack Implantation

For patients with vertebral fractures but no neurological deficits, the SpineJack system allows vertebral height restoration and accelerates functional recovery. Studies in traumatic and pathological fractures (mostly in the lower thoracic and upper lumbar regions) report [42, 43]:

- Significant reductions in pain intensity (VAS scores).
- Improved functional status and mobility.
- Reduction in the vertebral wedge angle, preventing kyphotic deformity [44–46].

Cornelis et al. evaluated SpineJack implantation in vertebral compression fractures related to cancer in 13 patients, demonstrating [47]:

- Restoration of vertebral height in 50% of treated levels.
- Significant pain improvement.
- No serious adverse events.
- In two patients, RFA was combined with SpineJack, enhancing tumor control and structural stabilization.

See Table 4.3. Results of RFA and of the combined treatment of bone fracture and impending fracture.

4.3.3 Efficacy Outcomes and Long-Term Benefits

The combination of RFA and vertebroplasty offers rapid pain relief and durable local tumor control, making it superior to either technique alone.

- Pain Relief (Table 4.3):
  - Preprocedure high VAS scores decrease significantly within weeks to months posttreatment [48].
  - Functional status and quality of life improve as pain diminishes.
- Local Tumor Control:
  - Tomasian et al. reported a 78.9% local control rate following RFA + vertebroplasty [49].
  - Wallace et al. found a 3-month tumor control rate of 89%, decreasing to 70% at 1 year [50].
  - Yang et al. observed a 66.67% progression-free survival rate, with a median PFS of ~330 days [51].
- Safety Profile:
  - Major complications are rare (~0.4% incidence) [49, 50].
  - Cementoplasty-related risks include:
    - Pulmonary embolism in multilevel thoracic vertebral procedures.
    - Transient motor deficits due to nerve root compression by cement leakage [49–52].

Table 4.3 Results of RFA and combined treatment of bone fracture and impending fracture [22, 40, 41, 72, 77–82]

Author	Year	Ablation modality	Title	N° of patients	Mean pain score (VAS)	Survival rate	Follow-up (months)	% Major complications
Pusceddu et al. [40]	2023	RFA + VP	Clinical Rationale of Using Steerable Technologies for Radiofrequency Ablation Followed by Cavity Creation and Cement Augmentation in the Treatment of Painful Spinal Metastases	16	7.75–0.5	94% 6 months	6	NR
Wang et al. [41]	2022	RFA + VP	The Combination of Radiofrequency Ablation and Vertebroplasty Shows Advantages Over Single Vertebroplasty in Treating Vertebral Neoplastic Lesions	35	8.46–1.7	NR	6	0
Senol et al. [77]	2022	RFA + VP	Radiofrequency Ablation and Augmentation in the Management of Spinal Metastases: Clinical Experience in 41 Patients	41	7.4–2.6	NR	6	7.3
Madani et al. [78]	2021	RFA + VP	Combined Local Treatments for Vertebral Metastases with Limited Epidural Extension	18	7.3–2	73% 2 years	16.7	0
Koo et al. [72]	2021	RFA	The Efficacy of Radiofrequency Ablation for Bone Tumors Unsuitable for Radical Excision	43	7.5–2.6	95.3% 1 year	NR	NR
Kastler et al. [79]	2021	RFA + VP	Bipolar Radiofrequency Ablation of Painful Spinal Bone Metastases Performed under Local Anesthesia: Feasibility Regarding Patients' Experience and Pain Outcome	25	8.4–1.8	100% 1 year	12	0
Pusceddu et al. [22]	2021	RFA + VP	The Role of a Navigational Radiofrequency Ablation Device and Concurrent Vertebral Augmentation for Treatment of Difficult-to-Reach Spinal Metastases	35	5.7–0.9	72% 1 year	19	0
Yildizhan. et al. [80]	2021	RFA + VP	Role of Radiofrequency Ablation and Cement Injection for Pain Control in Patients with Spinal Metastasis	40	7.44–2.31	nr	6	

Mayer et al. [24]	2021	RFA	Spinal Metastases Treated with Bipolar Radiofrequency Ablation with Increased (>70 °C) Target Temperature: Pain Management and Local Tumor Control	31	NR		5	2.7%
Levy et al. [81]	2020	RFA	Radiofrequency Ablation for the Palliative Treatment of Bone Metastases: Outcomes from the Multicenter OsteoCool Tumor Ablation Post-Market Study (OPuS One Study) in 100 Patients	218	70% 6 months	6	4	
De Marini et al. [82]	2020	RFA + CA	Percutaneous Image-Guided Thermal Ablation of Bone Metastases: A Retrospective Propensity Study Comparing the Safety Profile of Radiofrequency Ablation and Cryoablation	274	NR	99.64% 1 year	18.5	2.5

4.4 Procedures in Vertebral Metastases and Tumors

Minimally invasive procedures, including thermal ablation and vertebral augmentation, have revolutionized the management of vertebral metastases and primary bone tumors, particularly in patients with poor surgical candidacy or significant tumor burden. The goal of these interventions is to achieve local tumor control, pain relief, and structural stabilization, minimizing the risk of vertebral collapse and associated neurological complications.

4.4.1 Preprocedural Evaluation

A thorough preprocedural assessment is crucial to determine tumor extent, lesion accessibility, and the proximity of critical structures, allowing for optimal planning of probe placement, monitoring devices, and protective measures. Imaging studies should be recent, ideally within one month prior to the procedure, especially for aggressive tumors or patients with evolving symptoms [31].

- Computed Tomography (CT):
  - Noncontrast CT with fine-section acquisition (1–3 mm) and multiplanar reconstructions is essential for evaluating bony involvement, tumor margins, and cortical integrity [31].
- Magnetic Resonance Imaging (MRI):
  - Multiparametric MRI (including T1- and T2-weighted sequences, fat-saturation imaging, diffusion-weighted imaging (DWI), and dynamic contrast-enhanced sequences) provides superior soft-tissue contrast for assessing tumor infiltration, epidural extension, and spinal cord involvement [31].

4.4.2 Anesthesia and Preprocedural Preparation

All thermal ablation techniques involve significant procedural pain, necessitating adequate anesthesia management. The choice of anesthetic technique depends on [31]:

1. Tumor location (e.g., proximity to neural structures).
2. Patient characteristics (e.g., age, cardiovascular risk).
3. Institutional protocols (e.g., presence of an anesthesiologist).

- Anesthetic Protocols:
  - Local Anesthesia + Conscious Sedation: Suitable for peripheral vertebral lesions with no epidural involvement.
  - General Anesthesia (GA): Preferred for complex lesions requiring longer ablation times or multi-probe insertion.

  - Periosteal and Pedicle Block: Local anesthetic infiltration up to the cortical bone enhances intraoperative pain control.
- Preprocedural Checklist:
  - Informed consent and detailed neurological examination.
  - Laboratory Workup: Complete blood count, coagulation profile, renal function, blood typing.
  - Vital sign monitoring throughout the procedure.

4.4.3 Procedural Guidance and Imaging Modalities

Ablative procedures require precise lesion targeting and real-time monitoring, achieved using advanced imaging modalities [31]:

- Fluoroscopy-Guided Techniques: Rapid probe positioning but limited soft-tissue contrast.
- CT-Guided Procedures: Superior bony detail and probe localization, often combined with fluoroscopy for real-time tracking.
- MRI-Guided Interventions: Ideal for soft-tissue tumors and spinal cord monitoring, though less commonly available.
- 3D Navigation and Image Fusion Systems: Enhances precision, particularly in complex vertebral lesions.

Patient positioning is optimized to ensure the shortest, most direct access route while avoiding critical structures. Supine or lateral positioning is most commonly used, depending on lesion location.

- Antibiotic prophylaxis is recommended when cement augmentation or hardware fixation is planned in conjunction with ablation.

4.4.4 Thermal Ablation Procedure

Ablation Protocol [31]

The standard approach for vertebral tumor ablation involves:

- Approach Selection:
  - Transpedicular or parapedicular access is preferred.
  - An 11- or 13-gauge trocar is inserted into the target vertebra under imaging guidance.
  - Probe deployment is confirmed in multiple planes.
- Ablation Phase:
  - The radiofrequency (RF) or microwave ablation probe is introduced via the trocar.

  - The trocar is withdrawn ~1 cm outside the ablation zone to prevent heat transmission and soft-tissue burns.
  - Ablation is performed at 90 °C for 10–20 min, adjusted based on tumor volume and tissue response.
- Neuroprotection Strategies:
  - Epidural thermocouples for real-time temperature monitoring at the neural foramina and spinal canal.
  - Injection of CO_2 or 5% dextrose-cooled fluid for thermal insulation of nerve structures [17].

Lesion-Specific Considerations [31]:

- Ipsilateral Vertebral Body Tumors: A unipedicular approach is sufficient.
- Midline-Extending or Contralateral Tumors: A bipedicular approach ensures complete tumor coverage.

4.4.5 Combination of Radiofrequency Ablation (RFA) and Vertebroplasty

Ablation may be combined with vertebral augmentation (vertebroplasty or kyphoplasty) in a single-session approach, providing both tumor control and mechanical stabilization.

- Technical Approach:
  - A 10/11-G vertebroplasty needle is inserted into the tumor.
  - A bipolar RF electrode is coaxially introduced for controlled tumor ablation.
  - Thermocouple monitoring (distal at 10 mm, proximal at 15 mm) prevents excessive heat spread.
  - Ultra-high viscosity bone cement is injected at low pressure to minimize extravasation risk.
- Indications for Vertebroplasty-First Strategy:
  - Predominantly lytic lesions with high fracture risk.
  - Extensive osteolysis predisposing to vertebral collapse.
  - Secondary stabilization before adjuvant radiotherapy.

This combined approach has demonstrated superior pain relief and structural reinforcement compared to ablation or vertebroplasty alone.

4.4.6 Postprocedural Monitoring and Follow-Up [31]

Immediate postprocedural imaging (CT or MRI) is performed to:

Evaluate treatment response (nonperfused tumor volume).
Identify potential complications (e.g., cement leakage, hemorrhage, nerve injury).

Thermal Monitoring Techniques:
- Epidural fiber-optic thermosensors (for MRI guidance).
- Real-time electrophysiological monitoring (SSEPs, MEPs) for neuroprotection.

Postprocedure Pain Management:
- Local periosteal infiltration with ropivacaine (5–10 ml, 2 mg/ml).
- Non-Steroidal Anti-Inflammatory Drugs (NSAIDs) and acetaminophen for routine pain control.
- Opioids and antiemetics in selected cases.

Follow-Up Imaging (MRI or CT):
- Perfusion MRI and apparent diffusion coefficient (ADC) mapping confirm successful tumor ablation.
- Complete ablation is defined by a nonperfused tumor volume encompassing the lesion and intended margins.

4.5 Practical Tips and Tricks: Optimizing Radiofrequency Ablation (RFA) Outcomes [31]

Although minimally invasive, these procedures carry certain risks, including:

- Vertebral fractures (especially in structurally compromised vertebrae).
- Thermal injury to adjacent neurovascular structures.
- Cement extravasation leading to nerve compression.
- Infections and bleeding complications.

Strict preprocedural planning, intraoperative monitoring, and meticulous technique significantly mitigate these risks, optimizing patient safety and clinical outcomes.

Successful radiofrequency ablation (RFA) for bone tumors requires precise procedural execution, careful thermal protection, and structured postprocedural monitoring to ensure optimal efficacy and patient safety. The following subsections outline key strategies to improve treatment precision, minimize complications, and enhance long-term outcomes.

4.5.1 Optimize Imaging Guidance for Needle Placement and Tumor Targeting [31]

Accurate needle placement and tumor targeting are critical for maximizing ablation effectiveness while minimizing injury to adjacent structures.

Multimodal imaging guidance using computed tomography (CT), ultrasound (US), or magnetic resonance imaging (MRI) enhances real-time visualization of tumor margins and needle trajectory.

Fluoroscopy-assisted procedures provide continuous real-time feedback, particularly for vertebral metastases and bone lesions.

3D navigation and augmented reality (AR) systems, when available, improve spatial orientation and targeting accuracy for complex cases.

4.5.2 Use Thermal Protection Measures Proactively [31]

When treating lesions near critical neural structures, thermal protection techniques must be applied to prevent collateral damage and ensure procedural safety.

Epidural or neuroforaminal thermocouples provide real-time temperature monitoring, reducing the risk of nerve damage.

Injectable insulation techniques include:

Cold CO_2 injection which creates an insulating gas barrier around sensitive tissues.
5% dextrose in water (D5W) infusion, acting as a heat sink without interfering with ablation energy transmission.
Hydrodissection techniques using saline or contrast agents can also be employed to displace and protect critical structures.

4.5.3 Monitor Ablation Temperatures Carefully [31]

Maintaining precise thermal control is essential for maximizing ablation efficacy while preventing damage to adjacent organs and neurovascular structures.

Ablation parameters should be set between 15 and 30 W, with an optimal tissue temperature of 80–100 °C at the tumor site.

Thermal sensors at the probe tip ensure that the desired temperature is reached without excessive heat propagation.

Temperature monitoring in adjacent tissues, particularly the spinal canal, nerve roots, and vascular structures, prevents complications such as nerve injury, vascular occlusion, or unintended tissue necrosis.

4.5.4 Plan Multimodal Pain Management [31]

Postprocedural inflammatory pain is a common side effect of RFA and should be proactively managed to ensure patient comfort and recovery.

Preprocedural Analgesia: Administer NSAIDs or acetaminophen to preemptively reduce postablation inflammation.

Postprocedural pain control strategies:

Local anesthetic injection (e.g., ropivacaine at the periosteal level) to reduce immediate postprocedure pain.
NSAIDs and acetaminophen as first-line agents.
Opioids for breakthrough pain, especially in cases of large-volume ablation or extensive tumor burden.

Adjunct pain relief strategies such as nerve blocks or corticosteroid injections may be considered for high-risk patients.

4.5.5 Integrate Follow-Up Imaging Protocols [31]

Regular postprocedural imaging is essential to assess treatment durability, detect complications, and monitor for early recurrence.

Immediate postprocedure CT scans should be performed to confirm:

Complete tumor coverage within the ablation zone.

Absence of significant procedural complications (e.g., hemorrhage, nerve injury, cement leakage if vertebroplasty was performed).

Follow-up MRI or CT at 1–3 months is recommended to:

Evaluate treatment response and detect residual tumor activity.

Identify early recurrence for potential retreatment.

Assess perfusion changes and apparent diffusion coefficient (ADC) values, which correlate with tumor viability postablation.

4.5.6 Use a Lateral-Positioned C-Arm During CT-Guided Ablation [31]

For spinal tumors or lesions near critical structures, a lateral-positioned C-arm fluoroscopy setup can significantly enhance procedural accuracy.

This approach allows:

Simultaneous monitoring of ablation precision (CT-guided) and controlled cement injection (fluoroscopy-guided).

Improved visualization of thermal protection measures, such as hydrodissection or insulation techniques.

Real-time confirmation of structural integrity reduces the risk of thermal spread beyond the target zone.

This setup is particularly beneficial for vertebral metastases adjacent to the spinal canal, where thermal protection and cementation control are critical for preventing neurological complications.

4.5.7 Consider a Contralateral Vertebroplasty Needle Approach [31]

When vertebroplasty is combined with RFA, a contralateral needle placement strategy can optimize cement distribution and structural stability.

A bipedicular approach using a contralateral vertebroplasty needle ensures:

Balanced cement filling reduces excessive unilateral injection that could increase leakage risk.
Improved mechanical reinforcement, particularly in osteolytic lesions with significant cortical thinning.
Reduced cement extrusion toward the ablation site, maintaining vertebral body symmetry and biomechanical integrity.

This approach is particularly useful in cases where the primary ablation site is adjacent to the vertebral canal, preventing posterior cement leakage and spinal cord compression.

4.6 Limitations and Future Directions

Radiofrequency ablation (RFA) is an effective treatment for malignant bone tumors but faces limitations, primarily the accessibility and cost of steerable devices, which can hinder its widespread use, especially in resource-limited settings. Additionally, emerging technologies such as artificial intelligence (AI) and advanced robotics offer potential advantages in precision, treatment customization, and risk reduction. AI can improve tumor localization, while robotics enhances needle placement accuracy. As these technologies advance, they may challenge RFA's role in bone tumor treatment. However, RFA remains a valuable option, particularly when newer technologies are unavailable or not suitable [53–56].

4.6.1 Other Applications

Other Tumors

Radiofrequency (RF) ablation has emerged as a well-established, minimally invasive therapeutic option for various solid tumors, particularly in patients who are not candidates for surgical resection. In the hepatic setting, RF is widely used in the treatment of hepatocellular carcinoma (HCC) and hepatic metastases, particularly from colorectal cancer, offering local tumor control and improved survival rates in appropriately selected cases. Similarly, in the pulmonary context, RF ablation has been successfully applied in early-stage non-small cell lung carcinoma (NSCLC) and pulmonary metastases, particularly in lesions measuring ≤ 3 cm, where it serves as an alternative to surgical resection or stereotactic body radiotherapy (SBRT) [57, 58].

In the renal setting, RF ablation has been established as an effective nephron-sparing alternative to partial nephrectomy, particularly in patients with small renal tumors (<4 cm), underlying comorbidities, or solitary kidneys. It provides durable oncologic control with a favorable safety profile compared to surgery, making it an attractive option in select patients [59–61].

Osteoid Osteoma (Fig. 4.9)

Osteoid osteoma is a benign osteogenic tumor characterized by a small (<2 cm) central nidus surrounded by reactive bone sclerosis. It predominantly affects the metaphysis or diaphysis of long bones, with the highest incidence between 5 and 40 years of age. The hallmark clinical symptom is persistent pain, which is often nocturnal and exhibits a dramatic response to salicylates and NSAIDs due to the tumor's overproduction of prostaglandins [62].

Historically, surgical en bloc resection was the primary treatment modality; however, it has largely been replaced by percutaneous image-guided techniques,

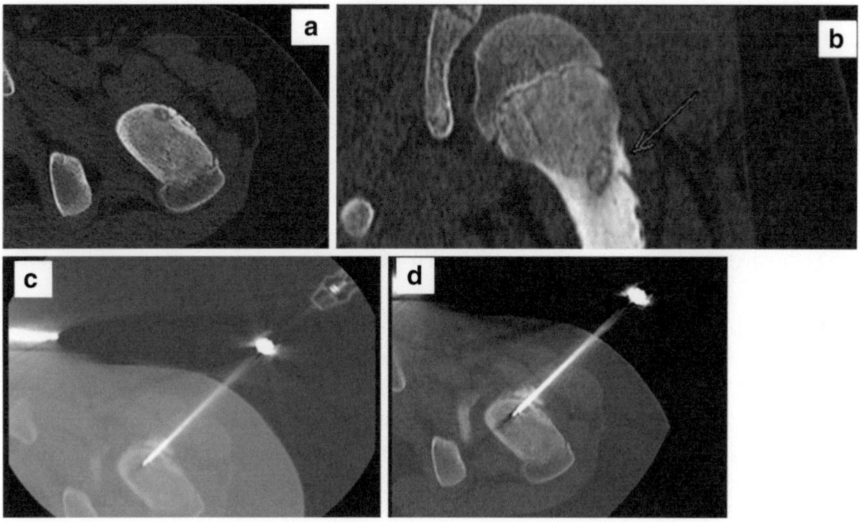

Fig. 4.9 In this case, we have a 12-year-old boy. Clinical consultation with left hip pain of more than 1 year's duration. He presents with progressive, nocturnal pain, which improves with NSAIDs. (**a**, **b**) These axial CT images, reconstructed with a bone filter, show at the left lower illustrates at the left lower extremity was performed, which showed a lytic lesion in the femoral neck with a sclerotic halo compatible with osteoma osteoide. 1. Preprocedure: A CT scan was used to locate the lesion and plan the puncture before the procedure. 2. Placement, sedation, and percutaneous access: Asepsis and local anesthesia and sedation by an anesthesiologist. Serum and intraarticular contrast are also infiltrated to further distend the joint capsule. 3. Procedure: Puncture with a 12G needle, 17G radiofrequency needle, and ablation is carried out for 6 min at 90°. The lesion area is then infiltrated with 0.5–0.6 cc bupivacaine (Fig. 4.2 and 4.3). (**c**, **d**) (Axial TC): Both show the RF needle optimal placement on the lesion. 4. Postprocedure: Rest for 24 h is recommended. Constant monitoring of the puncture site and analgesia regimen should be carried out, as there may be significant pain after the procedure. After the first 24–48 h, the patient was asymptomatic and did not present with pain

particularly radiofrequency ablation (RFA) and cryoablation, which provide comparable efficacy with significantly lower morbidity. These techniques offer a minimally invasive alternative that allows for precise tumor ablation, shorter recovery times, and lower complication rates [62, 63].

The choice between RFA and cryoablation is often based on lesion location. RFA remains the first-line therapy in most cases due to its high success rate and rapid procedural time. However, in lesions adjacent to neurovascular structures or articular surfaces, cryoablation may be preferred due to its controlled ice-ball formation and real-time visualization, reducing the risk of thermal injury. In cases of larger osteoid osteomas, multiple RFA applications may be required to ensure complete tumor ablation and prevent recurrence [64–67].

Facet Syndrome

Lumbar facet joint syndrome is a common etiology of chronic low back pain, estimated to account for 15–31% of all cases. The underlying pathophysiology involves degeneration and inflammation of the facet joints, leading to chronic mechanical back pain, which is often exacerbated by rotation, flexion-extension movements, and hyperextension [68].

While conservative treatment (physical therapy, NSAIDs, and intraarticular corticosteroid injections) remains the first-line approach, radiofrequency (RF) ablation has emerged as an effective intervention for patients with refractory facet syndrome. RF ablation of the medial branch nerves supplying the facet joints has demonstrated comparable or superior outcomes relative to intraarticular corticosteroid injections, with longer-lasting pain relief.

There are two principal RF techniques for facet syndrome treatment:

1. Continuous RF Ablation (CRF): This method delivers sustained high-temperature energy (>70 °C), causing permanent thermal coagulation of the targeted nerves.
2. Pulsed RF (PRF): Unlike CRF, PRF applies short, high-voltage pulses while maintaining a lower tissue temperature (<45 °C). This technique is nondestructive and is thought to exert its effects via neuromodulation rather than ablation, making it a preferred option in patients at risk of neural damage [69].

Several studies have shown that RF denervation of the facet joints provides superior pain relief compared to conservative treatments, with some patients experiencing symptom relief for up to 12 months postprocedure. The selection of CRF vs. PRF depends on patient factors, procedural goals, and anatomical considerations [70].

4.7 Future Directions

One of the primary challenges in minimally invasive procedures is the accurate navigation and placement of needles, which traditionally relies on two-dimensional (2D) imaging. Operators must mentally reconstruct the anatomy in three-dimensional (3D) space, a process that requires significant expertise and can lead to variability in accuracy [53]. Augmented reality (AR) has emerged as an innovative technological advancement that enhances procedural precision by directly visualizing 3D anatomical structures, enabling real-time guidance for more efficient and accurate needle placement [1, 54].

Several advanced navigation platforms and commercially available AR-integrated devices, such as PercuNav, XR90, and OpenSight, have been developed to incorporate ultrasound (US), computed tomography (CT), and magnetic resonance imaging (MRI) into AR-based guidance systems. These technologies enhance spatial orientation, providing operators with real-time 3D overlays of patient anatomy, thereby reducing the cognitive burden associated with transitioning from 2D imaging to 3D spatial awareness [55, 56]. Clinical studies have demonstrated that AR-assisted interventions can lead to improved depth perception, reduced procedure time, and greater accuracy in needle placement, ultimately enhancing the safety and efficacy of image-guided interventions [53].

Despite its promising advantages, barriers to widespread adoption remain. Key challenges include seamless integration into clinical workflows, the need for real-time, automated image segmentation, and the cost of implementation. Further technological advancements in artificial intelligence-driven segmentation, hardware miniaturization, and AR device ergonomics are essential to fully harness the potential of AR-assisted navigation in interventional radiology and other minimally invasive procedures. As these challenges are addressed, AR is poised to revolutionize image-guided interventions, enhancing procedural accuracy, reducing complications, and improving patient outcomes [71].

4.8 Conclusion

Radiofrequency ablation (RFA) has emerged as a minimally invasive, nonionizing thermal therapy that provides effective tumor cytoreduction and rapid, durable pain relief in patients with primary and metastatic bone lesions. By generating localized tissue heating through alternating electrical currents, RFA induces coagulative necrosis, effectively reducing tumor burden and alleviating pain within hours to days. This rapid response is attributed to sensory nerve destruction, reduced inflammatory mediator release, and decreased tumor mass effect, making it an invaluable tool in palliative and adjunctive oncologic treatment.

RFA is particularly beneficial in patients where conventional therapies are limited or insufficient. It serves as an effective alternative when radiotherapy is no longer feasible due to dose limitations or when severe pain restricts a patient's ability to tolerate the prone positioning required for radiation therapy planning and treatment delivery. Additionally, RFA complements external beam radiation therapy (EBRT), offering immediate pain relief while waiting for the delayed effects of radiation, which may take 4–6 weeks to achieve a full palliative response. In cases of radiation-resistant tumors such as renal cell carcinoma, melanoma, and sarcoma, where stereotactic body radiation therapy (SBRT) may not be available or suitable, RFA provides an alternative approach to local tumor control.

A crucial advantage of RFA is its ability to be combined with cementoplasty, particularly in weight-bearing bones and vertebral metastases, where mechanical stabilization is essential. Vertebral augmentation with cement following RFA not only prevents pathological fractures but also enhances pain relief by reinforcing osteolytic, structurally compromised lesions. The synergy between thermal ablation and cementoplasty ensures both oncologic control and biomechanical stability, reducing the risk of skeletal-related events and improving overall functional outcomes and quality of life.

As scientific evidence continues to support its safety and efficacy, RFA is solidifying its role as a key therapeutic modality in interventional oncology, offering tumor control, symptom relief, and structural stabilization in a single, image-guided percutaneous procedure. Its integration into multimodal cancer care strategies represents a significant advancement in the minimally invasive management of bone tumors, providing durable symptom relief and improving patient outcomes in both curative and palliative settings.

References

1. Dalili D, Isaac A, Cazzato RL, Åström G, Bergh J, Mansour R, Weber MA, Garnon J, Gangi A. Interventional techniques for bone and musculoskeletal soft tissue tumors: current practices and future directions – part II. Stabilization. Semin Musculoskelet Radiol. 2020;24(6):710–25. https://doi.org/10.1055/s-0040-1719104. Epub 2020 Dec 11. PMID: 33307586
2. Ridouani F, Srimathveeravalli G. Percutaneous image-guided ablation: from techniques to treatments. Presse Med. 2019;48(7–8 Pt 2):e219–31. https://doi.org/10.1016/j.lpm.2019.06.005. Epub 2019 Aug 22. PMID: 31447333
3. Mansur A, Garg T, Shrigiriwar A, Etezadi V, Georgiades C, Habibollahi P, Huber TC, Camacho JC, Nour SG, Sag AA, Prologo JD, Nezami N. Image-guided percutaneous ablation for primary and metastatic tumors. Diagnostics (Basel). 2022;12(6):1300. https://doi.org/10.3390/diagnostics12061300. PMID: 35741109; PMCID: PMC9221861
4. Pusceddu C, De Francesco D, Ballicu N, Santucci D, Marsico S, Venturini M, Fior D, Moramarco LP, Faiella E. Safety and feasibility of steerable radiofrequency ablation in combination with cementoplasty for the treatment of large extraspinal bone metastases. Curr Oncol. 2022;29(8):5891–900. https://doi.org/10.3390/curroncol29080465.
5. Glazer ES, Curley SA. The ongoing history of thermal therapy for cancer. Surg Oncol Clin N Am. 2011;20(2):229–35. https://doi.org/10.1016/j.soc.2010.11.001. vii. Epub 2010 Dec 13. PMID: 21377580; PMCID: PMC3061441
6. Grabnar M, Mueller M, Kim C. History of radiofrequency ablation (RFA). 2024. https://doi.org/10.1016/B978-0-323-87063-4.00010-2.
7. O'Connor JL, Bloom DA, William T. Bovie and electrosurgery. Surgery. 1996;119(4):390–6. https://doi.org/10.1016/s0039-6060(96)80137-1. PMID: 8644002
8. Rosenthal DI, Alexander A, Rosenberg AE, Springfeld D. Ablation of osteoid osteomas with a percutaneously placed electrode: a new procedure. Radiology. 1992;183(1):29–33.
9. Chu KF, Dupuy DE. Thermal ablation of tumours: biological mechanisms and advances in therapy. Nat Rev Cancer. 2014;14(3):199–208. https://doi.org/10.1038/nrc3672. PMID: 24561446

10. Andrade JG, Deyell MW, Macle L. Biophysics of ablation – radiofrequency and cryoablation. In: Encyclopedia of cardiovascular research and medicine. Amsterdam: Elsevier; 2018. p. 334–49.
11. Strand NH, Hagedorn JM, Dunn T, Johnson B, Abd-Elsayed A, Covington S, Freeman J, Dawodu A, Maloney J. M Advances in radiofrequency ablation: mechanism of action and technology. Ann Palliat Med. 2024;13(4):1028–34. https://doi.org/10.21037/apm-23-457.
12. Knavel EM, Brace CL. Tumor ablation: common modalities and general practices. Tech Vasc Interv Radiol. 2013;16(4):192–200. https://doi.org/10.1053/j.tvir.2013.08.002. PMID: 24238374; PMCID: PMC4281168
13. De Vita E, Lo Presti D, Massaroni C, Iadicicco A, Schena E, Campopiano S. A review on radiofrequency, laser, and microwave ablations and their thermal monitoring through fiber Bragg gratings. iScience. 2023;26(11):108260. https://doi.org/10.1016/j.isci.2023.108260. PMID: 38026224; PMCID: PMC10660479
14. Klimek K, Mader N, Happel C, Sabet A, Grünwald F, Groener D. Heat sink effects in thyroid bipolar radiofrequency ablation: an ex vivo study. Sci Rep. 2023;13(1):19288. https://doi.org/10.1038/s41598-023-45926-2. PMID: 37935715; PMCID: PMC10630443
15. Thakur S, Lavito S, Grobner E, Grobner M. Radiofrequency thermal ablation heat energy transfer in an ex-vivo model. Am Surg. 2017;83(12):1373–80. PMID: 29336757
16. Ghomashchi S, Whyne CM, Chinnery T, Habach F, Akens MK. Impact of radiofrequency ablation (RFA) on bone quality in a murine model of bone metastases. PLoS One. 2021;16(9):e0256076. https://doi.org/10.1371/journal.pone.0256076. PMID: 34495961; PMCID: PMC8425524
17. Rybak LD. Fire and ice: thermal ablation of musculoskeletal tumors. Radiol Clin North Am. 2009;47(3):455–69. https://doi.org/10.1016/j.rcl.2008.12.006. PMID: 19361670
18. Buy X, Tok CH, Szwarc D, Bierry G, Gangi A. Thermal protection during percutaneous thermal ablation procedures: interest of carbon dioxide dissection and temperature monitoring. Cardiovasc Intervent Radiol. 2009;32:529–34.
19. Pillai K, Akhter J, Chua TC, Shehata M, Alzahrani N, Al-Alem I, Morris DL. Heat sink effect on tumor ablation characteristics as observed in monopolar radiofrequency, bipolar radiofrequency, and microwave, using ex vivo calf liver model. Medicine (Baltimore). 2015;94(9):e580. https://doi.org/10.1097/MD.0000000000000580. PMID: 25738477; PMCID: PMC4553952
20. Ma Y, Wallace AN, Madaelil TP, Jennings JW. Treatment of osseous metastases using the Spinal Tumor Ablation with Radiofrequency (STAR) system. Expert Rev Med Devices. 2016;13:1137–45.
21. Reyes M, Georgy M, Brook L, Ortiz O, Brook A, Agarwal V, Muto M, Manfre L, Marcia S, Georgy BA. Multicenter clinical and imaging evaluation of targeted radiofrequency ablation (t-RFA) and cement augmentation of neoplastic vertebral lesions. J Neurointerv Surg. 2018;10:176–82.
22. Pusceddu C, De Francesco D, Melis L, Ballicu N, Fancellu A. The role of a navigational radiofrequency ablation device and concurrent vertebral augmentation for treatment of difficult-to-reach spinal metastases. Curr Oncol. 2021;28(5):4004–15. https://doi.org/10.3390/curroncol28050340. PMID: 34677258; PMCID: PMC8534768
23. Mulier S, Possebon R, Jiang Y, Jamart J, Wang C, Miao Y, Yu T, Jiang K, Feng Y, Marchal G, Michel L, Ni Y. Radiofrequency ablation with four electrodes as a building block for matrix radiofrequency ablation: ex vivo liver experiments and finite element method modelling. Influence of electric and activation mode on coagulation size and geometry. Surg Oncol. 2020;33:145–57. https://doi.org/10.1016/j.suronc.2020.02.005. Epub 2020 Feb 10. PMID: 32561081
24. Mayer T, Cazzato RL, De Marini P, Auloge P, Dalili D, Koch G, Garnon J, Gangi A. Spinal metastases treated with bipolar radiofrequency ablation with increased (>70°C) target temperature: Pain management and local tumor control. Diagn Interv Imaging. 2021;102(1):27–34. https://doi.org/10.1016/j.diii.2020.04.012. Epub 2020 May 29. PMID: 32482583
25. Anchala PR, Irving WD, Hillen TJ, Friedman MV, Georgy BA, Coldwell DM, Tran ND, Vrionis FD, Brook A, Jennings JW. Treatment of metastatic spinal lesions with a navigational

bipolar radiofrequency ablation device: a multicenter retrospective study. Pain Physician. 2014;17(4):317–27. PMID: 25054391

26. Ben-David E, Nissenbaum I, Gurevich S, Cosman ER, Goldberg SN. Optimization and characterization of a novel internally-cooled radiofrequency ablation system with optimized pulsing algorithm in an ex-vivo bovine liver. Int J Hyperth. 2019;36(2):81–8. https://doi.org/10.1080/02656736.2019.1617901.
27. Solbiati L, Ierace T, Gennaro N, Muglia R, Cosman ER, Goldberg SN. Percutaneous radiofrequency ablation of HCC: reduced ablation duration and increased ablation size using single, internally cooled electrodes with an optimized pulsing algorithm. Int J Hyperth. 2020;37(1):861–7. https://doi.org/10.1080/02656736.2020.1790678.
28. Snijders RAH, Brom L, Theunissen M, van den Beuken-van Everdingen MHJ. Update on prevalence of pain in patients with cancer 2022: a systematic literature review and meta-analysis. Cancers (Basel). 2023;15(3):591. https://doi.org/10.3390/cancers15030591. PMID: 36765547; PMCID: PMC9913127
29. Nakamura T, Asanuma K, Takao M, Yamanaka T, Koike H, Chen-Yoshikawa TF, Tsukushi S, Kuroda H, Kozawa E, Sano M, Aiba H, Nakanishi R, Nagano A, Yamada K, Shido Y, Kawanami K, Izubuchi Y, Sudo A, Nishida Y. Clinical outcome in soft tissue sarcoma patients with lung metastasis who received metastasectomy and/or radiofrequency ablation: Tokai musculoskeletal oncology consortium study. Cancer Manag Res. 2021;13:8473–80. https://doi.org/10.2147/CMAR.S333721. PMID: 34785953; PMCID: PMC8590959
30. Ruiz-Alva SK, Cortes-Cerda R, Mora-Ríos FG, Benítez-Romero A, Isunza-Ramírez A, Mejía-Rohenes LC. Tumors that cause bone metastases. Acta Ortop Mex. 2021;35(2):201–5. Spanish. PMID: 34731924
31. Ryan A, Byrne C, Pusceddu C, Buy X, Tsoumakidou G, Filippiadis D. CIRSE standards of practice on thermal ablation of bone tumours. Cardiovasc Intervent Radiol. 2022;45(5):591–605. https://doi.org/10.1007/s00270-022-03126-x. Epub 2022 Mar 29. PMID: 35348870; PMCID: PMC9018647
32. Fourney DR, Schomer DF, Nader R, et al. Percutaneous vertebroplasty and kyphoplasty for painful vertebral body fractures in cancer patients. J Neurosurg. 2003;98(1 suppl):21–3.
33. Alcorn S, Cortés ÁA, Bradfield L, Brennan M, Dennis K, Diaz DA, Doung YC, Elmore S, Hertan L, Johnstone C, Jones J, Larrier N, Lo SS, Nguyen QN, Tseng YD, Yerramilli D, Zaky S, Balboni T. External beam radiation therapy for palliation of symptomatic bone metastases: an ASTRO clinical practice guideline. Pract Radiat Oncol. 2024;14(5):377–97. https://doi.org/10.1016/j.prro.2024.04.018. Epub 2024 May 22. PMID: 38788923
34. Gazeloglu AO, Yilmaz A, Caglar O, Atilla B, Ayvaz M, Tokgozoglu AM. Effectiveness of RF ablation and cementoplasty in enhancing functional capacity in pelvic malignant bone metastases. Eur J Orthop Surg Traumatol. 2024;34(7):3609–18. https://doi.org/10.1007/s00590-024-04081-8. Epub 2024 Aug 21. PMID: 39167205
35. Coleman R, Hadji P, Body JJ, Santini D, Chow E, Terpos E, Oudard S, Bruland Ø, Flamen P, Kurth A, Van Poznak C, Aapro M, Jordan K, ESMO Guidelines Committee. Electronic address: clinicalguidelines@esmo.org. Bone health in cancer: ESMO clinical practice guidelines. Ann Oncol. 2020;31(12):1650–63. https://doi.org/10.1016/j.annonc.2020.07.019. Epub 2020 Aug 12. PMID: 32801018
36. Wray JK, Dixon B, Przkora R. Radiofrequency ablation. [Updated 2023 Jun 12]. In: StatPearls [Internet]. Treasure Island (FL): StatPearls Publishing; 2025. Available from: https://www.ncbi.nlm.nih.gov/books/NBK482387/
37. Barzilai O, Bilsky MH, Laufer I. The role of minimal access surgery in the treatment of spinal metastatic tumors. Glob Spine J. 2020;10(2 Suppl):79S–87S. https://doi.org/10.1177/2192568219895265. Epub 2020 May 28. PMID: 32528811; PMCID: PMC7263343
38. Dalili D, Isaac A, Bazzocchi A, Åström G, Bergh J, Lalam R, Weber MA, Fritz J, Mansour R. Interventional techniques for bone and musculoskeletal soft tissue tumors: current practices and future directions – part I. Ablation. Semin Musculoskelet Radiol. 2020;24(6):692–709. https://doi.org/10.1055/s-0040-1719103. Epub 2020 Dec 11. PMID: 33307585

39. Tian QH, Wu CG, Gu YF, He CJ, Li MH, Cheng YD. Combination radiofrequency ablation and percutaneous osteoplasty for palliative treatment of painful extraspinal bone metastases: a single-center experience. J Vasc Interv Radiol. 2014;25:1094–100. https://doi.org/10.1016/j.jvir.2014.03.018.
40. Pusceddu C, Marsico S, Derudas D, Ballicu N, Melis L, Zedda S, De Felice C, Calabrese A, Santucci D, Faiella E. Clinical rationale of using steerable technologies for radiofrequency ablation followed by cavity creation and cement augmentation in the treatment of painful spinal metastases. Curr Oncol. 2023;30(4):4257–68. https://doi.org/10.3390/curroncol30040324. PMID: 37185437; PMCID: PMC10136743
41. Wang F, Gu J, Xu C, Li G, Lv P. The combination of radiofrequency ablation and vertebroplasty shows advantages over single vertebroplasty in treating vertebral neoplastic lesions. Skeletal Radiol. 2022;51(3):565–71. https://doi.org/10.1007/s00256-021-03788-7. Epub 2021 Jul 10. PMID: 34247255
42. Sowa D, Guzik G, Bronisz M, Merkiel D, Pyrka D, Pyrka Z. Outcomes of treatment of spinal fractures with the SpineJack system. Ortop Traumatol Rehabil. 2023;25(1):1–8. https://doi.org/10.5604/01.3001.0053.4025. PMID: 38078347
43. Pusceddu C, Faiella E, Derudas D, Ballicu N, Melis L, Zedda S, Marsico S. Re-expansion of vertebral compression fractures in patients with multiple myeloma with percutaneous vertebroplasty using spinejack implants: a preliminary and retrospective study. Front Surg. 2023;10:1121981. https://doi.org/10.3389/fsurg.2023.1121981. PMID: 37288134; PMCID: PMC10242080
44. England RW, Gong A, Li T, Botros D, Manupipatpong S, Pang S, Hui F, Khan M. Clinical outcomes and safety of the SpineJack vertebral augmentation system for the treatment of vertebral compression fractures in a United States patient population. J Clin Neurosci. 2021;89:237–42. https://doi.org/10.1016/j.jocn.2021.04.031. Epub 2021 May 13. PMID: 34119274
45. Filippiadis DK, Marcia S, Ryan A, Beall DP, Masala S, Deschamps F, Kelekis A. New implant-based technologies in the spine. Cardiovasc Intervent Radiol. 2018;41(10):1463–73. https://doi.org/10.1007/s00270-018-1987-z. Epub 2018 May 22. PMID: 29789873
46. Bonaldi G, Cianfoni A. Percutaneous treatment of lumbar compression fracture with canal stenosis and neurogenic intermittent claudication: combining kyphoplasty and interspinous spacer. J Vasc Interv Radiol. 2012;23(11):1437–41. https://doi.org/10.1016/j.jvir.2012.06.023. PMID: 23101915
47. Cornelis FH, Razakamanantsoa L, Ben Ammar M, Najdawi M, Gardavaud F, El-Mouhadi S, Barral M. Expandable intravertebral implant in cancer-related vertebral compression fractures: a retrospective review of 36 implantations. J Vasc Interv Radiol. 2022;33(1):14–8. https://doi.org/10.1016/j.jvir.2021.10.002. PMID: 34980450
48. Faiella E, Vaccarino F, Pacella G, Santucci D, Vergantino E, Bruno A, Ragone R, Zobel BB, Grasso RF. Exploring the efficacy of combining radiofrequency thermal ablation or microwave ablation with vertebroplasty for pain control and disease management in metastatic bone disease-a systematic review. Curr Oncol. 2024;31(9):5422–38. https://doi.org/10.3390/curroncol31090401. PMID: 39330029; PMCID: PMC11430811
49. Tomasian A, Marlow J, Hillen TJ, Jennings JW. Complications of percutaneous radiofrequency ablation of spinal osseous metastases: an 8-year single-center experience. Am J Roentgenol. 2021;216:1607–13.
50. Wallace A, Tomasian A, Vaswani D, Vyhmeister R, Chang R, Jennings J. Radiographic local control of spinal metastases with percutaneous radiofrequency ablation and vertebral augmentation. Am J Neuroradiol. 2015;37:759–65.
51. Yang P-L, He X-J, Li H-P, Zang Q-J, Wang G-Y. Image-guided minimally invasive percutaneous treatment of spinal metastasis. Exp Ther Med. 2017;13:705–9.
52. Al-Nakshabandi NA. Percutaneous vertebroplasty complications. Ann Saudi Med. 2011;31(3):294–7. https://doi.org/10.4103/0256-4947.81542. PMID: 21623061; PMCID: PMC3119972
53. Evans M, Kang S, Bajaber A, Gordon K, Martin C 3rd. Augmented reality for surgical navigation: a review of advanced needle guidance systems for percutaneous tumor ablation. Radiol

Imaging Cancer. 2025;7(1):e230154. https://doi.org/10.1148/rycan.230154. PMID: 39750112; PMCID: PMC11791678
54. Kadkhodamohammadi A, Gangi A, de Mathelin M, Padoy N. Articulated clinician detection using 3D pictorial structures on RGB-D data. Med Image Anal. 2017;35:215–24.
55. Fritz J, U-Thainual P, Ungi T, et al. Augmented reality visualization using image overlay technology for MR-guided interventions: cadaveric bone biopsy at 1.5 T. Investig Radiol. 2013;48(06):464–70.
56. Issenhuth T, Srivastav V, Gangi A, Padoy N. Face detection in the operating room: comparison of state-of-the-art methods and a self-supervised approach. Int J CARS. 2019;14(06):1049–58.
57. Prud'homme C, Deschamps F, Moulin B, Hakime A, Al-Ahmar M, Moalla S, Tselikas L. Image-guided lung metastasis ablation: a literature review. Int J Hyperth. 2019;36(2):37–45. https://doi.org/10.1080/02656736.2019.1647358.
58. Wang H, Wu Z, Cui D, Shi Y, Zhai B. Radiofrequency ablation of hepatocellular carcinoma: current status, challenges, and prospects. Liver Res. 2023;7(2):108–15. https://doi.org/10.1016/j.livres.2023.05.002. PMID: 39958948; PMCID: PMC11791925
59. Xie GL, Zhong ZH, Ye TW, Xiao ZQ. Radiofrequency ablation combined with immunotherapy to treat hepatocellular carcinoma: a comprehensive review. BMC Surg. 2025;25(1):47. https://doi.org/10.1186/s12893-025-02778-z. PMID: 39875933; PMCID: PMC11776151
60. Park J, Lee MW, Ahn SH, Han S, Min JH, Cha DI, Song KD, Kang TW, Rhim H. Treatment outcomes of percutaneous radiofrequency ablation for hepatocellular carcinomas: effects of the electrode type and placement method. Korean J Radiol. 2023;24(8):761–71. https://doi.org/10.3348/kjr.2023.0022. PMID: 37500577; PMCID: PMC10400371
61. Wood BJ, Ramkaransingh JR, Fojo T, Walther MM, Libutti SK. Percutaneous tumor ablation with radiofrequency. Cancer. 2002;94(2):443–51. https://doi.org/10.1002/cncr.10234. PMID: 11900230; PMCID: PMC2408948
62. Dookie AL, Joseph RM. Osteoid Osteoma. 2023 Aug 14. In: StatPearls [Internet]. Treasure Island (FL): StatPearls Publishing; 2025. PMID: 30725964.
63. Lindquester WS, Crowley J, Hawkins CM. Percutaneous thermal ablation for treatment of osteoid osteoma: a systematic review and analysis. Skeletal Radiol. 2020;49(9):1403–11. https://doi.org/10.1007/s00256-020-03435-7. Epub 2020 Apr 8. PMID: 32270226
64. Noordin S, Allana S, Hilal K, Nadeem N, Lakdawala R, Sadruddin A, et al. Osteoid osteoma: contemporary management. Orthop Rev (Pavia). 2018;10(3):7496.
65. Ghanem I. The management of osteoid osteoma: updates and controversies. Curr Opin Pediatr. 2006;18:36–41.
66. Singh DK, Katyan A, Kumar N, Nigam K, Jaiswal B, Misra RN. CT-guided radiofrequency ablation of osteoid osteoma: established concepts and new ideas. Br J Radiol. 2020;93(1114):20200266. https://doi.org/10.1259/bjr.20200266. Epub 2020 Jun 24. PMID: 32520586; PMCID: PMC7548372
67. Cazzato RL, De Marini P, Leonard-Lorant I, Dalili D, Koch G, Autrusseau PA, Mayer T, Weiss J, Auloge P, Garnon J, Gangi A. Percutaneous thermal ablation of sacral metastases: assessment of pain relief and local tumor control. Diagn Interv Imaging. 2021;102(6):355–61. https://doi.org/10.1016/j.diii.2020.12.008. Epub 2021 Jan 22. PMID: 33487588
68. Ambrosio L, Vadalà G, Russo F, et al. Interventional minimally invasive treatments for chronic low back pain caused by lumbar facet joint syndrome: a systematic review. Glob Spine J. 2022;13(4):1163–79. https://doi.org/10.1177/21925682221142264.
69. Sansone P, Giaccari LG, Lippiello A, Aurilio C, Paladini A, Passavanti MB, Pota V, Pace MC. Pulsed radiofrequency for lumbar facet joint pain: a viable therapeutic option? A retrospective observational study. Pain Ther. 2020;9(2):573–82. https://doi.org/10.1007/s40122-020-00187-z. Epub 2020 Aug 8. PMID: 32770486; PMCID: PMC7648804
70. Chen YS, Liu B, Gu F, Sima L. Radiofrequency denervation on lumbar facet joint pain in the elderly: a randomized controlled prospective trial. Pain Physician. 2022;25(8):569–76. PMID: 36375186
71. Booher G, Vardiman A. Navigated robotic assisted thoracic pedicle screw placement for metastatic renal cell carcinoma. Neurosurg Focus. 2018;45(VideoSuppl1):V5.

72. Koo JS, Chung SH. The efficacy of radiofrequency ablation for bone tumors unsuitable for radical excision. Clin Orthop Surg. 2021;13:278–85.
73. Luigi Cazzato R, Auloge P, De Marini P, Rousseau C, Chiang JB, Koch G, Caudrelier J, Rao P, Garnon J, Gangi A. Percutaneous image-guided ablation of bone metastases: local tumor control in oligometastatic patients. Int J Hyperth. 2018;35(1):493–9. https://doi.org/10.1080/02656736.2018.1508760. Epub 2018 Oct 11. PMID: 30307346
74. Ma Y, Wallace AN, Waqar SN, Morgensztern D, Madaelil TP, Tomasian A, Jennings JW. Percutaneous image-guided ablation in the treatment of osseous metastases from non-small cell lung cancer. Cardiovasc Intervent Radiol 2018;41(5):726–733. doi: https://doi.org/10.1007/s00270-017-1843-6. Epub 2017 Dec 4. PMID: 29204695.
75. Vaswani D, Wallace AN, Eiswirth PS, Madaelil TP, Chang RO, Tomasian A, Jennings JW. Radiographic local tumor control and pain palliation of sarcoma metastases within the musculoskeletal system with percutaneous thermal ablation. Cardiovasc Intervent Radiol. 2018;41(8):1223–32. https://doi.org/10.1007/s00270-018-1932-1. Epub 2018 Mar 14. PMID: 29541840
76. Erie AJ, Morris JM, Welch BT, Kurup AN, Weisbrod AJ, Atwell TD, Schmit GD, Kwon ED, Callstrom MR. Retrospective review of percutaneous image-guided ablation of oligometastatic prostate cancer: a single-institution experience. J Vasc Interv Radiol. 2017;28(7):987–92. https://doi.org/10.1016/j.jvir.2017.03.012. Epub 2017 Apr 21. PMID: 28434661
77. Senol N, Oguzoglu AS, Goksel HM. Radiofrequency ablation and augmentation in the management of spinal metastases: clinical experience in 41 patients. World Neurosurg. 2022;163:e420–5. https://doi.org/10.1016/j.wneu.2022.03.140. Epub 2022 Apr 5. PMID: 35395426
78. Madani K, Najafi A, Boticella A, et al. Combined local treatments for vertebral metastases with limited epidural extension. Support Care Cancer. 2022;30:337–45. https://doi.org/10.1007/s00520-021-06443-y.
79. Kastler A, Barbé DA, Alemann G, Hadjidekov G, Cornelis FH, Kastler B. Bipolar radiofrequency ablation of painful spinal bone metastases performed under local anesthesia: feasibility regarding patient's experience and pain outcome. Medicina (Kaunas). 2021;57(9):966. https://doi.org/10.3390/medicina57090966. PMID: 34577889; PMCID: PMC8466129
80. Yildizhan S, Boyaci MG, Rakip U, Aslan A, Canbek I. Role of radiofrequency ablation and cement injection for pain control in patients with spinal metastasis. BMC Musculoskelet Disord. 2021;22(1):912. https://doi.org/10.1186/s12891-021-04799-0. PMID: 34715849; PMCID: PMC8556885
81. Levy J, Hopkins T, Morris J, Tran ND, David E, Massari F, Farid H, Vogel A, O'Connell WG, Sunenshine P, Dixon R, Gangi A, von der Höh N, Bagla S. Radiofrequency ablation for the palliative treatment of bone metastases: outcomes from the multicenter Osteocool tumor ablation post-market study (OPuS One Study) in 100 patients. J Vasc Interv Radiol. 2020;31(11):1745–52. https://doi.org/10.1016/j.jvir.2020.07.014. PMID: 33129427
82. De Marini P, Cazzato RL, Auloge P, Koch G, Dalili D, Garnon J, Gangi A. Percutaneous image-guided thermal ablation of bone metastases: a retrospective propensity study comparing the safety profile of radio-frequency ablation and cryo-ablation. Int J Hyperth. 2020;37(1):1386–94. https://doi.org/10.1080/02656736.2020.1859628. PMID: 33322960

Microwave Ablation

5

Alberto Solano López, Igor Radalov,
Helena Puigderrajols Vehils, Jesús Ares Vidal,
Salvatore Marsico, and Claudio Pusceddu

5.1 Introduction

Tumor ablation is defined as the direct application of chemical or thermal therapies to a tumor to achieve eradication or substantial tumor destruction [1, 2]. The first references to this technique date back to the late 1970s and originate from studies by Taylor, Douple, and Strohbehn [3].

The various ablative techniques used for tumor ablation include chemical ablation with alcohol, hyperthermic energy-based methods such as radiofrequency ablation (RFA), microwave ablation (MWA), cryoablation (CO), and high-intensity focused ultrasound (HIFU), as well as nonthermal modalities like irreversible electroporation (IRE). Ablative procedures can be performed via open surgery, laparoscopy, percutaneous, transcutaneous routes, or using catheter-based applicators.

Bone is the third most common site for cancer metastases, affecting approximately 50% of patients with metastatic disease. Among these patients, 80% experience pain, with 50% being severe and 30% refractory [4–7].

A. S. López (✉) · I. Radalov · H. P. Vehils · J. A. Vidal
Department of Radiology Hospital del Mar, Barcelona, Spain
e-mail: igor.radalov.radalov@hmar.cat

S. Marsico
Department of Radiology Hospital del Mar, Barcelona, Spain

Interventional Oncology Institute, Barcelona, Spain

C. Pusceddu
Department of Radiology Mater Olbia Hospital, Olbia, Cagliari, Italy

Interventional Oncology Institute, Barcelona, Spain

C. Pusceddu, S. Marsico (eds.), *Malignant Bone Lesions and Beyond*,
https://doi.org/10.1007/978-3-032-00018-7_5

Image-guided tumor ablation offers several advantages over surgical treatment, including faster recovery, reduced morbidity and mortality, lower procedural costs, accurate targeting under ultrasound or CT scan guidance, immediate effects, a favorable safety profile, synergy with other cancer treatments, and the ability to perform procedures in an outpatient setting. This reduces hospital stays and allows for easy repetition if residual lesions are present [1–2].

5.2 Basic Physical Principles of Microwave Ablation

5.2.1 Microwave Energy for Tissue Ablation

Microwaves occupy a distinct segment of the electromagnetic spectrum, ranging from 300 MHz to 300 GHz. The frequencies most used for microwave ablation are 915 MHz and 2.45 GHz, due to their optimal penetration and heating characteristics. Ongoing research is exploring other frequencies for therapeutic microwave applications, including 433 MHz, as well as broadband pulses with the highest spectral energy density typically within the range of 1 GHz to 10 GHz [8].

5.2.2 Electromagnetic Interactions with Tissue

The most significant effect of an electromagnetic field on biological tissue is the conversion of microwave energy into thermal energy. This thermal energy transfer within tissues can be effectively modeled using the bioheat equation developed by Pennes, which provides a comprehensive framework for understanding heat distribution and thermal effects in the biological system.

In simpler terms, this process can be described as:

Coagulation necrosis = Energy deposited interacting with local tissue conditions minus the heat loss.

Note that penetration depth is inversely related to conductivity, while the heating rate is proportional to conductivity. Specific values have been determined for the relationship between temperature and cell viability [9].

The term "coagulation necrosis" is used to describe irreversible thermal damage to cells, even though the final manifestations of cell death may not strictly meet the histological criteria for coagulative necrosis. A direct correlation exists between the temperature achieved at the cellular level, the duration of this temperature increase, and the resultant cellular effects, as illustrated in Fig. 5.1.

TEMPERATURE	EFFECT ON CELLS	DURATION/OUTCOME
Up to 40°C	Cellular homeostasis maintained	No damage observed
42–45°C (Hyperthermia)	Increased susceptibility to chemotherapy and radiation	Prolonged exposure does not kill all. cells
46°C	Irreversible cellular damage	60 minutes
50–52°C	Rapid induction of cytotoxicity	4–6 minutes
60–100°C	Near instantaneous protein coagulation	Immediate damage
>105°C	Tissue boiling, vaporization, and carbonization	Instantaneous

Fig. 5.1 Correlation between cellular damage and temperature

5.2.3 Dielectric Properties of Biological Tissues

The transmission of electromagnetic energy is determined by the dielectric permittivity and magnetic permeability of the media through which the waves propagate. In biological tissues, the magnetic permeability is approximately equal to that of a vacuum. However, the dielectric permittivity is significantly larger and encompasses concepts such as relative permittivity and conductivity.

Permittivity is a material property that influences the Coulomb force between two point charges within the material. Relative permittivity, often referred to as the "dielectric constant," is the factor by which the electric field between charges is reduced relative to a vacuum. It measures how effectively a material can support an electric field and is quantified relative to the permittivity of a vacuum. A dielectric is an insulating material, and its dielectric constant reflects the ability of the insulator to store electric energy in an electric field.

Relative permittivity determines the wavelength of an applied electromagnetic field at a given frequency, which affects how efficiently energy will propagate through the tissue and influences the design of the antenna. Higher permittivities result in shorter wavelengths.

5.2.3.1 Effective Conductivity

The effective conductivity of a material is defined from the imaginary part of the complex permittivity and is used to describe how well a material absorbs microwave energy. Tissues with high conductivity have a high water content and readily absorb microwaves, while tissues with low conductivity have a low water content and readily allow microwave propagation.

It is important to note that effective conductivity differs from electrical conductivity. Electrical conductivity refers to an alternating flow of electrons, whereas effective conductivity encompasses effects related to the rotation of dipoles [10].

Effective conductivity describes contributions from both moving charges (electrical current) and time-varying electric fields (displacement current), specifically the rotation of dipoles in the material as they attempt to align with an alternating electric field.

5.2.3.2 Physical Influences

Both relative permittivity and conductivity depend on various physical factors, including water content, cellular composition, and temperature. Tumor tissue, which is rich in water, relatively anaerobic, and has a low pH value, is more sensitive to heat than normal tissue.

5.2.4 Microwaves Compared to Other Sources of Thermal Therapy

Microwaves are capable of propagating through and effectively heating various types of tissue, even those with low electrical conductivity, high impedance, or low thermal conductivity. Unlike radiofrequency (RF) (Fig. 5.2) and laser energy, microwaves can readily penetrate through charred or desiccated tissues. Additionally, microwaves may offer more direct heating than other ablation energies, making them particularly effective in organs with high blood perfusion or near vascular heat sinks.

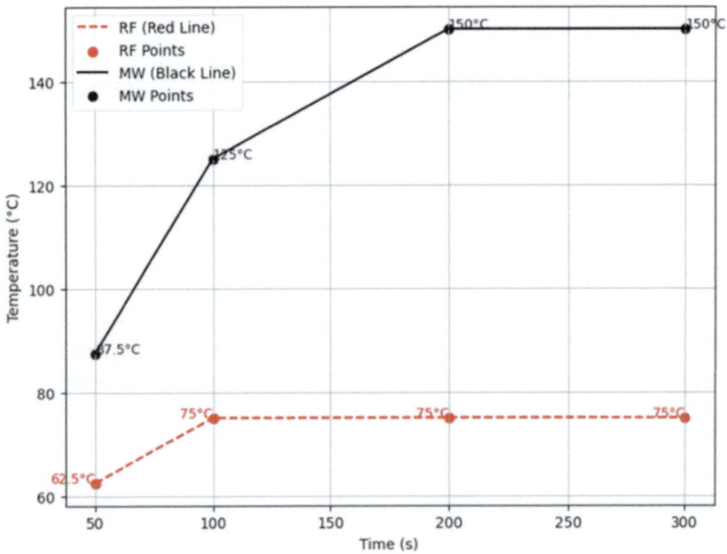

Fig. 5.2 Temperature-time profiles for microwave ablation (MWA) and radiofrequency ablation (RFA): a comparative analysis

5.2.5 Mechanism of Thermal Energy Production via Microwave Ablation

Microwave electromagnetic waves heat matter by agitating water molecules in the surrounding tissue, generating friction and heat, which induces cellular death through coagulation necrosis. Microwave ablation operates based on two primary mechanisms [1, 10–12]:

5.2.5.1 Dipole Rotation Theory (Fig. 5.3)

Water molecules are polar due to their asymmetric distribution of electric charges. The water molecule has a V-shape, with two hydrogen atoms bonded to a single oxygen atom. Because of oxygen's high electronegativity, this atom attracts electrons from the covalent bonds with hydrogen, resulting in a transfer of charge toward the oxygen. This creates a partially negative charge on the oxygen and a partially positive charge on the hydrogen atoms.

This asymmetric distribution of charges gives rise to a dipole moment in the water molecule, which is why water molecules are polar. The dipole moment is a measure of the separation between the centers of the positive and negative charges within the molecule [22]. Electromagnetic radiation possesses an oscillating electric field, which interacts with water molecules, causing them to rotate. Microwave radiation is specifically tuned to the natural frequency of water molecules to maximize this interaction. As a result, the electric dipole moment of the water molecule oscillates back and forth approximately 2–5 billion times per second, depending on the microwave frequency. Since temperature reflects molecular motion, the vigorous

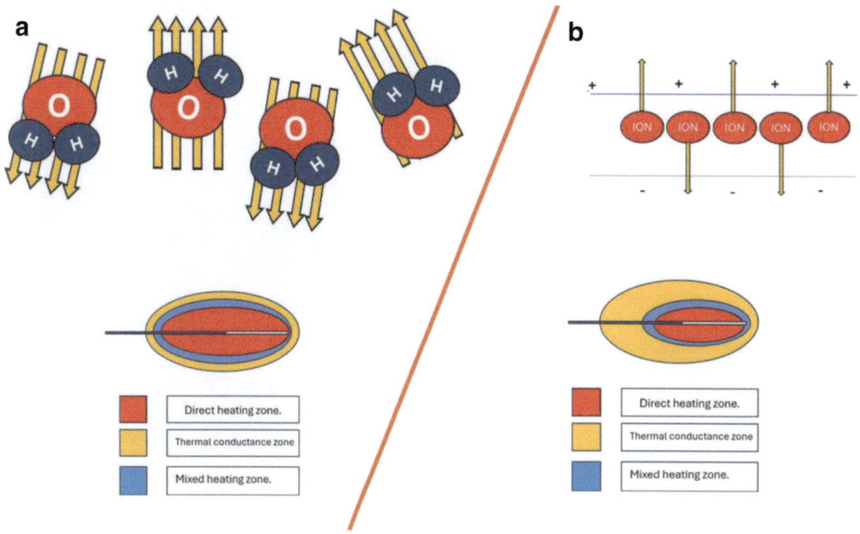

Fig. 5.3 Mechanism of action and heat transfer for microwave ablation (**a**) and radiofrequency ablation (**b**)

movement of water molecules increases the temperature of the water. Microwave ablation is a special case of dielectric heating, where tissue acts as the dielectric material.

5.2.5.2 Ionic Polarization Theory (Fig. 5.4)

In tissue, the application of an electromagnetic field displaces ions, causing them to collide with other ions. This process converts kinetic energy into heat, although it is significantly less important than dipole rotation in terms of heat generation during microwave ablation.

The rate of heat generation (Qh) in microwave ablation is directly proportional to the square of the magnitude of the applied electric field (E). This relationship is governed by the effective conductivity (σ) of the tissue, which is a measure of how efficiently the tissue absorbs microwave energy. The equation describing this process is $Qh = \frac{\sigma E^2}{2.}$ where

- Qh is the rate of heat generation per unit volume.
- σ is the effective conductivity of the tissue (in S/m).
- E is the magnitude of the applied electric field.

This equation highlights that tissues with higher effective conductivity generate more heat under the same electric field strength, making conductivity a critical factor in determining the efficiency of microwave ablation procedures. Due to their high water content, most biological tissues exhibit high conductivity, which enables them to readily absorb microwave energy and convert it into heat.

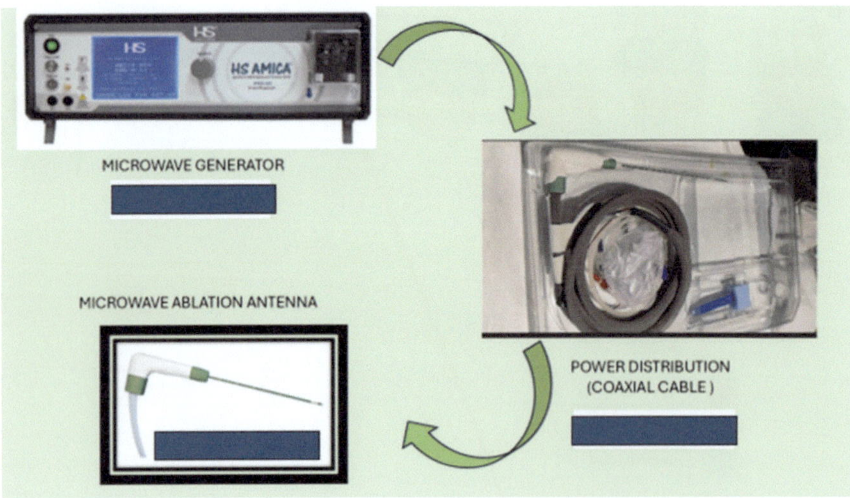

Fig. 5.4 Detailed illustration of the key components in a microwave ablation system

5.3 Components of a Microwave Ablation System

The most general design for microwave ablation (MWA) systems typically involves an interstitial antenna or an array of antennas, which receive power from a microwave generator via a distribution system. However, due to variations in intellectual property among manufacturers, no two MWA systems are identical (Fig. 5.4). This diversity in design can lead to differences in performance and applicability across various clinical scenarios. The antenna used in MWA is often informally referred to as a "needle," but for precision, the terms "applicator," "antenna," and "probe" are commonly used to describe energy-based devices. Understanding these differences is crucial for selecting the most appropriate MWA system for specific medical applications [8–14].

5.3.1 Microwave Generators

Microwave ablation generators utilize one of two basic power sources: a magnetron or a solid-state amplifier.

A magnetron generates electromagnetic energy by accelerating electrons through a magnetic field within a resonant cavity. The continuous wave (CW) magnetron, pioneered by Albert Hull [15] at General Electric in 1921, is the oldest thermoelectric vacuum device to produce microwaves. This design was later refined by Hans Hollmann at Telefunken, who developed the resonant cavity version 14 years later, which remains widely used today due to its improved efficiency and stability.

Operating a magnetron involves two primary aspects:

The Power Supply Level: This includes the anode and filament voltage parameters necessary to maintain the magnetron within its active oscillation range.

The Microwave (MW) Level: This encompasses propagation characteristics throughout the entire microwave circuit.

The power supply parameters significantly influence the MW output spectrum, affecting both its bandwidth and the stability of the central frequency. Additionally, the magnetron waveguide parameters impact the amplitude of the MW energy transmitted to the load, with potential reflections back to the magnetron.

The fundamental principle of microwave solid-state generators involves utilizing the nonlinear properties of semiconductor devices to convert direct current (DC) power into microwave power. In semiconductor generators, a quartz crystal determines the frequency of the initial signal, which is then significantly amplified by a series of transistor stages. To achieve power outputs of several kilowatts, multiple semiconductor amplifiers can be combined until the desired power level is reached.

The output of microwave generators can be controlled relatively independently of tissue type, avoiding the impedance spikes or reduced power output typically associated with RF ablation in high-impedance tissues. This feature is particularly

	MAGNETRON	SOLID-STATE MICROWAVE GENERATORS
TECHNOLOGY	Vacuum tube-based	Semiconductor components
POWER	Up to thousands of watts	Up to thousands of watts, more efficient at lower levels
ENERGY EFFICIENCY	Less efficient, especially at lower power levels	More efficient, precise control and power modulation
RELIABILITY	Short lifespan	Longer lifespan and more dependable
SIZE AND WEIGHT	Larger and heavier	Compact and lightweight
FREQUENCY RANGE	Fixed frequency	Greater versatility in the frequency range
ENVIRONMENTAL BENEFITS	Not mentioned	Reduced energy consumption, more sustainable
INNOVATION	Established technology	Continuously evolving, improving performance and reducing costs

Fig. 5.5 Schematic representation of the basic components of a coaxial cable

advantageous in medical procedures where consistent power delivery is crucial. The generator frequencies are generally either 915 MHz or 2.45 GHz, as permitted by the Federal Communications Commission (FCC).

The key differences between the two microwave generator models are summarized in Fig. 5.5.

5.3.2 Power Distribution

In electromagnetics, the term "transmission line" refers to a structure specifically designed to support a guided wave [16]. A guided wave is an electromagnetic wave that is confined within or bound to a line, preventing it from radiating away. This condition is typically satisfied when the length and cross-sectional dimensions of the transmission line are small compared to the wavelength.

Transmission lines utilize specialized construction and impedance matching to transmit electromagnetic signals with minimal reflections and power losses. The distinguishing feature of most transmission lines is their uniform cross-sectional dimensions along their length, which provide a uniform impedance known as the characteristic impedance. This characteristic impedance helps prevent reflections by ensuring that the signal is properly matched to the line's properties, thereby maintaining signal integrity and reducing power losses. Types of transmission lines include parallel lines, coaxial cables, and planar transmission lines, each suited to different applications based on their unique properties and advantages. For instance,

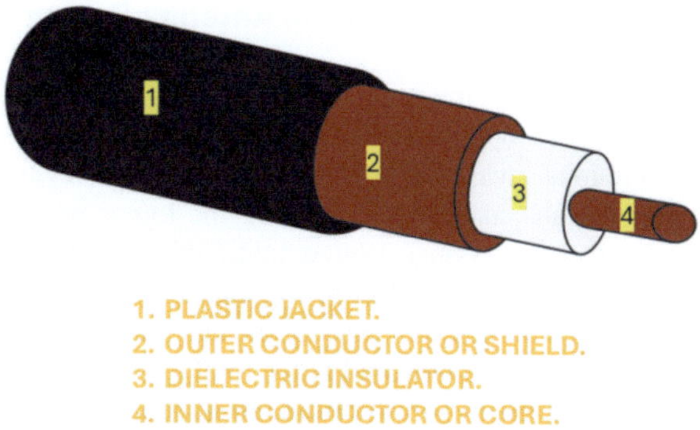

Fig. 5.6 Relationship between power rating in watts and antenna size in gauges

coaxial cables are often used for high-frequency applications, while planar transmission lines are preferred in integrated circuits for their compact size and ease of fabrication.

Electromagnetic energy is transmitted through transmission lines [17]. One of the most popular types is the coaxial transmission line, commonly known as a coaxial cable, which consists of metallic inner and outer conductors separated by a spacer material (Fig. 5.6). The spacer material is typically a low-loss dielectric material with a permeability approximately equal to that of free space. This design ensures that electromagnetic energy is efficiently transmitted with minimal loss, making coaxial cables ideal for applications requiring high signal integrity. Coaxial lines are particularly well-suited for connecting single-ended circuits in widely separated locations and for connecting antennas to receivers and transmitters due to their excellent shielding properties and ability to minimize signal interference.

Despite their numerous strengths, coaxial cables have limitations in their ability to carry substantial amounts of power at microwave frequencies. As the cable diameter decreases, the power handling capability, the ability to safely transfer power without overheating or failure, decreases significantly [8]. Power handling is closely related to both the cable diameter and the construction material, as well as the frequency of the applied microwave power. For instance, cables with larger diameters and materials with high thermal conductivity can handle more power. There is a limit to how small and flexible cables can be without resulting in dangerous overheating of the cable [12]. This limitation necessitates careful design considerations to ensure that coaxial cables are used within safe operating parameters, especially in high-power microwave applications.

Other components that may be part of the power distribution system include power splitters, phase shifters, and amplitude modulation or switches [12]. Power splitters utilize a specific transmission line geometry to divide an input power into multiple output channels, typically in equal proportions. Although it is theoretically possible to split a single input into as many output channels as needed, a typical microwave ablation system usually has no more than four output channels. Switches or continuous amplitude modulation may also be used in the power distribution system to selectively activate antennas.

5.3.3 Microwave Ablation Antenna Design

In microwave ablation, an ideal antenna is one that achieves the desired ablation zone pattern—both in size and shape—with high efficiency in energy transmission and minimal invasiveness for patients [18]. Achieving the expected ablation zone pattern means successfully ablating the tumor while minimizing damage to surrounding normal tissues. Both omnidirectional and directional radiation patterns are used in the literature for delivering microwave energy.

The transmission efficiency of the antenna represents how much energy is transferred into tissues compared to the total energy. The lowest return loss is desirable to maximize energy transfer from the antenna into the tissue [8]. This energy reflection is typically caused by impedance mismatching, which can increase the heating of the antenna itself and the tissues in proximity. Furthermore, with the concept of minimally invasive ablation, an antenna with a small size is more desirable when considering patient comfort and safety during MWA procedures [18].

One major technical challenge for microwave ablation is the antenna diameter. There is an inherent trade-off between power handling and invasiveness with all microwave ablation antennas. However, it is well understood that increasing power is the most straightforward way to increase the ablation zone size with a given antenna design. This trade-off necessitates careful consideration in clinical settings, as larger antennas may be more invasive but can handle higher power levels, while smaller antennas are less invasive but may require more precise power control to achieve the desired ablation zone (Fig. 5.7).

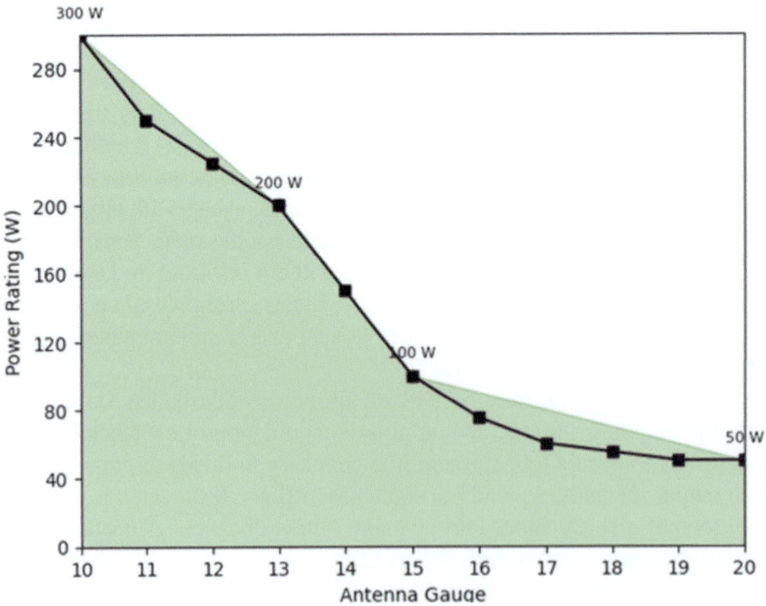

Fig. 5.7 Parameters to consider in the antenna of the bone microwave ablation system. (**a**) Evaluation of the short and long axes of the ablation zone. (**b**) Heating mechanism in the ablation zone. (**c**) Relationship between power and time on the size of the ablation zone

MWA applicators are evaluated based on three primary criteria [20] (Fig. 5.8)

Short-Axis Diameter: This is the maximum radial width of the thermal ablation zone measured perpendicular to the applicator shaft. Achieving a consistent short-axis diameter is crucial for ensuring uniform tissue heating and minimizing damage to surrounding tissues.

Axial ratio: This ratio compares the short-axis diameter to the long-axis diameter of the ablation zone, providing insight into its shape.

Shaft Diameter: A smaller diameter reduces invasiveness, enhancing patient comfort and minimizing the risk of complications. Clinically used MWA applicators typically range from 13-gauge to 17-gauge.

Informed by in vivo and ex vivo models, leading medical companies provide detailed guidelines for the optimal protocol, specifying power output (watts) and duration to achieve the desired ablation area size. For the ablation area, a safety margin of 5–10 mm is strongly recommended. As a result, rigorous pretreatment planning is essential to ensure thorough ablation of the lesion while adhering to the recommended safety margin, thus minimizing the risk of complications.

Comparing ex vivo and in vivo parameters in Microwave Ablation (MWA) technology is challenging due to differences in physiological environment, tissue variability, and biological responses. Key factors include [11]:

Blood Circulation: In ex vivo settings, the absence of blood circulation eliminates the "heat-sink effect," which reduces ablation effectiveness near large blood vessels. MWA is less susceptible to this effect than Radiofrequency Ablation (RFA).

Imaging Challenges: Ex vivo ablation volumes are easier to quantify, but in vivo assessment is complicated by the hyperemic zone, unclear cell death margins, and dynamic changes over time. Techniques like CT scans underestimate ablation volumes compared to MRI.

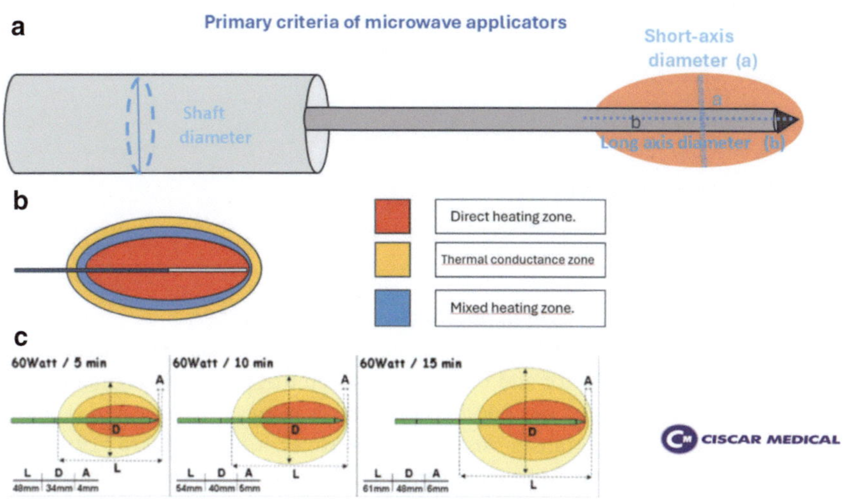

Fig. 5.8 Fundamental antenna designs for microwave ablation applications. (**a**) awt, (**b**) dwt, (**c**) dipole, (**d**) slot, (**e**) sleeve, (**f**) choke, (**g**) cap

Tissue Variability: Living tissues have diverse physical and biological properties, such as thermal conductivity and electrical impedance, affecting ablation effectiveness.

Biological Response: In vivo, the body responds with inflammation and scarring, absent in ex vivo studies.

Tissue Contraction: Tissue contraction, caused by dehydration and architectural collapse during MWA, affects short-axis diameter assessment and depends on tissue type and MWA protocol.

Ideally, the applicator should be made from echogenic materials to enhance visibility on ultrasound imaging and minimize streak artifacts on CT scans. This is particularly important for procedures where precise placement is crucial. Furthermore, MR compatibility is beneficial for treating tumors that are only visible on MRI, allowing for more precise targeting and monitoring during the procedure.

During microwave ablation (MWA) procedures, two key factors are used to assess the performance of microwave antennas: the reflection coefficient (S11) and the specific absorption rate (SAR) [19].

Reflection Coefficient (S11): S11 measures the amount of electromagnetic power reflected to the source, indicating the antenna's power transmission efficiency. A low S11 value ensures efficient energy transfer to tissues, as it signifies minimal reflection and optimal power delivery [19].

Specific Absorption Rate (SAR): SAR quantifies the energy absorbed by tissue from microwaves, which is crucial for understanding tissue interaction and temperature increase. It helps identify radiation exposure and electric field propagation, thereby optimizing ablation while minimizing damage to healthy tissues. The SAR pattern also evaluates tumor ablation performance. Ideally, the heating pattern should be spherical, but most interstitial antennas produce ellipsoid or teardrop-shaped patterns due to their design and interaction with surrounding tissues [19].

Technically, the specific absorption rate (SAR) is calculated using the formula:

$$\mathrm{SAR} = \frac{\sigma E^2}{\rho}$$

where

- σ is the tissue conductivity.
- E is the electric field intensity.
- ρ is the tissue density.

Basic types of antennas used in microwave ablation (Fig. 5.9)

Dielectric Wrapped Tip (DWT) Monopole Antenna: This antenna is created by extending the inner conductor and dielectric of a semi-rigid coaxial cable outward while keeping the length of the outer conductor unchanged. This design helps in achieving efficient energy transmission and a controlled heating pattern [19].

Air Wrapped Tip (AWT) Monopole Antenna: This antenna is formed by extending the inner conductor all the way to the tip, without any additional dielectric

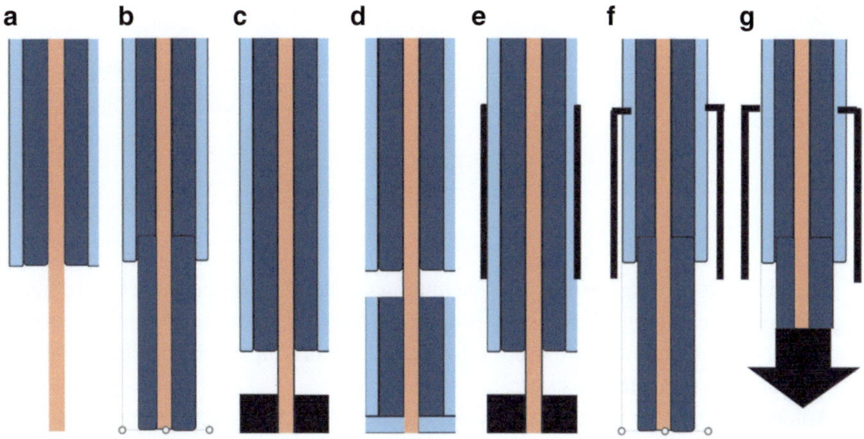

Fig. 5.9 Thermal synergy in microwave ablation refers to the enhanced effect achieved when multiple microwave antennas are used simultaneously. This technique results in larger ablation zones than would be expected from the sum of each antenna's effect

material. The absence of dielectric material can affect the antenna's impedance matching and heating pattern, potentially leading to variations in ablation zone shape and size.

The dipole antenna was proposed by adding a metal block to the distal end of the coaxial cable and electrically connecting it to the inner conductor. This configuration can enhance the antenna's radiation efficiency and ablation zone characteristics.

The slot antenna is another fundamental microwave antenna, distinguished by a soldered connection between the inner and outer conductors at the distal end of the semi-rigid coaxial cable. This design allows for specific radiation patterns.

While these three basic antennas can concentrate electromagnetic energy around the active tip and heat target tissues to a lethal level, they are hindered by the issue of backward heating caused by leaking currents. Researchers have found that incorporating a choke or a metal sleeve into microwave antennas can significantly reduce unwanted electrical currents [19, 20]. A metal cap at the antenna tip also plays a crucial role in enhancing performance. By combining these approaches, such as using a cap with a choke, the overall efficiency and effectiveness of the antenna are improved. Additionally, the inclusion of a second choke can further decrease these unwanted currents, resulting in better control over the ablation zone and enhanced safety. This improved control not only enhances the precision of the ablation but also reduces the risk of complications, making microwave ablation a safer and more reliable treatment option.

Recent techniques also enable the reduction of antenna diameter by integrating chokes within coaxial cables. Additionally, increasing the number of slots in slot antennas helps minimize backward heating [19].

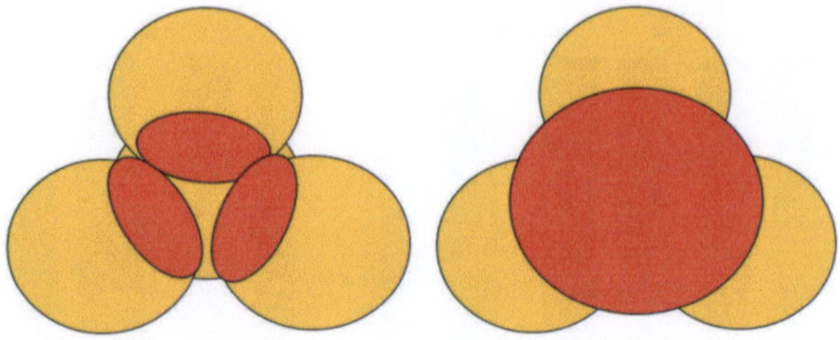

Fig. 5.10 Comparative analysis of microwave ablation: advantages and limitations versus other ablative modalities

Integrating a cooling system into the antenna effectively reduces backward heating but poses a challenge due to size limitations. In clinical settings, both gas-cooled and water-cooled antennas are used; however, incorporating a cooling channel inevitably increases the antenna's size.

Antenna Arrays for Microwave Ablation: Researchers are exploring the use of antenna arrays due to power limitations in single antennas. Studies, such as those by Laeseke et al. [21], highlight that arrays enhance power distribution efficiency and create larger ablation zones through "thermal synergy," where simultaneous heating exceeds the sum of individual effects (Fig. 5.10). This synergy allows for more efficient and effective ablation procedures.

To enhance microwave ablation (MWA) efficiency, several strategies can be employed. These include using magnetic nanoparticles and liposomes as localized heat sources [23], which help reduce the required input power while maintaining treatment outcomes.

Optimizing the internal structure of the antenna improves power transmission, thereby increasing tissue energy deposition.

Additionally, integrating matching networks further enhances the overall performance of the system by ensuring efficient impedance matching and minimizing energy loss.

5.4 Directional Microwave Ablation (DMWA): A New Era in Cancer Treatment [20]

DMWA represents a groundbreaking advancement in microwave ablation therapies, providing unparalleled precision and control in the treatment of complex tumors. By leveraging directional antennas with reflectors, DMWA precisely focuses electromagnetic energy in specific directions, thereby significantly enhancing the efficacy and safety of the procedure. Although this technology is still in the laboratory phase, it holds great promise to revolutionize minimally invasive cancer treatments by offering new possibilities for effective tumor management and improved patient outcomes.

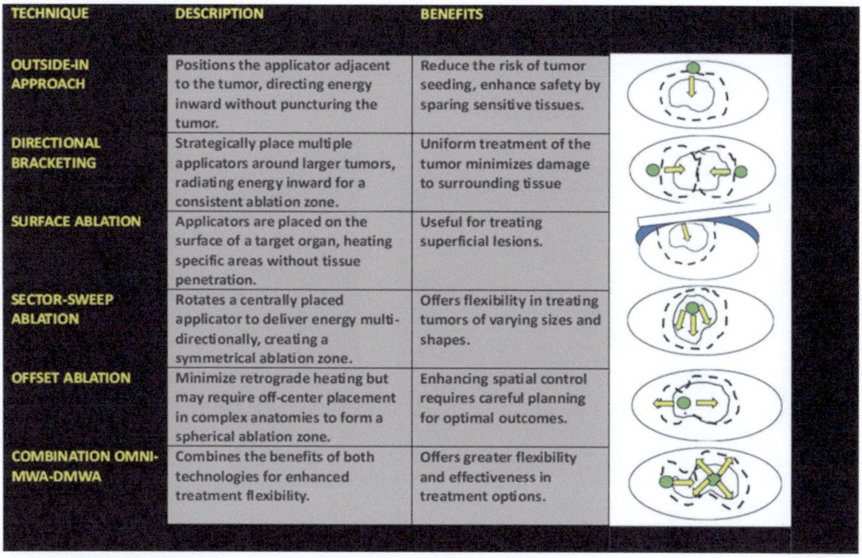

TECHNIQUE	DESCRIPTION	BENEFITS
OUTSIDE-IN APPROACH	Positions the applicator adjacent to the tumor, directing energy inward without puncturing the tumor.	Reduce the risk of tumor seeding, enhance safety by sparing sensitive tissues.
DIRECTIONAL BRACKETING	Strategically place multiple applicators around larger tumors, radiating energy inward for a consistent ablation zone.	Uniform treatment of the tumor minimizes damage to surrounding tissue
SURFACE ABLATION	Applicators are placed on the surface of a target organ, heating specific areas without tissue penetration.	Useful for treating superficial lesions.
SECTOR-SWEEP ABLATION	Rotates a centrally placed applicator to deliver energy multi-directionally, creating a symmetrical ablation zone.	Offers flexibility in treating tumors of varying sizes and shapes.
OFFSET ABLATION	Minimize retrograde heating but may require off-center placement in complex anatomies to form a spherical ablation zone.	Enhancing spatial control requires careful planning for optimal outcomes.
COMBINATION OMNI-MWA-DMWA	Combines the benefits of both technologies for enhanced treatment flexibility.	Offers greater flexibility and effectiveness in treatment options.

Fig. 5.11 Characteristics of microwave generators

DMWA offers several key advantages that significantly improve treatment outcomes. One of its primary benefits is the precise targeting of tumors, which minimizes damage to surrounding healthy tissues. The integration of DMWA with real-time imaging technologies further optimizes treatment results by allowing for more accurate and dynamic adjustments during the procedure. Additionally, DMWA expands treatment options by enabling the successful treatment of tumors that were previously inaccessible due to their location or complexity.

Comparative differences between directional microwave ablation (DMWA) and standard microwave ablation techniques (Fig. 5.11) [20]

5.5 Benefits and Drawbacks of Microwave Ablation Relative to Other Ablative Methods

Figure 5.12 provides a schematic summary of the advantages and disadvantages of this technique.

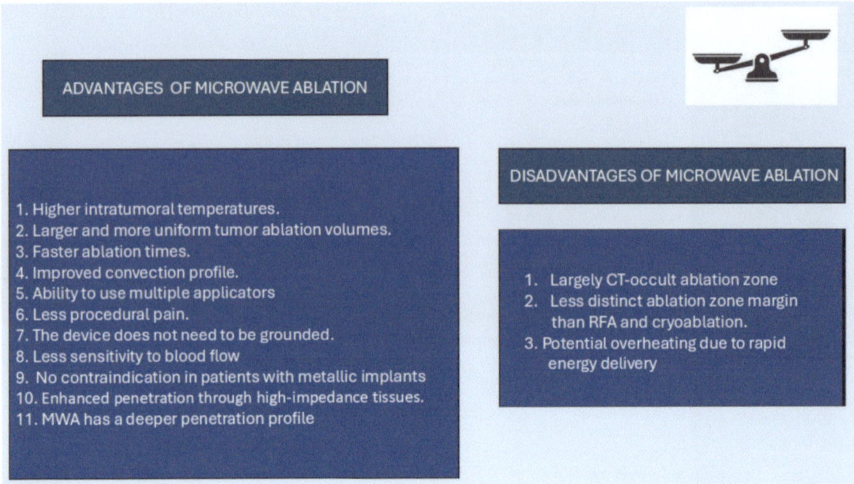

Fig. 5.12 Overview of different approaches in directional microwave ablation

5.6 General Principles of Indications for Microwave Ablation in Bone Lesions

Microwave ablation (MWA) offers a key advantage compared to other ablation therapies by achieving higher temperatures within tumors and being less affected by tissue conductivity and impedance. This makes MWA more effective for sclerotic lesions compared to radiofrequency ablation (RFA), which is impaired by sclerotic bone's high impedance.

Similar to other ablation therapies, the indications for bone lesions can be categorized based on curative or palliative treatment intent (Table 5.1). In the case of curative intent, microwave ablation can be used for benign bone tumors, primary malignant bone tumors in carefully selected cases, or in patients with oligometastatic, oligorecurrent, or oligoprogressive disease. For palliative purposes, ablation is offered to manage painful metastases that are refractory to, or not suitable for, pharmacological management, radiotherapy, or surgery [24].

In this chapter, we will delve into the current and potential applications of microwave ablation (MWA) for both curative and palliative treatment of bone lesions, focusing on each type of lesion separately. The analysis will primarily draw on systematic reviews and meta-analyses published over the past decade, up to the current year. Since MWA is a relatively recent therapy, it is important to note that there is limited knowledge and, while constantly improving, most evidence is still based on retrospective, limited case series. The current Cardiovascular and Interventional Radiological Society of Europe (CIRSE) Standards of Practice for Thermal Ablation of Bone Tumors provide a useful starting point and overview.

Table 5.1 Current established indications for curative and palliative treatment of bone lesions (based on CIRSE Standards of Practice on Thermal Ablation of Bone Tumors)

	Curative intent	Palliative intent
Goals	Eradicate the tumor and restore the patient's health to a pre-disease state	Local control of tumor extension, pain alleviation, pathological fracture, and spinal canal stenosis prevention
Established indications	Osteoid osteoma Primary malignant bone tumors in carefully selected cases of small (<3 cm), slow-growing lesions in nonsurgical candidates or in patients refusing surgery Selected patients presenting with oligometastatic, oligorecurrent, and oligoprogressive disease	Painful metastases refractory to, or unsuitable for, pharmacologic management, RT, or surgery

5.7 Indications by Type of Lesion (Table 5.2)

5.7.1 Benign Tumors

5.7.1.1 Osteoid Osteoma (OO)

Osteoid osteoma is a benign, relatively common lesion typically found in the cortical region of long bones, characterized by a radiolucent nidus surrounded by reactive osteosclerosis. This condition predominantly affects young male patients, who experience characteristic nocturnal pain that is relieved by salicylates or non-steroidal anti-inflammatory drugs (NSAIDs).

Osteoid osteoma is a well-established indication for the treatment of bone lesions with microwave ablation, demonstrating high efficacy and success rates. Recent evidence consistently shows near-complete pain relief shortly after ablation, with sustained symptom resolution in the vast majority of patients, resulting in significant and lasting pain reduction [25]. It is safe and has low complication rates comparable to other thermal ablation techniques, with no significant difference in serious adverse events compared to radiofrequency ablation, laser ablation, or cryoablation.

Complications are generally minor and self-limiting. The most common issues reported are skin burns or transient nerve irritation near the ablation zone, particularly when the lesion is close to the skin or neurovascular structures [26]. To mitigate these risks, thorough planning and careful safety considerations are crucial to protect adjacent joints, growth plates, and neurovascular structures from thermal damage. Techniques such as hydrodissection or cooling methods may be employed when necessary.

Table 5.2 Summary of current indications (established and potential) of MWA for the treatment of bone lesions

Bone lesion	Indications	References
Osteoid osteoma	Curative treatment and pain reduction	Prud'homme et al. [27], Shanmugasundaram et al. [25], Bianchi et al. [26]
Enchondroma	Possible curative treatment when combined with endoscopic curettage	Wu et al. [30]
Giant cell tumor of the bone	Intraoperative adjuvant to intralesional curettage	Jiang et al. [32], Cui et al. [33]
Aneurysmal bone cysts	Curative intent in anatomically challenging locations Pre-curettage to reduce bleeding and improve resection safety (alternative to preop embolization)	Zheng et al. [34]
Primary sarcomas of the bone (osteosarcoma, chondrosarcoma, Ewing's sarcoma)	Carefully selected cases of small (<3 cm), slow-growing lesions in nonsurgical candidates or in patients refusing surgery Selected patients presenting with oligometastatic, oligorecurrent, and oligoprogressive disease Adjuvant to intralesional curettage for central atypical cartilaginous tumors (ACT) or grade I chondrosarcomas in long bones	Gennaro et al. [35], Deckers et al. [37], Bourgouin et al. [36], Ryan et al. [24]
Metastatic bone lesions	Symptomatic pain relief Local tumor control through debulking to prevent further growth, skeletal complications, or neurological compromise	Gennaro et al. [35], Coleman et al. [42], Sagoo et al. [40], Papalexis et al. [41], Ryan et al. [24]

When compared to radiofrequency ablation (RFA), the traditional gold standard for osteoid osteoma treatment over the past few decades, recent evidence suggests that microwave ablation yields similar outcomes [25]. Notably, MWA generates higher temperatures within lesions than RFA, creating larger and more uniform ablation zones, as it operates independently of impedance. This advantage allows for effective treatment with a single needle insertion, which does not require precise positioning at the nidus center [27]. Consequently, MWA may be particularly valuable for treating lesions in difficult-to-reach or concealed locations. However, in practice, the choice between RFA and MWA often depends on equipment availability or operator preference. In summary, MWA is a safe and effective treatment for osteoid osteoma, offering significant and durable pain relief with low recurrence and complication rates.

5.7.1.2 Enchondroma

Enchondromas are benign intramedullary cartilaginous tumors often discovered incidentally and typically asymptomatic. Treatment is generally reserved for symptomatic lesions, which may present pain or have an increased risk of pathological fracture, or those that appear radiologically aggressive. Traditionally, surgical curettage has been the standard management approach. However, percutaneous ablation techniques are emerging as less invasive adjunctive therapies and, in some cases, complete alternatives to surgery. Most of the existing evidence focuses on radiofrequency ablation, where mid- to long-term data indicate high success rates in eradicating low-grade and atypical cartilaginous tumors [28, 29].

Unfortunately, published outcomes specifically focusing on microwave ablation for enchondromas are limited. However, data from related contexts, such as low-grade chondrosarcomas and other benign bone tumors, can be extrapolated. Early studies suggest that MWA can effectively eradicate cartilaginous tumor tissue when used in conjunction with curettage [30].

5.7.1.3 Giant Cell Tumor of the Bone (GCTB)

Giant cell tumor of bone is a locally aggressive, benign bone tumor that typically affects the epiphyses of long bones in young adults. Standard treatment is intralesional curettage with local adjuvants or en bloc resection in select cases, but curettage alone yields high recurrence rates, which makes adjuvant therapies necessary [31].

The predominant use of MWA in GCTB is specifically as an intraoperative adjuvant to intralesional curettage. After surgical removal of the tumor, a microwave probe is inserted into the cavity to thermally destroy residual tumor cells in situ (often called "microwave in situ inactivation") [32]. Systematic reviews indicate this combined approach is highly effective, achieving excellent local control and function in short- to mid-term follow-up with low recurrence rates. In most series, after MWA inactivation, the defect is filled with cement, often augmented with subchondral bone graft or internal fixation for additional support [33].

Pure standalone use of MWA (without open surgery) in GCTB has been reported only in limited cases, and current evidence is mostly extrapolated from other bone tumor applications. While it may be potentially effective, this approach remains experimental and off-protocol, typically reserved for recurrent or anatomically challenging cases.

5.7.1.4 Aneurysmal Bone Cysts (ABCs)

Aneurysmal bone cysts are benign, osteolytic bone lesions that can be locally aggressive and expansile. They commonly affect children and adolescents but can also occur in adults of all ages. Traditional management, as it happens with most locally aggressive lesions, has centered on surgical curettage (often with bone grafting or cement) to remove the cyst and prevent recurrence. In the past decade, minimally invasive treatments (including percutaneous sclerotherapy, cryoablation, and, more recently, microwave ablation) have gained traction as alternatives or adjuncts to surgery. These methods are particularly useful in anatomically challenging locations where complete surgical resection is not feasible.

Microwave ablation generates higher temperatures and larger ablation zones compared to other percutaneous procedures, making it less susceptible to the "heat-sink" effect caused by blood flow cooling the tissue. This makes MWA particularly suitable for highly vascular lesions like aneurysmal bone cysts (ABCs). MWA can be applied percutaneously as a standalone treatment, often followed by osteoplasty to fill the cavity, or adjunctively during surgery to coagulate the cyst before or after limited curettage. It is also well-suited for lesions in high-risk locations (e.g., pelvis, sacrum, spine, or deep pelvic bones) or recurrent ABCs where previous surgeries have failed. The application of heat at approximately 60–100 °C causes instant tissue coagulation, destruction of the cyst's vascular lining, and vessel sealing, providing hemostasis. Clinical guidelines suggest that pre-curettage MWA can significantly reduce tumor bleeding and improve resection safety [34]. Therefore, MWA is a valuable option for highly vascular ABCs, offering an alternative to preoperative embolization.

5.8 Primary Malignant Bone Tumors

5.8.1 Osteosarcoma

Osteosarcoma is the most common primary malignant bone tumor. It typically develops in the metaphysis of long bones, especially the femur, proximal tibia, and humerus. Treatment typically involves a combination of surgery and chemotherapy, although MWA is being explored in specific scenarios to improve local control or preserve function.

In primary osteosarcoma, standalone microwave ablation is uncommon. It has been explored as a local treatment option for primary osteosarcoma in anatomically challenging locations or when limb-sparing surgery is difficult to achieve.

There is increasing potential for MWA in metastatic osteosarcoma, particularly at bone and lung sites, which are the most common locations. It is known that thermal ablation is well-established as a method for relieving pain and stabilizing bone in patients with skeletal metastases from various cancers. In clinical practice, percutaneous MWA can be used to ablate tumors and alleviate symptoms in osteosarcoma patients with painful bone metastases or residual skeletal lesions. This procedure often provides immediate or rapid pain relief and can be combined with cement injections to prevent fractures in weight-bearing sites [35]. For lung metastases, MWA and similar ablation techniques can achieve high local control rates with minimal morbidity [36], can be repeated as needed, and result in little loss of lung function compared to surgery. While surgical metastasectomy remains the standard for resectable pulmonary disease, MWA offers an evidence-based alternative for patients who are not candidates for surgery or have recurrent metastatic nodules.

5.8.2 Chondrosarcoma

Chondrosarcoma is a malignant bone tumor arising from cartilaginous tissue. Unlike many other sarcomas, it is largely resistant to chemotherapy and radiotherapy due to its hypovascular, cartilage-rich matrix, making surgery the mainstay of treatment. For low-grade central chondrosarcomas in extremities, less radical approaches such as intralesional curettage with adjuvant therapies are often employed to preserve function. Like other primary bone tumors, like osteosarcoma, the role of MWA in managing chondrosarcoma is increasingly defined by specific clinical scenarios.

In low-grade intramedullary chondrosarcoma of extremities, MWA is indicated as an adjuvant to intralesional curettage for central atypical cartilaginous tumors (ACT) or grade I chondrosarcomas in long bones. MWA-assisted curettage has demonstrated excellent local control and functional outcomes in these cases [37]. Patients with tumors in accessible locations (e.g., metaphysis of humerus, femur, or tibia) and without soft tissue extension are ideal candidates for this approach.

In situations where chondrosarcoma is in anatomically difficult sites (such as pelvis or sacrum) and is of low to moderate grade, or when the patient is a poor surgical candidate, MWA may be considered for tumor debulking or cytoreduction. Although definitive data are limited, there is precedent for using ablative therapies when wide resection is not feasible. Multidisciplinary tumor boards may recommend MWA in borderline cases to avoid amputation or significant disability, recognizing it as a measure to control the tumor when conventional surgery is contraindicated.

In oligometastatic disease, MWA is an established option for lung metastases from chondrosarcoma, particularly when there are a limited number of metastases (typically up to 3 in number) and each is relatively small ($\leq$3 cm) [34]. Clinical series have demonstrated durable local control in most ablated lung nodules with survival outcomes comparable to those achieved with surgery in sarcoma patients, as is also the case with osteosarcoma [36].

In the context of bone metastases, MWA is indicated for palliation in patients with symptomatic bone metastases or residual/recurrent chondrosarcoma where curative intent is not possible [35].

5.8.3 Ewing's Sarcoma

Ewing sarcoma is a rare and aggressive malignant tumor that predominantly affects children and adolescents. The standard treatment is multimodal, typically combining intensive multi-agent chemotherapy with local control measures such as surgical resection and/or radiotherapy. Despite this aggressive treatment approach, achieving local tumor control and managing metastases or recurrences remains a significant challenge.

Similar to other types of sarcomas discussed above, such as osteosarcoma and chondrosarcoma, MWA is particularly relevant for tumors in anatomically complex locations (e.g., pelvis, sacrum, or spine) where wide resection would be exceedingly morbid or technically difficult [38]. It is essential to note that MWA in this scenario would serve as an adjunctive treatment, and all Ewing sarcoma patients should receive standard neoadjuvant chemotherapy as per established protocols, consistent with other sarcomas.

Like other sarcomas, MWA can also be applied to metastases as a technique for local control and pain relief, offering a less invasive alternative to surgery for eradicating limited, small lung metastases [36, 39].

5.8.4 Metastatic Bone Lesions

Bone metastases are a common complication of advanced cancers, affecting a significant percentage of patients with metastatic disease, most frequently originating from breast, prostate, lung, and kidney (Figs. 5.13a and 5.13b).

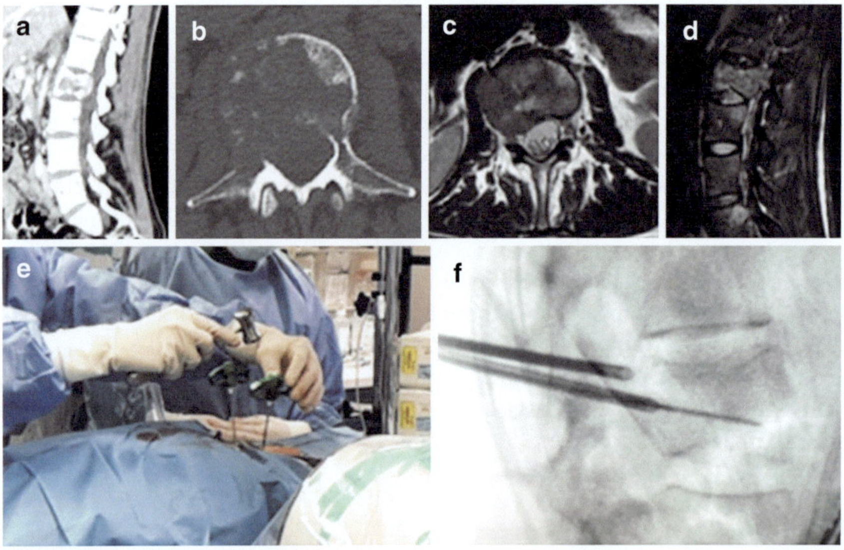

Fig. 5.13a A 50-year-old patient with a history of breast cancer presented with acute lumbar pain (**a**, **b**) Sagittal and axial CT images revealed a pathological fracture of the L2 vertebral body with a soft tissue component in the medullary canal. (**c**, **d**) MRI images in the axial plane using T1 TSE sequence (**c**), and in the sagittal plane with Short Tau Inversion Recovery (STIR) sequence (**d**), confirmed the presence of an active vertebral fracture, associated with a posterior soft tissue component and involvement of the right pedicle, leading to compression in the medullary canal. A CT-guided procedure was performed, combining diagnostic and therapeutic approaches: percutaneous biopsy, bilateral microwave ablation, placement of a SpineJack® implant, and cementation. (**e**) A photograph shows two bone cannulas inserted via bi-pedicle access. (**f**) A lateral fluoroscopy view illustrates the use of a semi-automatic 16G coaxial biopsy needle for percutaneous biopsy

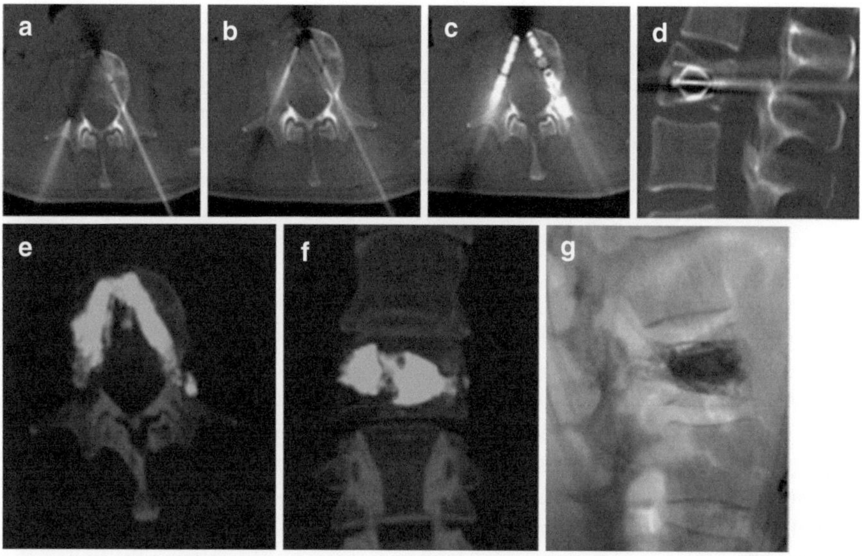

Fig. 5.13b Axial CT images. (**a**) The microwave antenna is inserted coaxially through the cannulas postablation. (**b**) Preparation for inserting expandable intravertebral titanium implants on both sides. (**c**) Two SpineJack® implants are inserted into the vertebral body via working cannulas. (**d**) A sagittal CT image with maximal intensity projection (MIP) shows the expansion of the SpineJack® implants. (**e**, **f**) Axial and coronal CT images with MIP reveal complete cementoplasty of the bilateral SpineJack® implants without immediate complications. (**g**) A lateral fluoroscopy image confirms correct vertebral expansion with homogeneous cement distribution

These lesions may cause severe pain, reduced mobility, pathological fractures, and neurological compression, all of which drastically impair quality of life. Conventional management has traditionally focused on external beam radiotherapy (RT) as the gold standard for pain palliation and local tumor control, largely due to its noninvasive nature and ability to provide meaningful pain relief in the majority of patients.

However, radiotherapy has limitations: pain relief can take weeks to manifest and may be insufficient for some patients. Another drawback is that certain tumors are relatively radioresistant, such as renal cell carcinoma, sarcoma, and melanoma. Also, prior radiation exposure limits further doses due to normal tissue tolerance. Systemic therapies, including chemotherapy, hormonal therapy, and analgesics like opioids, are often employed. However, they may not provide rapid control of local bone pain, and opioids have significant side effects and often offer incomplete relief.

Over the past two decades, minimally invasive thermal ablation techniques have emerged as valuable adjuncts or alternatives for treating painful bone metastases. Two key indications for MWA in this context are pain relief and local tumor control. Current clinical guidelines, notably those from the National Comprehensive Cancer Network (NCCN) and the European Society of Medical Oncology (ESMO), incorporate percutaneous ablation as a treatment option for bone metastases. This is particularly relevant for patients experiencing persistent or refractory pain despite radiation therapy, those who cannot undergo further radiation therapy, or in oligometastatic scenarios where definitive local control is sought.

Pain relief is the primary indication for ablation of bone metastases. Current evidence indicates that MWA provides rapid and substantial pain reduction, lasting for at least up to 3 months [35]. Similar results are observed in spinal metastases, demonstrating substantial analgesia lasting up to 6 months in most cases [40]. Pain relief typically begins within days following ablation and continues to improve over several weeks, allowing reduction in opioid use and rapid improvement in function [41].

Beyond symptomatic relief, another key indication for ablative therapy is local tumor control through debulking to prevent further growth, skeletal complications, or neurological compromise. MWA can achieve high local control rates with minimal recurrence, comparable to other focal percutaneous therapies in oligometastatic disease [41]. Maintaining local control is crucial not only for preventing tumor progression but also for avoiding skeletal-related adverse events and allowing patients to continue with other cancer treatments.

Ablation can prevent the progression of bone metastases that might otherwise lead to pathological fracture or spinal cord compression. By ablating the tumor, the structural integrity of the bone can be preserved for a longer period and, when combined with adjunctive cement augmentation or fixation in weight-bearing bones, ablation helps stabilize impending fractures. This approach is particularly effective in spinal metastases, where MWA combined with vertebral cementoplasty is widely used.

It is essential to note that current evidence does not demonstrate a clear global survival advantage from ablation in patients with multiple metastases, as overall outcomes are typically determined by systemic disease burden. However, studies suggest that patients who undergo ablation can experience prolonged local progression-free survival. By preventing local progression, MWA may reduce the need for palliative surgeries or radiation and avoid interruptions of systemic therapy due to skeletal complications.

MWA and similar ablation treatments should be considered part of a multimodal strategy for managing metastatic bone disease. Systemic therapies, including chemotherapy, hormonal therapy, targeted agents, or immunotherapy, remain the cornerstone for treating widespread metastatic cancer. These therapies can stabilize or shrink bone metastases over time; however, they may take weeks or months to achieve their maximal effect on bone lesions. Some patients cannot tolerate high doses of analgesics in the interim. For patients experiencing severe pain from bone metastasis, MWA offers immediate local action by ablating the tumor to debulk it and denervate the periosteum, thereby disrupting the pain cycle.

This approach can bridge the gap for patients during the latency of systemic therapy or provide support when systemic options are failing. Interventional radiologists and oncologists often select patients for ablation when one or a few metastases are causing disproportionate symptoms or risk, such as a solitary metastasis threatening the spinal cord, while the rest of the disease is being managed medically. When comparing MWA to purely systemic approaches, they are not mutually exclusive but complementary. Ablation addresses problems that drugs often cannot:

it provides rapid pain relief, local tumor eradication, and prevention of further bone destruction. In contrast, systemic therapy treats the underlying disease process but might leave patients suffering from a specific lesion for too long. A multidisciplinary approach is ideal, where radiation oncologists, interventional radiologists, medical oncologists, surgeons, and other specialists work together to select the best combination of treatments for each patient.

In clinical practice, ideal candidates for ablation are patients with one or a few dominant bone metastases causing disproportionate pain or risk, who have a reasonable performance status to undergo a minor procedure. Successful treatment with MWA has been reported for metastases from various common origins: breast (Figs. 5.13a and 5.13b), prostate, lung (Fig. 5.14), kidney, thyroid, and myeloma (Figs. 5.15a and 5.15b), among others. The decision to use MWA should be made

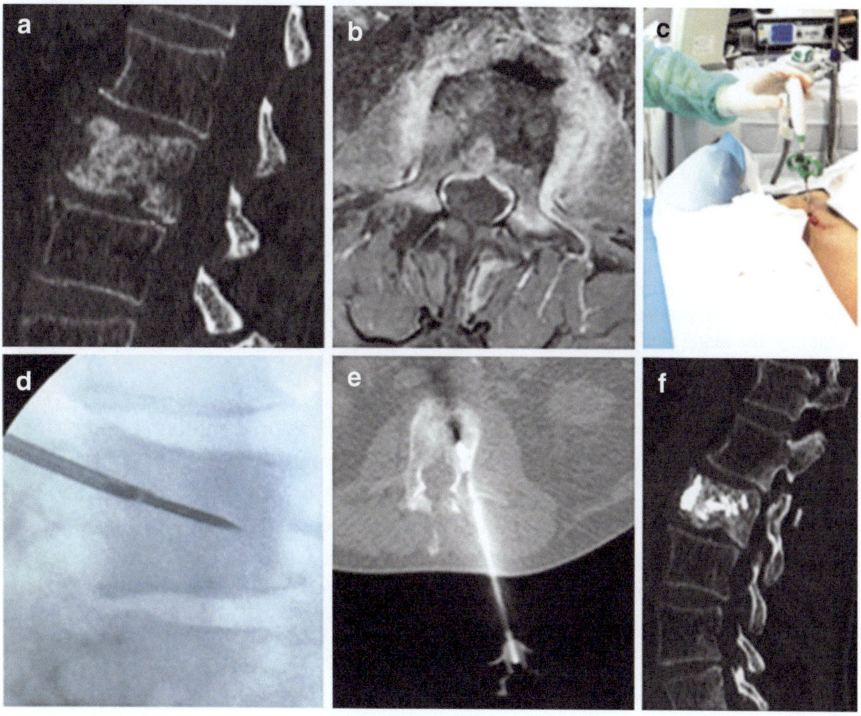

Fig. 5.14 A 74-year-old man with recurrent urothelial carcinoma of the renal pelvis and metastases to the lungs and retroperitoneal lymph nodes presented with sudden back pain. CT and MRI scans of the lumbar spine were performed (**a**) A sagittal CT image reveals osteolytic infiltration of the L2 vertebral body. (**b**) A contrast-enhanced MRI confirms vertebral infiltration with an associated soft tissue component, suggesting bone metastases. A CT-guided procedure combining diagnostic and therapeutic interventions was conducted. (**c**) A photograph shows the microwave antenna in place during ablation. (**d**) A lateral fluoroscopy view demonstrates the use of a semi-automatic 16G coaxial biopsy needle for percutaneous biopsy via a bone cannula. (**e**) An axial CT image shows the microwave antenna inserted coaxially through left pedicle access, precisely positioned at the ablation site. (**f**) A postprocedure sagittal CT image shows complete cementoplasty with substantial cement placement at the anterior column level

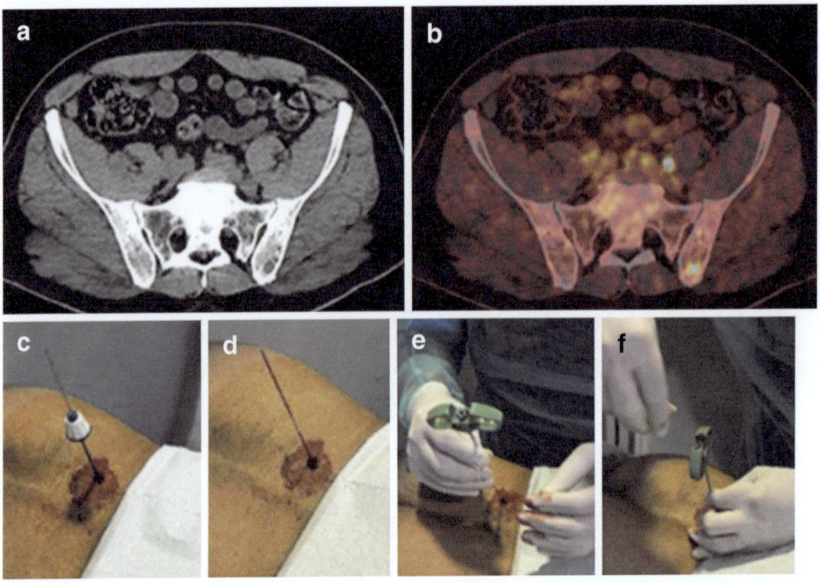

Fig. 5.15a A 53-year-old man with a history of scapular plasmacytoma, previously treated with chemotherapy with a favorable therapeutic response, presented with left hip pain five years later. Axial CT (**a**) and axial fused PET/CT (**b**) revealed a hypermetabolic lytic lesion in the left iliac bone, suggesting disease recurrence. A CT-guided procedure was performed, combining diagnostic and therapeutic approaches. Initially, a percutaneous bone biopsy using a 16G coaxial needle confirmed plasmacytoma/multiple myeloma. The external needle guided the insertion of a bone cannula to the target area

by a multidisciplinary team, considering factors such as prior radiation, tumor location, and overall disease status. Moving forward, ongoing prospective studies and potential randomized trials (e.g., versus radiotherapy or comparing ablation modalities) will further clarify the optimal use of MWA. Nonetheless, the recent literature and current ESMO (European Society for Medical Oncology) guidelines support that MWA is an indicated and effective therapy for painful or progressive bone metastases, offering significant pain relief, improved quality of life, and local tumor control when used in the appropriate clinical context [42–45].

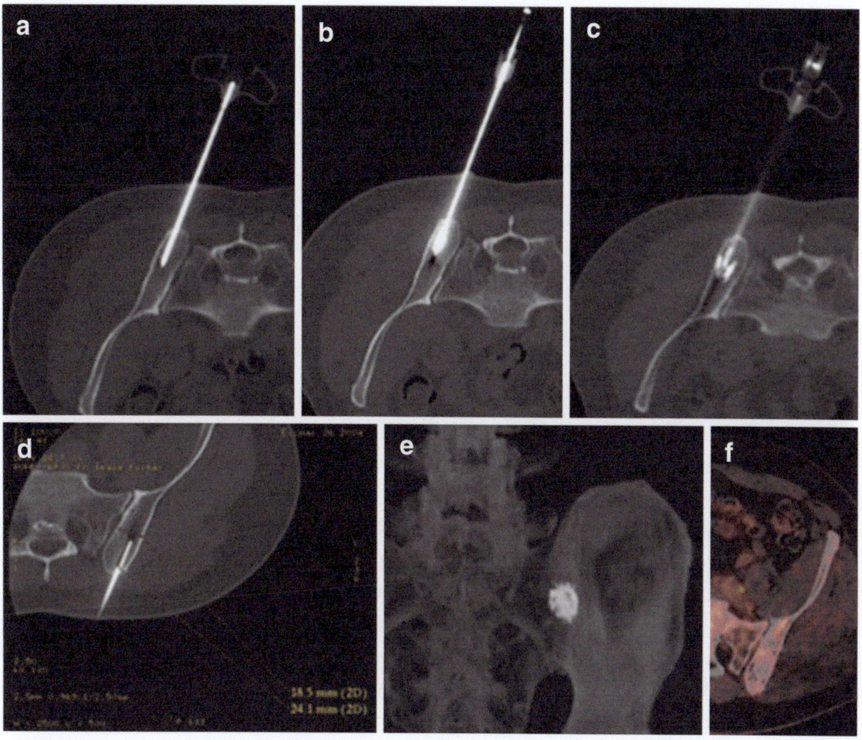

Fig. 5.15b Axial CT images with a bone filter illustrate the microwave ablation sequence. (**a**) The bone cannula is positioned at the target area. (**b**) The microwave ablation antenna is placed through this access to initiate ablation. (**c**) Cementoplasty is used to stabilize the lesion and provide pain relief, achieving optimal cement distribution without complications. (**d**) Axial CT images show the method for calculating the ablation area and simulating heat distribution. (**e**) A coronal CT with MIP demonstrates the postprocedure outcome, with well-distributed cement in the ablation zone. (**f**) A 6-month follow-up PET/CT scan shows complete metabolic resolution, indicating an excellent and sustained therapeutic response

5.9 Limitations and Contraindications (Table 5.3)

Absolute contraindications for microwave ablation are rare but include lack of a safe access route, acute immunosuppression, local or systemic infection, uncorrected coagulopathy, and patient refusal to provide informed consent [24].

Relative contraindications include key factors that a proceduralist should consider, such as tumor characteristics, proximity to vital structures, and patient characteristics.

Table 5.3 Summary of absolute and relative contraindications of MWA in bone lesions

Absolute contraindications	Relative contraindications
Lack of safe access Acute immunosuppression Local or systemic infection Uncorrected coagulopathy Patient refusal to consent	Likely damage to adjacent neurovascular structures, unless no other options exist, and the patient is informed of the risks Large soft-tissue extension, unless the goal is just partial debulking for palliation Extensive cortical destruction where ablation without immediate stabilization would likely lead to fracture. In such cases, a combined approach (ablation + cement or surgical hardware) is recommended

One major limitation of microwave ablation is when a lesion is located very close to critical nerves, the spinal cord, or major blood vessels. This is because microwave ablation produces high temperatures, which can cause irreversible damage to nerves or vessels if they are within the ablation zone. In such cases, alternative treatments such as cryoablation (which allows better control and monitoring of an ice ball) or surgery may be considered. Alternatively, special protective techniques can be employed. These techniques include using temperature monitoring probes near nerves (Fig. 5.16), hydrodissection with cool fluid to shield structures, and employing short ablation times to avoid overheating.

The size of the tumor is also a practical limiting factor. MWA typically ablates a roughly spherical area, and larger tumors may require multiple ablation probes or sessions to achieve complete treatment. In practice, malignant bone tumors >3–5 cm in diameter are challenging for percutaneous ablation to fully eradicate. Current evidence often cites 3 cm as an upper size for optimal results in a single ablation for metastases [34], although larger lesions have been treated using multiple overlapping ablations or by employing multiple antennas simultaneously. However, as tumor size increases, so do the risks: incomplete ablation, longer procedure times, and a greater likelihood of complications such as heat damage to a larger area. Additionally, if a tumor has a large extra-osseous soft tissue component, percutaneous ablation will only treat the part in or immediately around the bone. A bulky soft tissue mass may not be fully treated, and heating large soft tissue tumors can risk the skin or other organs.

Ablating a tumor can also weaken the bone structure. Weight-bearing bones with large lesions are particularly at risk if not stabilized. A limitation of MWA is that treating sizable lesions in the femur, acetabulum (Figs. 5.17a and 5.17b) or vertebral body may necessitate prophylactic internal fixation and/or cement injection to prevent collapse.

In certain locations, the proximity of vital organs can limit the use of MWA. For instance, a rib metastasis adjacent to the lung or pleura poses a risk of pneumothorax or lung injury due to heat. Lesions in the posterior pelvis near the colon or iliac vessels risk causing bowel injury or vessel perforation if not approached with

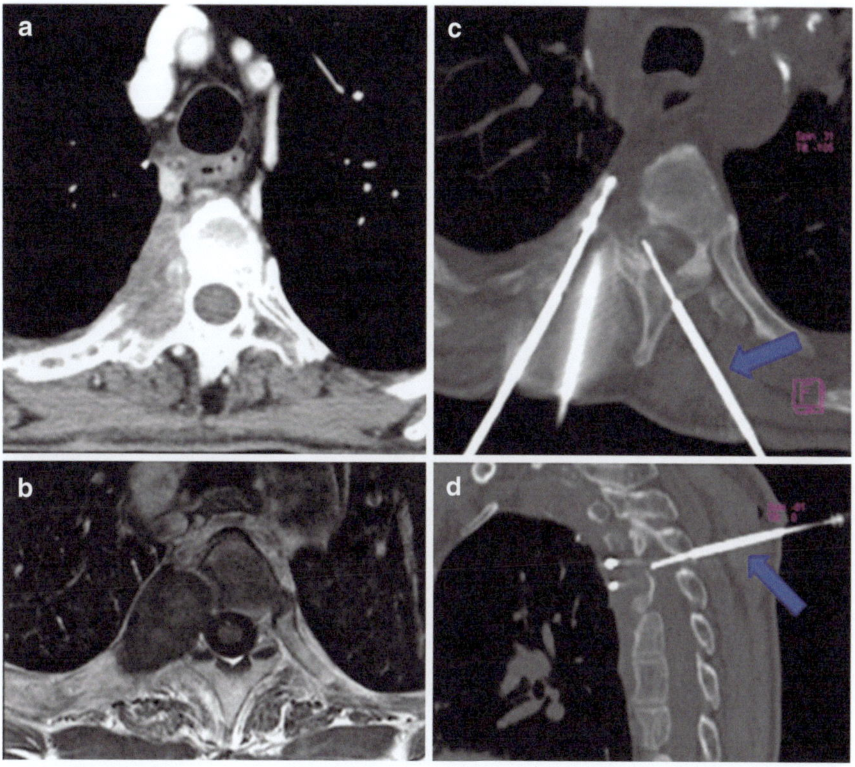

Fig. 5.16 An 83-year-old woman with lung cancer and bone metastases presented with dorsal pain and neurological symptoms. CT and MRI scans of the dorsolumbar spine were conducted (**a**) An axial CT image shows an osteolytic lesion in the D3 vertebral body, with a paravertebral soft tissue component extending to the right pedicle and protruding into the spinal canal. (**b**) An MRI axial T1 TSE sequence confirms a lytic metastatic lesion with an associated paravertebral soft tissue component on the right side and an intravertebral paramedian extension. (**c**, **d**) A CT-guided therapeutic microwave ablation was performed through the right pedicular approach, using temperature monitoring (blue arrows) to prevent overheating due to its proximity to the spinal cord

extreme caution. If no safe percutaneous path exists that avoids these organs, ablation is contraindicated. Additionally, the articular cartilage of joints is sensitive to heat; so, tumors very close to a joint surface must be treated with caution using shorter ablation times or considering cryoablation to avoid inducing osteoarthritis.

Known complications of MWA in bone reflect these limitations. A systematic review reported an overall significant complication rate of about 4% for percutaneous MWA of bone tumors [16]. The most frequent significant complication in tumor ablations is pathologic fracture. Cement leakage is another common issue when cement is used, especially in spine or pelvis cases, although it is often clinically insignificant (Fig. 5.18). Skin burns and nerve injuries can also occur.

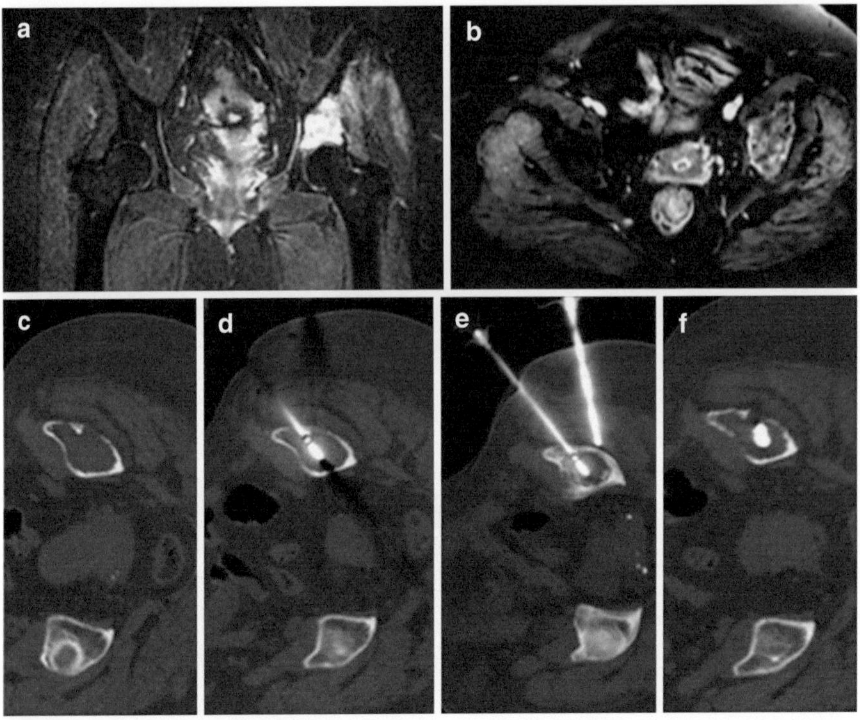

Fig. 5.17a 63-year-old woman with multiple myeloma presented with a persistent left supra-acetabular plasmacytoma and adjacent soft tissue involvement, despite previous treatments (**a**, **b**) Preablation contrast-enhanced MRI in coronal (**a**) and axial (**b**) planes revealed a soft tissue lesion in the left supra-acetabular region, along with adjacent soft tissue involvement. (**c**–**f**) Axial CT images show the microwave ablation sequence. (**c**) The lytic bone lesion is visible in the left supra-acetabular region. (**d**) The microwave antenna was inserted coaxially via the cannula to initiate ablation. (**e**) After ablation, cementoplasty was performed by inserting a second cannula to deliver cement. (**f**) Cement was well-distributed within the center of the ablation zone, providing structural reinforcement

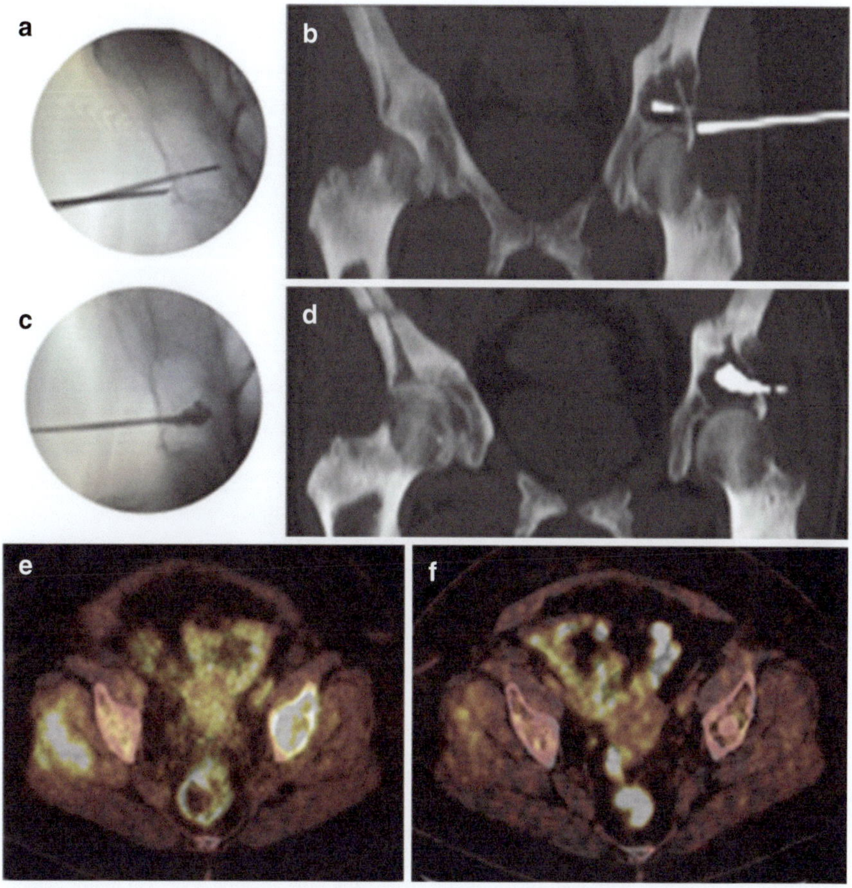

Fig. 5.17b A lateral fluoroscopy image and a coronal CT with MIP show the microwave antenna at the cavity's center, alongside the cementoplasty cannula, ready for cement injection. (**c**) A lateral fluoroscopy image captures cementation of the ablation cavity. (**d**) A postprocedure coronal CT with MIP image reveals well-distributed cement throughout the ablation zone. (**e**, **f**) Axial fused PET/CT images compare preablation and 12-month follow-up states. (**e**) A hypermetabolic lesion is visible in the left supra-acetabular region. (**f**) The lesion shows complete metabolic resolution, indicating an excellent and sustained treatment response

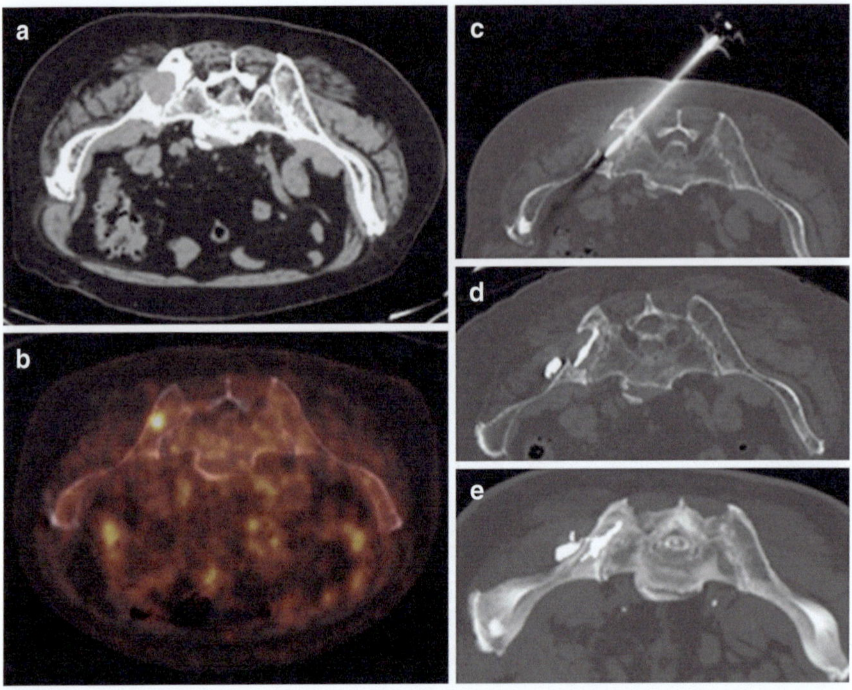

Fig. 5.18 A 75-year-old woman with multiple myeloma developed hypermetabolic osteolytic lesions despite undergoing multiple lines of chemotherapy. Because of persistent left hip pain, a PET/CT scan was performed (**a**, **b**) Axial CT (A) and axial fused PET/CT (**b**) images reveal a hypermetabolic lytic lesion in the left iliac bone, indicative of disease recurrence. A CT-guided microwave ablation (MWA) procedure was performed on this lesion. (**c**) An axial CT image shows the microwave antenna placed within the lytic lesion. (**d**, **e**) Postprocedure axial CT images and MIP show the outcome, with well-distributed cement filling the ablation zone and minor cement leakage into the periliac soft tissues, which was of no clinical significance

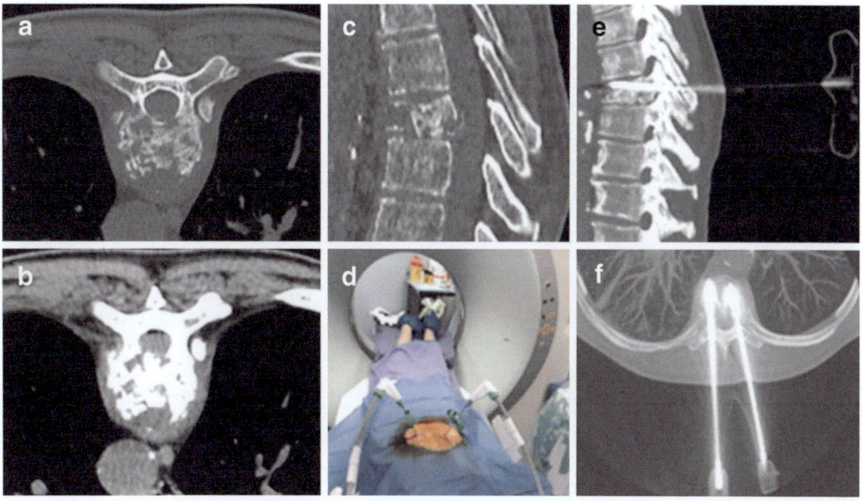

Fig. 5.19a A 56-year-old man with stage III lung cancer and bone metastases presented with worsening dorso-lumbar pain and neurological symptoms Axial (**a**, **b**) and sagittal (**c**) CT scans of the thoracic spine revealed a pathological fracture of T8 with vertebral collapse and an associated soft tissue component affecting the entire vertebral body and extending outside the vertebra. A CT-guided therapeutic procedure was performed, combining bilateral microwave ablation, placement of an expandable intravertebral titanium implant (SpineJack®), and subsequent cement injection. (**d**) A photograph showing the bilateral microwave antennas in place during the ablation procedure. Axial (**e**) and sagittal (**f**) CT images with a bone filter and maximal intensity projection (MIP) show the microwave antennas positioned at the center of the vertebral body during ablation, with bi-pedicular access achieved through coaxially inserted cannulas

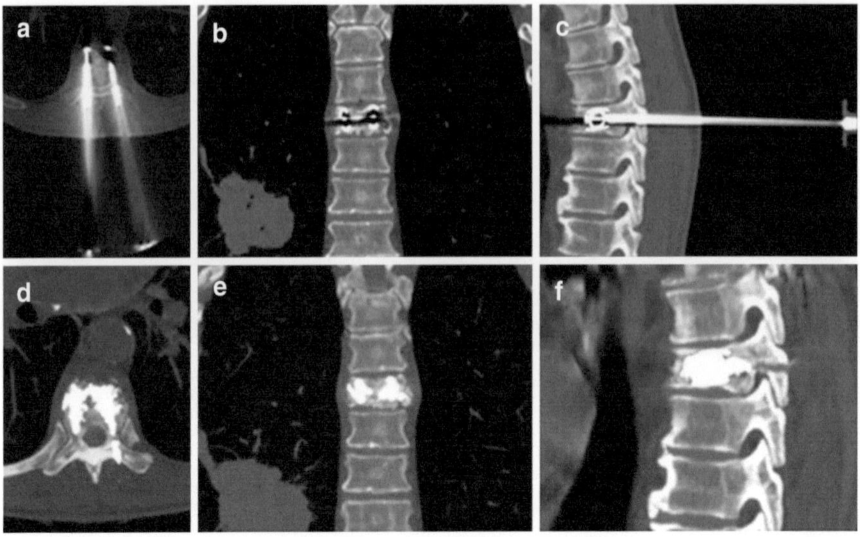

Fig. 5.19b CT images in different planes with a bone filter illustrate the final stages of the insertion of the expandable intravertebral titanium implants (SpineJack®). (**a**) Axial CT image obtained postablation demonstrates the placement of two SpineJack® implants within the vertebral body through the working cannulas. (**b, c**) Coronal and sagittal CT images confirm the successful expansion of both implants within the vertebra. (**d–f**) CT images in different planes with a bone filter and maximal intensity projection (MIP) depict the postprocedural outcome, showing complete cementoplasty surrounding the bilateral SpineJack® implants, with no immediate complications in the ablation zone

5.10 Conclusions

Throughout this chapter, we have delved into the fundamental principles of microwave ablation and its clinical applications in bone pathology. The cases presented here are derived from our institution's experience with this technique (Figs. 5.19a and 5.19b), underscoring our commitment to advancing its use in the management of bone lesions and tumors.

Our experience emphasizes the vital role of a multidisciplinary team in patient selection, where radiologists, oncologists, orthopedic surgeons, and other specialists collaborate to tailor treatment plans that meet the unique needs of each patient. A key component of this approach is meticulous preoperative planning, which involves advanced imaging studies and a thorough assessment of the tumor's location, size, and proximity to critical structures. This precise planning enables the optimization of the ablation procedure, ensuring that the treatment is both effective and safe.

The combination of this comprehensive planning, operator expertise, and rigorous post procedure follow-up is essential for achieving optimal outcomes. In summary, microwave ablation in bone pathology is a promising modality that can significantly enhance clinical outcomes and improve patients' quality of life.

References

1. Gala KB, Shetty NS, Patel P, Kulkarni SS. Microwave ablation: how we do it? Indian J Radiol Imaging. 2020;30(2):206–13.
2. Simon CJ, Dupuy DE, Mayo-Smith WW. Microwave ablation: principles and applications. Radiographics. 2005;25(Suppl 1):S69–83.
3. Ryan TP, Turner PF, Hamilton B. Interstitial microwave transition from hyperthermia to ablation: historical perspectives and current trends in thermal therapy. Int J Hyperth. 2010;26(5):415–33.
4. Tomasian A, Jennings JW. Percutaneous minimally invasive thermal ablation of osseous metastases: evidence-based practice guidelines. AJR Am J Roentgenol. 2020;215(2):502–10.
5. Ward RC, Healey TT, Dupuy DE. Microwave ablation devices for interventional oncology. Expert Rev Med Devices. 2013;10(2):225–38.
6. Yang Y, Ren B, Bian X, Li D, Xu C, Shi F, Zhao J, Tao M, Liang R. Effect of palliative microwave ablation on metastatic osseous pain: a single-center retrospective study. Ann Palliat Med. 2021;10(9):9725–31.
7. Kinczewski L. Microwave ablation for palliation of bone metastases. Clin J Oncol Nurs. 2016;20(3):249–52.
8. Brace CL. Microwave tissue ablation: biophysics, technology, and applications. Crit Rev Biomed Eng. 2010;38(1):65–78.
9. Goldberg SN, Gazelle GS, Mueller PR. Thermal ablation therapy for focal malignancy: a unified approach to underlying principles, techniques, and diagnostic imaging guidance. AJR Am J Roentgenol. 2000;174(2):323–31.
10. Brace CL. Radiofrequency and microwave ablation of the liver, lung, kidney, and bone: what are the differences? Curr Probl Diagn Radiol. 2009;38(3):135–43.
11. Kim C. Understanding the nuances of microwave ablation for more accurate post-treatment assessment. Future Oncol. 2018;14(17):1755–64.
12. Lubner MG, Brace CL, Hinshaw JL, et al. Microwave tumor ablation: mechanism of action, clinical results, and devices. J Vasc Interv Radiol. 2010;21(8 suppl):S192–203.
13. Brace CL. Microwave ablation technology: what every user should know. Curr Probl Diagn Radiol. 2009;38(2):61–7.
14. Vogl TJ, Nour-Eldin NA, Hammerstingl RM, Panahi B, Naguib NNN. Microwave ablation (MWA): basics, technique and results in primary and metastatic liver neoplasms – review article. Rofo. 2017;189(11):1055–66.
15. Surducan V, Surducan E, Ciupa R, Neamtu C. Microwave generator for scientific and medical applications. AIP Conf Proc. 2012;1425(1):89–92.
16. https://eng.libretexts.org/Bookshelves/Electrical_Engineering/Electro-Optics/Book%3A_Electromagnetics_(Ellingson)/03%3A_Transmission_Lines/3.01%3A_Introduction_to_Transmission_Lines
17. https://uk.rs-online.com/web/content/discovery/ideas-and-advice/coaxial-cable-guide
18. https://en.wikipedia.org/wiki/Transmission_line
19. Huang H, Zhang L, Moser MAJ, Zhang W, Zhang B. A review of antenna designs for percutaneous microwave ablation. Phys Med. 2021;84:254–64.

20. Pfannenstiel A, Iannuccilli J, Cornelis FH, Dupuy DE, Beard WL, Prakash P. Shaping the future of microwave tumor ablation: a new direction in precision and control of device performance. Int J Hyperth. 2022;39(1):664–74.
21. Laeseke PF, Frey TM, Brace CL, Sampson LA, Winter TC 3rd, Ketzler JR, Lee FT Jr. Multiple-electrode radiofrequency ablation of hepatic malignancies: initial clinical experience. AJR Am J Roentgenol. 2007;188(6):1485–94.
22. Sokhan VP, Jones AP, Cipcigan FS, Crain J, Martyna GJ. Signature properties of water: their molecular electronic origins. Proc Natl Acad Sci USA. 2015;112(20):6341–6.
23. Szwed M, Marczak A. Application of nanoparticles for magnetic hyperthermia for cancer treatment-the current state of knowledge. Cancers (Basel). 2024;16(6):1156.
24. Ryan A, Byrne C, Pusceddu C, Buy X, Tsoumakidou G, Filippiadis D. CIRSE standards of practice on thermal ablation of bone Tumours. Cardiovasc Intervent Radiol. 2022;45(5):591–605.
25. Shanmugasundaram S, Nadkarni S, Kumar A, Shukla PA. Percutaneous ablative therapies for the Management of Osteoid Osteomas: a systematic review and meta-analysis. Cardiovasc Intervent Radiol. 2021;44(5):739–49.
26. Bianchi G, Zugaro L, Palumbo P, Candelari R, Paci E, Floridi C, et al. Interventional radiology's osteoid Osteoma management: percutaneous thermal ablation. JCM. 2022;11(3):723.
27. Prud'homme C, Nueffer JP, Runge M, Dubut J, Kastler B, Aubry S. Prospective pilot study of CT-guided microwave ablation in the treatment of osteoid osteomas. Skeletal Radiol. 2017;46(3):315–23.
28. Nijland H, Overbosch J, Ploegmakers JJW, Kwee TC, Jutte PC. Long-term halo follow-up confirms less invasive treatment of low-grade cartilaginous tumors with radiofrequency ablation to be safe and effective. JCM. 2021;10(9):1817.
29. Dierselhuis EF, Overbosch J, Kwee TC, Suurmeijer AJH, Ploegmakers JJW, Stevens M, et al. Radiofrequency ablation in the treatment of atypical cartilaginous tumours in the long bones: lessons learned from our experience. Skeletal Radiol. 2019;48(6):881–7.
30. Wu M, et al. Use of percutaneous microwave ablation for the treatment of bone tumors: a retrospective study of clinical outcomes in 47 patients. Cancer Imaging. 2019;19(1):87.
31. Leng A, Gao H, Li J, Meng L, Wang Q, Xiang L. Intralesional curettage and surgical adjuvants in the treatment of giant cell tumor of bone: meta-analysis and systematic review. Chin Clin Oncol. 2024;13(2):20.
32. Jiang X, Xia P, Yu A. Microwave in situ inactivation technique for the treatment of giant cell tumor of bone: a systematic review and meta-analysis. J Cancer Res Clin Oncol. 2023;149(8):4653–61. https://doi.org/10.1007/s00432-022-04348-9.
33. Cui H, Li J, Zheng K, Xu M, Zhang G, Hu Y, et al. Microwave-assisted intralesional curettage combined with other adjuvant methods for treatment of Campanacci III giant cell tumor of bone in distal radius: a multicenter clinical study. Front Oncol. 2024;14:1383247.
34. Zheng K, Yu X, Hu Y, Zhang Y, Wang Z, Wu S, et al. Clinical guideline for microwave ablation of bone tumors in extremities. Orthop Surg. 2020;12(4):1036–44.
35. Gennaro N, Sconfienza LM, Ambrogi F, Boveri S, Lanza E. Thermal ablation to relieve pain from metastatic bone disease: a systematic review. Skeletal Radiol. 2019;48(8):1161–9.
36. Bourgouin PP, Wrobel MM, Mercaldo ND, Murphy MC, Leppelmann KS, Levesque VM, et al. Comparison of percutaneous image-guided microwave ablation and Cryoablation for sarcoma lung metastases: a 10-year experience. Am J Roentgenol. 2022;218(3):494–504.
37. Deckers C, De Leijer EM, Flucke U, De Rooy JWJ, Schreuder HWB, Dierselhuis EF, et al. Curettage and cryosurgery for enchondroma and atypical cartilaginous tumors of the long bones: oncological results of a large series. J Surg Oncol. 2021;123(8):1821–7.
38. Fan QY, Zhou Y, Zhang M, Ma B, Yang T, Long H, et al. Microwave ablation of primary malignant pelvic bone tumors. Front Surg. 2019;6:5.
39. Cazzato RL, Garnon J, Ramamurthy N, Koch G, Tsoumakidou G, Caudrelier J, et al. Percutaneous image-guided cryoablation: current applications and results in the oncologic field. Med Oncol. 2016;33(12):140.

40. Sagoo NS, Haider AS, Rowe SE, Haider M, Sharma R, Neeley OJ, et al. Microwave ablation as a treatment for spinal metastatic tumors: a systematic review. World Neurosurg. 2021;148:15–23.
41. Papalexis N, Parmeggiani A, Peta G, Spinnato P, Miceli M, Facchini G. Minimally invasive interventional procedures for metastatic bone disease: a comprehensive review. Curr Oncol. 2022;29(6):4155–77.
42. Coleman R, Hadji P, Body JJ, Santini D, Chow E, Terpos E, et al. Bone health in cancer: ESMO clinical practice guidelines. Ann Oncol. 2020;31(12):1650–63.
43. Pusceddu C, Sotgia B, Fele RM, Melis L. Treatment of bone metastases with microwave thermal ablation. J Vasc Interv Radiol. 2013;24(2):229–33. https://doi.org/10.1016/j.jvir.2012.10.009.
44. Pusceddu C, Sotgia B, Fele RM, Ballicu N, Melis L. Combined microwave ablation and Cementoplasty in patients with painful bone metastases at high risk of fracture. Cardiovasc Intervent Radiol. 2016;39(1):74–80. https://doi.org/10.1007/s00270-015-1151-y.
45. Pusceddu C, Marsico S, Derudas D, Ballicu N, Melis L, Zedda S, de Felice C, Calabrese A, De Francesco D, Venturini M, Santucci D, Faiella E. Percutaneous vertebral reconstruction (PVR) technique of pathological compression fractures: an innovative combined treatment of microwave ablation, bilateral expandable titanium SpineJack implants followed by Vertebroplasty. J Clin Med. 2023;12(13):4178. https://doi.org/10.3390/jcm12134178.

Cryoablation of Bone Tumors

6

Eliodoro Faiella, Domiziana Santucci, Elva Vergantino, and Rosario Francesco Grasso

6.1 Introduction

Cryoablation has emerged as a valuable tool in the minimally invasive management of bone lesions, offering both curative and palliative benefits across a wide spectrum of benign and malignant pathologies. Leveraging the biological effects of extreme cold, this technique allows for precise and controllable tissue destruction while minimizing collateral damage to surrounding structures. Originally used for soft tissue tumors, its application in the musculoskeletal system has grown rapidly due to advancements in probe technology, imaging guidance, and adjunctive protective strategies. Cryoablation is particularly advantageous in anatomically complex or functionally critical areas such as the spine, pelvis, and long bones, where conventional surgery or thermal ablation may be contraindicated or carry significant morbidity. This chapter provides a comprehensive overview of cryoablation for bone lesions, encompassing its mechanisms, procedural planning, technical execution, clinical indications, outcomes, and safety considerations. Emphasis is placed on its role in both curative settings—such as osteoid osteoma and select oligometastatic scenarios—and palliative contexts, where pain relief and functional preservation are paramount.

E. Faiella (✉) · D. Santucci · E. Vergantino · R. F. Grasso
Department of Radiology and Interventional Radiology, Fondazione Policlinico Universitario Campus Bio-medico di Roma, Rome, Italy
e-mail: e.faiella@policlinicocampus.it; d.santucci@policlinicocampus.it; elva.vergantino@unicampus.it; r.grasso@unicampus.it

C. Pusceddu, S. Marsico (eds.), *Malignant Bone Lesions and Beyond*,
https://doi.org/10.1007/978-3-032-00018-7_6

6.1.1 What Is Cryoablation

Cryoablation is an advanced therapeutic technique that induces tissue destruction through extreme cold. This modality is gaining prominence in the percutaneous management of various malignancies, including hepatic, renal, pulmonary, prostatic, and breast tumors, with particular relevance in the treatment of bone neoplasms.

6.1.1.1 Mechanisms of Cryoablation

Cryoablation has a longer historical precedent than other ablative modalities, originating in the mid-nineteenth century when James Arnott utilized extreme cold for tumor therapy [1]. The technique advanced considerably in the 1960s with the development of cryogenic systems that could administer liquid nitrogen via trocar-based probes, allowing for controlled percutaneous tumor ablation and solidifying its role in contemporary oncologic treatment [2].

Percutaneous cryoablation is conducted by placing cryoprobes into the tumor tissue with the aid of imaging techniques to ensure precise targeting. After positioning one or more cryoprobes within the target lesion, rapid cooling is initiated; this process is driven by the Joule-Thompson effect, in which the rapid expansion of a specific gas results in a significant temperature drop [3] (below −183 °C). Within the cryoprobe, high-pressure argon is forced through a throttle and expands to atmospheric pressure at the distal tip, causing a rapid decrease in temperature that is transferred to the probe's metallic walls, leading to tissue freezing. The depressurized gas is then vented out of the system, while thawing is achieved by introducing high-pressure helium, which, upon expansion, warms the probe and facilitates controlled tissue rewarming. [3, 4].

Cryoablation induces cell death by lowering tissue temperature to between −20 °C and − 40 °C, a range that is critical for cellular lethality.

The biological mechanisms responsible for cryoablative injury can be divided into four main categories: direct cell injury, vascular injury and ischemia, apoptosis, and immunomodulation [5]:

- Direct Cellular Injury: As temperature drops below 0 °C, extracellular ice forms, creating an osmotic gradient that draws water out of cells, leading to dehydration and shrinkage, particularly between 0 °C and − 20 °C. This dehydration can increase intracellular solute concentrations, causing damage, though it may not always be lethal. Below −20 °C, intracellular ice formation begins, disrupting organelles and membranes. This is lethal, especially below −40 °C, where rapid freezing accelerates ice formation inside cells. Upon thawing, the extracellular environment becomes hypotonic, causing water to reenter cells, leading to swelling and membrane rupture. Recrystallization of ice further damages cells by enlarging ice crystals [6].
- Vascular injury during cryoablation results from endothelial damage to the microvasculature, leading to platelet aggregation, microthrombosis, and vasoconstriction. This ultimately causes vascular stasis and ischemic tissue death, contributing to the coagulative necrosis seen at the center of the lesion. In con-

trast, apoptosis, a more controlled form of cell death, occurs in the peripheral regions of the lesion, where temperatures are sublethal [7].

- Immunomodulation is another key aspect of cryoablation. The technique has been shown to stimulate an immune response against tumor cells, possibly due to the release of tumor-specific antigens during tissue destruction. Unlike high-temperature methods, which denature antigens, cryoablation preserves cell structure, allowing for a more robust immune recognition [8]. Proinflammatory cytokines, such as IL-1, IL-6, and TNFα, are released in higher amounts following cryoablation compared to other ablative methods like radiofrequency ablation (RFA), suggesting that cryoablation elicits a stronger immune response [9, 10].
- This enhanced immunogenicity has been linked to an increase in tumor-specific antibodies and the activation of cytotoxic T lymphocytes (CTLs) [11]. Some studies have even reported the regression of metastatic tumors after the focal treatment of primary tumors with cryoablation [12]. Furthermore, cryoablation may promote a paradoxical immunosuppressive effect under certain conditions. The balance between necrosis and apoptosis, along with the type of cytokines released, can influence whether an immune-stimulatory or suppressive response is triggered. In some cases, the presence of regulatory T cells (Tregs) and immunosuppressive cytokines like TGFβ and IL-10 may lead to immune tolerance, potentially promoting tumor metastasis or worsening prognosis [13, 14].

Thus, while cryoablation can determine a potent immune, vascular, and necrotic response, its effects are complex and depend on several factors, including the extent of tissue ablation, the tumor type, and the tumor location.

6.1.2 Types of Cryoablation Systems

Cryoablation can be performed using two primary systems based on different gases: argon and liquid nitrogen. Each has unique characteristics that influence its suitability for different procedures.

The argon-based cryoablation system generally requires intravenous sedation, making it less ideal for office-based procedures. This system relies on multiple cryoprobes (up to 25) to achieve controlled and extensive tissue freezing and requires high-pressure argon gas (300 bar) for freezing and helium for thawing, both of which are expensive noble gases. Additionally, argon-based systems require dedicated storage space for large gas cylinders and must be used in specially equipped rooms with institutional safety validation. Despite these logistical challenges, the ability to use multiple probes allows for the treatment of larger or irregularly shaped lesions with greater precision and flexibility.

On the other hand, the liquid nitrogen-based cryoablation system is a more cost-effective and manageable alternative. This system typically utilizes a single cryoprobe, offering the benefit of a larger ablation zone and quicker freezing times compared to the argon-based system. Liquid nitrogen is stored in small, insulated flasks, which are easier to manage and transport than the large gas cylinders needed for argon. As a result, this system is more practical for many settings. It is particularly advantageous in treating larger lesions as it rapidly forms a larger iceball, enhancing the overall treatment efficiency. Although it tends to have fewer complications due to the use of a single cryoprobe, larger probes may sometimes be required, which could hypothetically increase the risk of complications [15–17].

In summary, while both systems are effective, the choice between them depends on factors like the lesion size, the required ablation zone, cost considerations, and the need for sedation or anesthesia.

6.1.3 Advantages of Cryoablations

Cryoablation offers several advantages over other thermal ablation techniques, with the primary benefit being the ability to monitor the ablation zone in real-time during the procedure: as tissue freezes, the water undergoes to solid phase, forming an iceball, which is visible under various imaging techniques, including ultrasound (US), computed tomography (CT), and magnetic resonance (MR) imaging.

Cryoablation is generally less painful than heat-based thermal ablation techniques, such as microwave or radiofrequency ablation, because it provides an anesthetic effect by cooling tissues and nerves. As a result, cryoablation often does not require general anesthesia and can be performed under moderate sedation.

Tumors near metallic implants can be safely treated without the risks of electrical conductivity or unwanted thermal effects associated with RFA and MWA. Cryoablation probes function independently, allowing multiple probes to be used simultaneously and positioned strategically to shape the iceball as needed, ensuring precise tumor ablation. [18, 19].

6.1.4 Procedure

6.1.4.1 Anesthesia and Periprocedural Management

Cryoablation is generally associated with lower levels of pain compared to heat-based techniques, due to the intrinsic anesthetic effect of freezing, which contributes to reduced procedural discomfort [18]. This unique property often allows procedures to be safely performed under local anesthesia and/or conscious sedation alone. Nevertheless, in selected scenarios—such as deep-seated lesions, anatomically sensitive sites, or in specific patient groups like pediatric populations—general anesthesia (GA) may still be necessary. This is particularly relevant in the treatment of osteoid osteoma in children, where patient immobility is critical to ensure safety and precision. Notably, recent evidence has shown that CT-guided percutaneous cryoablation of osteoid osteomas in pediatric patients can be effectively and safely performed under conscious sedation, offering a viable alternative to GA [20].

For lesions involving the spine, pelvis, or proximal lower limbs, neuraxial techniques such as spinal anesthesia may be considered. Similarly, regional nerve blocks can provide effective anesthesia for peripheral lesions, contributing to both intra- and postprocedural analgesia [21].

In anticipation of postoperative pain, it is advisable to initiate systemic analgesic therapy in the preprocedural phase. Routine administration of intravenous paracetamol, combined with nonsteroidal anti-inflammatory drugs (NSAIDs), is recommended starting prior to the procedure and continuing throughout the periprocedural period. This approach enhances patient comfort and reduces the need for stronger analgesics postintervention.

Postprocedural pain following cryoablation is typically mild to moderate and tends to peak within the first 24 h. Importantly, both the incidence and severity of pain are significantly lower compared to thermal ablation techniques [18]. The relative anesthetic effect of cold contributes to this favorable profile.

Nevertheless, appropriate pain control remains essential. The use of systemic analgesics, such as intravenous paracetamol and NSAIDs, should be continued in the immediate postoperative phase. In cases where stronger pain management is required, patient-controlled analgesia (PCA) systems delivering opioids and anti-emetic agents can be employed effectively.

Antibiotic prophylaxis is indicated when cement injection or screw placement is planned. In other cases, it may be considered based on operator or institutional protocols [18].

6.1.4.2 Planning

Preprocedural imaging (CT, magnetic resonance imaging (MRI), PET-CT) is essential for determining the type, number, and placement of cryoprobes within the lesion to ensure complete coverage, while also guiding the optimal approach to the target, identifying at-risk structures, and facilitating the precise positioning of probes and monitoring devices. Ideally, these imaging studies should be no older than one month. If the tumor exhibits aggressive behavior or if there have been changes in the patient's symptoms, updated imaging may be required closer to the procedure date [18].

For detailed assessment of osseous structures, noncontrast, thin-section (1–3 mm) CT with multiplanar reconstructions is the preferred imaging modality [18].

For malignant bone tumors, a multiparametric MRI (that includes T1- and T2- with and without fat saturation—and diffusion-weighted/apparent diffusion coefficient (ADC) sequences), with associated dynamic contrast-enhanced T1-weighted sequences in multiple planes, is recommended. Positron emission tomography-computed tomography (PET-CT) is essential for detecting oligometastatic disease and assessing important metabolic markers, such as standardized uptake value (SUV) and metabolic tumor volume; technetium-based imaging remains the more sensitive option for identifying bone metastases [22, 23].

6.1.4.3 Intraprocedural Guidance

Intraprocedural imaging techniques—such as fluoroscopy, computed tomography (CT), cone-beam CT (CBCT), and magnetic resonance imaging (MRI)—used either independently or in combination with advanced technologies like navigation systems or image fusion platforms, are essential for ensuring precise probe placement during percutaneous procedures. High-resolution multimodal imaging, particularly the integration of contrast-enhanced or noncontrast CT with fluoroscopy, allows for the planning and execution of adjunctive therapies such as embolization, percutaneous screw fixation, or cementoplasty when needed [21, 24, 25].

In selected cases—particularly when lesions are superficial and readily accessible—ultrasound (US) guidance for probe positioning may be sufficient, provided that adjacent critical structures are clearly identifiable and can be safely avoided [26]. Nevertheless, intraprocedural CT (with or without contrast) is often performed to confirm accurate cryoprobe placement and to document the iceball formation and its spatial extent.

Among all available imaging modalities, CT with and without contrast remains the most widely used technique for guiding percutaneous procedures involving bone lesions. However, it is limited by its high radiation exposure and the lack of real-time imaging capabilities [27].

To address these limitations, a variety of navigation systems have been developed, enhancing targeting accuracy while reducing procedure time and radiation dose. These systems employ electromagnetic (EM), optical, or hybrid tracking technologies, enabling real-time visualization of instruments during intervention [29 – 35].

EM-based navigation systems, which utilize field generators and sensors, have been effectively implemented in multiple settings, including thermal ablation of hepatic tumors and other surgical procedures, resulting in reduced radiation exposure [35]. Additionally, fusion imaging platforms based on flat-panel cone beam computerized tomography (CBCT)—used with or without contrast—have been proposed to assist in percutaneous biopsies of bone, offering simplified needle path planning and shorter procedure times [36].

Despite their advantages, these advanced systems have certain limitations. Not all procedural devices are compatible with EM fields; optical systems require an unobstructed line of sight between the tracking camera and the surgical tools, laser guidance may involve additional costs and setup time, and robotic-assisted systems often necessitate bulkier instrumentation [28].

Demonstrating the clinical potential of these emerging technologies, augmented reality EM-navigation systems have shown significant benefits in the context of percutaneous bone interventions. Compared to standard CT-guided techniques, the use of EM-navigation systems has been associated with reduced procedure time, fewer CT scans, and lower radiation doses, particularly in small bone lesions (<2 cm). Furthermore, a higher diagnostic accuracy has been observed in EM navigation-assisted biopsies. These findings support the growing integration of advanced navigation systems into clinical practice, promoting safer, more efficient, and more accurate percutaneous procedures [37, 38] (Figs. 6.1, 6.2, 6.3, and 6.4).

6.1.4.4 Treatment

Prior to probe insertion, local anesthesia should be administered to the skin, subcutaneous tissues, and periosteum to minimize procedural discomfort and reduce postoperative pain. Under imaging guidance, a coaxial 17-gauge gas-driven cryoprobe

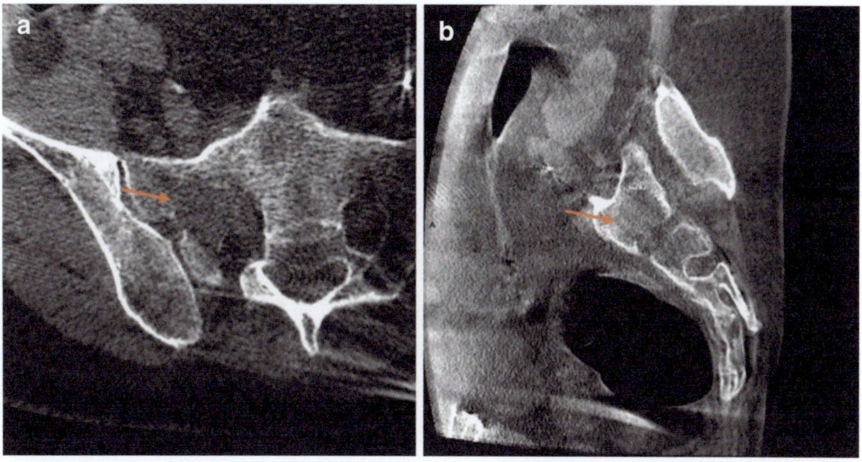

Fig. 6.1 (**a, b**) Intraprocedural axial (**a**) and reconstructed sagittal (**b**) CT images of the pelvis showing a lytic bone metastasis involving the right hemisacrum at the level of S1. The lesion demonstrates cortical destruction and irregular margins, with early invasion of the adjacent right S1 neural foramen

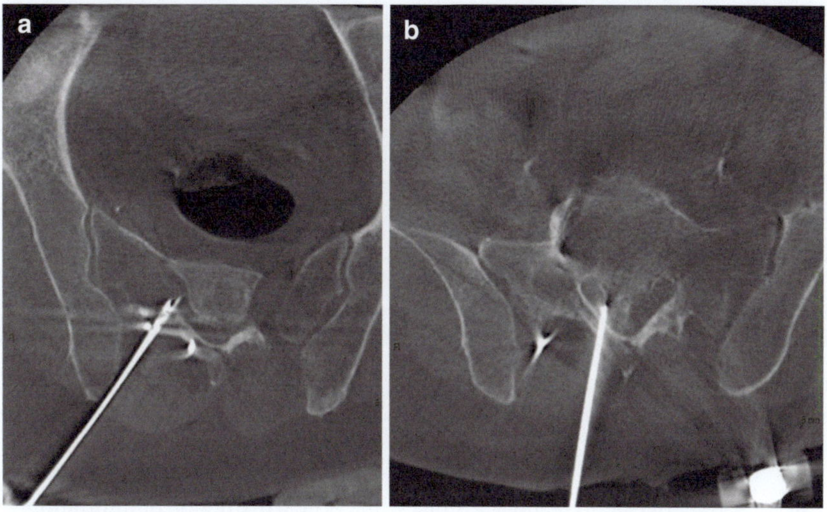

Fig. 6.2 (**a, b**) Fluoroscopy-guided procedure assisted by the robotized tracking system for intraoperative targeting (SIRIO) infrared navigation system. (**a**) Placement of the thermocouple probe at the proximal segment of the right S1 neural foramen, adjacent to the metastatic lesion and within the anticipated iceball margin. (**b**) Positioning of a 19G Chiba needle at the distal portion of the S1 foramen to allow hydrodissection of the adjacent nerve root, providing thermal protection during the ablative procedure

is then inserted through an 11G or 13G trocar, which is subsequently retracted approximately 1 cm outside the anticipated ablation zone [18]. If clinically indicated, a biopsy may be performed before cryoprobe placement by introducing a biopsy needle coaxially through the same 11G or 13G trocar.

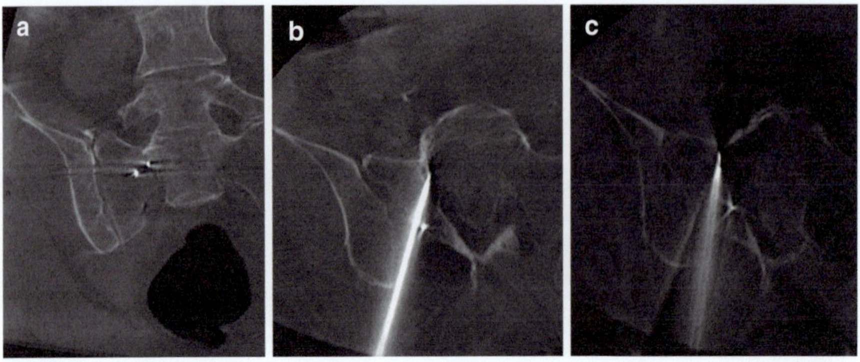

Fig. 6.3 (**a, b, c**) Coronal (**a**) and axial (**b, c**) CT images show the accurate placement of IceRod cryoablation needles within the lytic sacral metastasis with fluoroscopy and SIRIO infrared navigation system guide

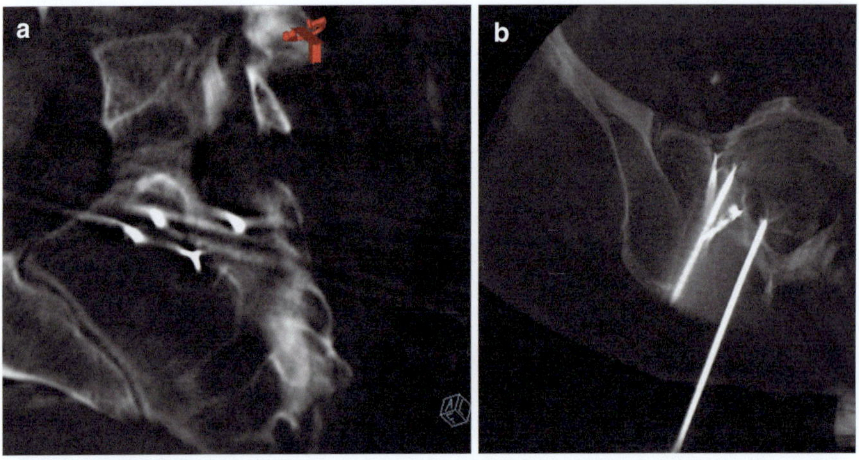

Fig. 6.4 (**a, b**) Images showing the configuration of the four positioned needles, ensuring comprehensive coverage of the lesion and optimizing the anticipated iceball formation while preserving adjacent neural structures

In the setting of osteolytic bone lesions with cortical disruption or infiltration, the cryoprobe can often be inserted directly into the lesion without the need for a coaxial guiding trocar (e.g., 11G or 13G needle). The lytic nature of the lesion typically results in reduced bone density and structural integrity, facilitating direct probe advancement through the compromised cortical bone (Figs. 6.1 and 6.3). This approach may simplify the procedural steps, particularly in cases where the cortical breach provides a natural access route.

Superficial lesions can be treated without penetrating the bone by positioning the probe next to the target, making sure the iceball fully encompasses the lesion.

Ablation applicators are placed only after all tumor access points have been established; a variety of cryoprobes are available, allowing for the simultaneous activation of multiple probes to generate iceballs of different sizes and shapes, conforming to the lesion's morphology. The treatment protocol requires multiple freeze-thaw cycles, involving a 10-min freezing phase, a 9-min passive thaw, and a subsequent 10-min freeze to achieve effective cellular destruction within the −20 °C to −40 °C range [39].

Iceball formation is monitored through periodic CT imaging to ensure complete tumor coverage while maintaining a safe margin from adjacent critical structures.

After completing a full ablation cycle, active thawing is briefly performed to release the probe, which invariably adheres to the tissue. If needed, the probe can also be heated during withdrawal to achieve tract cauterization [18].

Two critical aspects of the procedure—protection of adjacent structures and posttreatment consolidation to prevent fractures—will be discussed in detail in the following sections.

6.1.4.5 Postprocedural Follow-Up and Assessment of Treatment Efficacy

Postprocedural follow-up after bone cryoablation is structured into two main phases: an early phase focused on the timely detection of complications and the initial evaluation of clinical benefit, and a later phase, tailored according to the nature of the treated lesion and the therapeutic intent.

– Early Follow-Up

In the immediate postprocedural period, clinical evaluations are typically performed at 4 h, 1 day, and 1 week following treatment. The goal of this early phase is to rule out acute complications—such as hemorrhage, infection, fracture, or cement leakage—and to monitor the initial analgesic response.

Patients are generally observed overnight to ensure adequate recovery from anesthesia and optimal pain control, which is particularly important in pediatric patients. Most patients are discharged on the first postoperative day. Even when cryoablation is combined with augmentation techniques in weight-bearing regions, early mobilization is encouraged, though patients should be advised to avoid excessive loading and strenuous activity for 2–3 weeks.

– Long-Term Follow-Up

Long-term follow-up depends on the type of lesion treated, with different strategies applied for benign versus malignant tumors. In malignant disease, further distinction is made between curative and palliative settings.

For benign lesions, the frequency and duration of follow-up depend on histologic subtype. In most cases, a single clinical and radiological assessment at 1–3 months posttreatment is sufficient. In conditions such as osteoid osteoma or osteoblastoma, treatment success is evaluated not only by the disappearance of the lesion on imaging but also by the resolution of pain and reduction or discontinuation of analgesic medications. To objectively assess pain control and quality of life, validated tools such as the Visual Analogue Scale (VAS) and the Brief Pain Inventory should be used, with assessments at days 1, 3, 7, and 14 postprocedure, followed by monthly evaluations for up to one year. This approach is particularly relevant in cases of malignant lesions infiltrating the cortical bone, where the aim of the treatment is primarily or also analgesic. In such scenarios, clinical response, changes in analgesic use, and patient-reported outcomes should all be documented.

In malignant lesions treated with curative intent, follow-up is aimed at assessing local control and identifying systemic progression. This includes periodic clinical visits, laboratory tests (including tumor markers), and imaging. MRI and PET-CT are the preferred modalities for detecting residual or recurrent disease and metachronous metastases.

In the palliative setting, clinical follow-up may suffice unless symptoms suggest complications or disease progression, in which case targeted imaging is indicated.

Across all settings, bone remineralization observed on CT is considered an indirect but meaningful sign of successful ablation [18].

6.1.5 Complications

Complications may result from unintended thermal damage to adjacent critical structures during probe insertion or ablation, as well as from the effects of bone injury. The specific risks depend on the treatment site and the surrounding anatomical features.

Normal structures may be injured either by the applicator passing through them during placement or by its proximity to the ablation zone; for example, for spinal lesions, transpedicular and parapedicular approaches can be used, with the parapedicular route posing a higher risk of bleeding or injury to radicular arteries, including the artery of Adamkiewicz, which can lead to paraplegia if occluded; myelographic contrast helps identify neural structures to guide the safest approach [40].

The overall complication rate for cryoablation procedures is reported at 9.1%. Several risk factors have been associated with an increased likelihood of complications, including an eastern cooperative oncology group – performance status (ECOG-PS) greater than 2, cryoablation of long bones, and the use of more than three cryoprobes [17].

Major complications occur in 2.5% of cases, with secondary fractures being the most frequent (1.25%), typically after a mean delay of 71 days, especially in weight-bearing bones; for this reason, in bones such as the hip or spine, ablation is often combined with bone reinforcement to reduce the risk of fractures [17, 18]. Ablation in the periacetabular region carries a risk of accidental osteochondral injury, including avascular necrosis, leading to collapse of the hip joint, which may require hip replacement, as seen 8 months after cryoablation of a periacetabular chondrosarcoma metastasis. Inclusion of these structures in the ablation zone can cause varying degrees of osteochondral damage. Ablation applicators should be directed away from the joint space, and the procedure should be closely monitored radiographically, with termination if the hip joint is encroached [41].

Other severe but rare complications include infection at the cryoablation site, tumor seeding, bleeding, and severe hypotension, each observed in 0.3% of cases [17].

Minor complications are more common and include postprocedural pain (2.2%), peripheral neuropathy (0.9%), and temporary paresthesia (0.9%) [17].

In rare cases, complications reported in the literature for lesions treated with cryoablation in the rib and sternum include pleural effusion in 18.2% of patients (6 out of 33), and pulmonary embolism in 6.1% of patients (2 out of 33) [42].

One important consideration is the treatment of large bone lesions, such as solitary plasmacytomas or desmoid tumors, as ablating a significant volume of tumor and surrounding bone tissue can cause a substantial release of proteins from tissue breakdown, similar to rhabdomyolysis or tumor lysis, potentially leading to acute tubular necrosis, requiring hemodialysis, and electrolyte imbalances. Although no formal guidelines define the maximum tissue volume for ablation in a single session, in cases where large tumors are ablated, patients undergo intensive hydration during and after the procedure, with close monitoring of urine output [40].

A rare but serious complication is high-pressure argon gas leakage from a fractured cryoprobe, potentially causing life-threatening embolism. If resistance occurs during insertion through intact bone, immediate CT imaging can help detect gas escape early for prompt intervention [40]. Cryoshock, a rare inflammatory response triggered by the release of necrotic material into circulation, has not been reported in osseous cryoablation [43].

6.1.5.1 Neural Complications

Cryoablation can induce nerve injury when temperatures drop to approximately 10 °C or lower [5, 44–47] with temporary neuropraxia occurring around −20 °C and permanent neurological damage at temperatures below −40 °C.

Cold exposure initially slows neuronal conduction, eventually causing conduction blockade. This is accompanied by neuronal and perineural edema, demyelination, and axonal degeneration. In extreme cases, direct cellular damage may occur due to dehydration and membrane disruption. Additionally, endothelial injury and vasa nervorum occlusion can lead to ischemia, increasing the risk of permanent nerve impairment [44, 48, 49].

A key advantage of cryoablation is the clear visualization of the ablation zone, enabling precise control over tissue destruction. The iceball's outer margin, visible on CT, aligns with the 0 °C isotherm, indicating the threshold for nerve injury [48, 50]. In contrast, heat-based ablation relies on MR thermometry for temperature monitoring, which offers less anatomical detail. Additionally, freezing is generally less painful than heating [51], allowing the procedure to be performed with lower levels of anesthesia. This may enable the patient to remain alert and responsive, facilitating an intraoperative neurological examination to detect early signs of nerve involvement. The safety margin for cryoablation near critical nerves is not fixed and varies based on factors such as the precision in defining the ablation zone, the feasibility of repositioning the nerve, and the operator's expertise. Damage to a single nerve with overlapping innervation may have little clinical impact, but if the contralateral nerve is already compromised, the risk of significant functional impairment increases. Furthermore, nerves in previously irradiated areas may be more vulnerable to injury due to reduced microvascular integrity [52, 53].

Ablation procedures for bone lesions can lead to unintended nerve injuries, resulting in sensory and motor deficits of varying severity. The impact of these complications depends on the nerve involved, its anatomical location, and the extent of the damage (Table 6.1) [53].

Table 6.1 Common nerve ablation sites and their potential complications

Nerve	Ablation site	Potential complications
Intercostal and subcostal nerves	Ribs	Usually asymptomatic; minor sensory deficits; rarely, abdominal wall laxity perceived as a "hernia"
Long thoracic nerve	Lateral ribs	Winged scapula. Often asymptomatic
Dorsal scapular nerve	Scapula	Mild lateral scapular displacement, usually of little clinical significance
Suprascapular nerve	Superior and lateral scapula	Weakness in arm abduction and loss of lateral humeral rotation if injured above the suprascapular notch
Lumbar plexus	Deep or medial to the psoas muscle	Lower extremity motor dysfunction due to injury of major nerve branches
Femoral nerve	Iliopsoas muscle or iliac bone	Loss of hip flexion and knee extension; sensory deficits in the anterior and medial thigh, knee, and leg
Obturator nerve	Periacetabular or pubic bone	Loss of hip adduction, causing gait instability
Sacral nerve roots	Sacrum or medial iliac bone	Severe lower extremity dysfunction, urinary and anal sphincter dysfunction, saddle anesthesia
Sciatic nerve	Periacetabular, ischium, or femur	Significantly lower extremity motor loss; the peroneal branch injury causes foot drop
Pudendal nerve	Periacetabular region (near ischial spines, Alcock canal)	Genital paresthesias and dysesthesias; bilateral injury (or unilateral in preirradiated patients) may cause urinary and fecal incontinence

6.1.6 Supportive Interventions

6.1.6.1 Thermal Insulation

Cryoablation of bone lesions requires careful thermal protection of adjacent sensitive structures, particularly nerves, cartilage, skin, viscera, and joint capsules. Thermoprotective strategies are essential to avoid iatrogenic injury and are generally categorized into passive monitoring and active protection techniques.

– Passive Monitoring

Passive monitoring plays a vital role in reducing the risk of injury during cryoablation procedures. This technique involves the strategic placement of thermocouples or thermistors—sometimes fiber-optic when under MR guidance—near critical anatomical structures that may be vulnerable to extreme temperatures. In spinal applications, one or more temperature probes are commonly inserted into the epidural space using sublaminar or transforaminal approaches (Fig. 6.2a). This allows for continuous real-time assessment of the thermal dose delivered to nearby neural structures, including those within the spinal canal and neural foramina. If the temperature near these vital areas approaches critical thresholds (typically below 10 °C in cryoablation), the ablation must be immediately halted to prevent irreversible damage [40].

Additionally, thermocouples may be placed near periarticular regions to monitor temperatures adjacent to articular cartilage, helping to prevent chondrolysis or joint dysfunction in lesions with subchondral extension. The thermal feedback provided by these sensors enables precise control of the ablation zone and enhances procedural safety, especially in anatomically complex or joint-adjacent locations.

Peripheral nerve integrity can also be evaluated, under GA, using intraoperative electrophysiologic monitoring techniques such as somatosensory and motor evoked potentials (SSEP and MEP). These involve delivering transcranial electrical impulses and recording responses via electrodes placed over target muscle groups. A stable response indicates intact neural conduction; however, diminishing signals suggest early nerve compromise and necessitate immediate interruption of the ablation to prevent irreversible injury. To ensure accurate monitoring, neuromuscular blocking agents should be avoided during general anesthesia, as they inhibit muscle responsiveness and confound real-time assessments [54, 55].

Alternatively, when procedures are conducted under conscious sedation, patient feedback becomes a valuable diagnostic tool. The operator may conduct targeted neurologic evaluations during ablation or ask the patient to report unusual sensations or pain, which can serve as early indicators of neural involvement. Pain perception, especially during heat-based techniques, may signal impending nerve injury and should prompt immediate cessation of the ablation, followed by implementation of additional protective measures [40].

In some cases, direct peripheral nerve stimulation has been used as a supplementary technique. Electrodes are placed adjacent to major nerves, and reduced muscular response during stimulation may signal impending dysfunction [56]. While these approaches provide functional information about the neuromotor pathway, a limitation is that signal loss may occur after irreversible injury has begun, underscoring the importance of real-time monitoring and rapid operator response [40].

– Active Protection

Active protection strategies are employed to modify the local anatomy or thermal environment, thereby reducing the risk of injury to critical structures.

- *Hydrodissection*

Hydrodissection is a widely adopted method for thermal protection during cryoablation, particularly in anatomically complex or high-risk locations. It involves the controlled injection of sterile fluid—commonly normal saline or 5% dextrose—into the tissue planes between the ablation zone and adjacent vulnerable structures. A fine needle (typically 20G or 22G) is positioned under imaging guidance (CT, ultrasound, or MRI), and fluid is administered until sufficient separation, usually around 1 cm, is achieved. The extent and direction of fluid spread depend heavily on the local anatomical planes, requiring a thorough understanding of the surrounding tissue architecture.

This technique offers both passive and active protection. Passive protection is achieved by the insulating effect of the fluid and the increased physical distance between the cryoprobe and the organ at risk. Active protection can be added by using continuous infusion of cooled or warmed fluid during the ablation, helping to modulate local temperatures. Thermocouples may be placed adjacent to the protected structures to monitor temperature in real time and ensure safety thresholds are maintained.

In the epidural or periradicular space, particularly when neural elements are located within 8 mm of the lesion, continuous irrigation with room-temperature saline is recommended. This is especially important in spinal interventions, where thermal spread must be tightly controlled (Fig. 6.2b).

In thoracic procedures, such as sternal cryoablation, hydrodissection can also be employed in the retrosternal space to safely displace the pericardium and reduce cardiopulmonary risk [57]. In periarticular lesions, intraarticular fluid instillation can displace the joint capsule and synovial membrane from the ablation zone, reducing the risk of cartilage damage.

The amount of fluid used is highly variable and depends on the location and complexity of the procedure, ranging from a few milliliters to several liters. For improved visibility under CT, the fluid can be diluted with a small amount of nonionic contrast medium at a ratio of approximately 1:50, enhancing delineation of the dissection plane without generating artifacts [58].

- *Carbodissection*

Carbodissection is another thermal protection modality that involves the percutaneous injection of carbon dioxide (CO_2) into specific anatomical planes to physically displace vulnerable structures from the ablation zone. CO_2 is preferred over room air because of its significantly reduced risk of symptomatic gas embolism if inadvertently introduced into the vascular system. The technique is especially useful for creating insulation in anterior compartments, given that gas tends to accumulate in nondependent areas of the anatomy. For this reason, carbodissection is most effective when the structure to be protected lies anterior to the target lesion.

CO_2 is delivered via a spinal needle placed under imaging guidance, and because the gas is rapidly reabsorbed by the body, repeated injections are often required. Intermittent CT monitoring throughout the procedure is essential to ensure that the gas pocket remains sufficient for effective protection. An example of this technique is the injection of CO_2 into the intervertebral foramen to mechanically separate the dural sac and nerve roots, which has proven effective in managing sacral and foraminal lesions.

In complex clinical scenarios, carbodissection may be combined with hydrodissection to optimize spatial separation and enhance thermal safety, particularly when multiple critical structures surround the treatment site [58].

For superficial lesions, subcutaneous injection of an anesthetic or dextrose solution, combined with external protection using warm saline-filled surgical gloves, has been shown to prevent frost injury to the skin. Contemporary cryoablation systems incorporate probes with thermally insulated shafts. This design feature minimizes the risk of ice formation along the insertion path, offering added protection to superficial soft tissues, especially when the access route passes close to the skin [18].

6.1.6.2 Consolidation

In osseous sites that are biomechanically critical—particularly weight-bearing structures such as vertebral bodies, the femoral head and neck, and the acetabulum—cryogenic tumor ablation is frequently integrated with percutaneous structural reinforcement to achieve both oncologic and orthopedic objectives. This dual-modality approach is essential not only for local tumor control and analgesia but also to prevent biomechanical compromise that may culminate in pathological fracture, especially in the presence of extensive osteolysis [21].

When cryoablation is performed with curative or durable palliative intent, subsequent consolidation should be planned as part of the same procedural session or in close temporal proximity. In such cases, percutaneous osteoplasty with polymethylmethacrylate (PMMA) is the most commonly used method of reinforcement. PMMA injection may be performed via the same coaxial access used for probe placement, ensuring procedural efficiency and minimizing additional tissue trauma [59].

Cementoplasty has demonstrated a consistent and rapid analgesic effect, with pain reduction reported in up to 90% of treated cases. The mechanisms are likely multifactorial, involving stabilization of microfractures and possible neurolytic effects from the exothermic polymerization process. Despite its stabilizing role, its consolidative effect remains variable and context-dependent, particularly influenced by cement volume, distribution, and the extent of cortical involvement [60].

Critical technical parameters must be observed during the transition from cryoablation to consolidation:

- Thermal Recovery of Tissue: Following cryoablation, the target tissue must be allowed to passively thaw until the temperature exceeds −20 °C. Injecting PMMA into hypothermic tissue carries a significant risk of rapid polymerization, incomplete interdigitation, and insufficient mechanical integration with the host bone.
- Timing of Cement Augmentation: Immediate cement injection postthaw may be feasible, but delayed augmentation—up to 24 h later—is often preferred in anatomically sensitive regions (e.g., posterior vertebral body or acetabular dome) to reduce thermal mismatch and the risk of cement leakage due to residual cryo-induced tissue brittleness.
- Risk Mitigation for Compression Fracture: In spinal metastases or lesions involving the acetabular roof, PMMA injection following cryoablation is particularly indicated to prevent microstructural collapse. The cryo-induced necrotic zone can weaken trabecular architecture, and prompt cement reinforcement reduces the likelihood of delayed mechanical failure.
- Adjunctive Stabilization: In cases where lesion size, cortical disruption, or load transmission exceeds the mechanical capabilities of cement alone, augmentation with percutaneous screws, expandable implants, or other internal fixation systems may be warranted to enhance axial and torsional stability.

Ultimately, the integration of cryoablation with bone consolidation requires a careful balance between oncologic efficacy and orthopedic safety. Real-time imaging, thermometry (when available), and procedural staging are all critical for optimizing outcomes and minimizing complications [18, 61].

6.1.7 Combined Treatments

6.1.7.1 Embolization

In the interventional management of osseous neoplasms, particularly those with hypervascular features or located in anatomically critical areas such as the sacrum, spine, and pelvis, transarterial embolization (TAE) plays a pivotal role in augmenting the safety and efficacy of image-guided cryoablation. When performed prior to thermal ablation, embolization reduces blood flow to the lesion, thereby minimizing the cold-sink effect that could impair complete tumor necrosis and decreasing the risk of hemorrhagic complications during subsequent cryoablation or cementoplasty [61, 62].

TAE is particularly indicated in:

- Hypervascular lesions, such as those arising from renal cell carcinoma (RCC), thyroid, and some sarcomas
- Lesions in proximity to critical neural structures, where reduction of vascularity can help define safer ablation margins
- Large tumors with soft tissue extension, to reduce intraprocedural bleeding and augment the thermal field coverage during cryoablation

Embolization is typically performed 1–3 days prior to cryoablation. Vascular access is obtained via the femoral artery, followed by selective catheterization of tumor-feeding arteries.

Embolic agents include:

- Polyvinyl alcohol (PVA) particles (150–500 μm) [62, 63]
- N-butyl cyanoacrylate (NBCA) mixed with Lipiodol, to achieve capillary-level devascularization, was employed in the preablation management of an aneurysmal bone cyst (ABC) located at the cervicothoracic junction, adjacent to the costocervical trunk [61]

Neuromonitoring and provocative testing (e.g., Brevital challenge) may be employed intraoperatively to reduce the risk of nontarget embolization and to ensure functional preservation of adjacent neurovascular structures [63].

Clinical evidence supports the use of embolization prior to cryoablation in complex bone lesions.

A retrospective study by Sundararajan et al. involving 15 patients with osseous metastases showed that the combination of TAE followed by cryoablation—with or without osteoplasty—led to a statistically significant reduction in pain scores (mean NRS-11 reduced from 8.7 pretreatment to 3.9 postintervention; $p = 0.0015$), and all patients reported decreased analgesic use [63]. No complications were reported, demonstrating the safety of sequential therapy in palliative care. Griauzde et al. achieved long-term control (16 months) of a spinal aneurysmal bone cyst in a pediatric case using NBCA embolization [61]. Lee et al. described a sacral metastasis from RCC treated with PVA embolization, followed by cryoablation, alcohol ablation, and sacroplasty. The combined approach resulted in rapid pain relief and preserved neurologic function, with no major intra- or post-procedural complications [62].

6.2 When Cryoablation

6.2.1 Indications

The clinical indications for cryoablation of bone lesions largely overlap with those of radiofrequency ablation. However, cryoablation is particularly advantageous for large (>4 cm) or morphologically complex lesions, as well as tumors located near critical structures. It provides precise ablation while minimizing damage to surrounding tissues and is also safer for tumors adjacent to metallic implants, avoiding the risks of electrical conductivity and heat-related complications associated with radiofrequency (RFA) and microwave ablation (MWA). The treatment approach varies based on intent, either curative or palliative [18].

Curative Cryoablation

For curative treatment, the iceball must extend 5–8 mm beyond the tumor margins to compensate for reduced freezing efficacy at the periphery [18].

- Benign Bone Tumors: Cryoablation has been successfully applied to conditions such as osteoid osteoma [64], osteoblastoma, chondroblastoma [65], aneurysmal bone cysts [66], and chondromyxoid fibroma [67].
- Primary Malignant Bone Tumors: These are primarily managed through surgical resection, frequently in combination with systemic therapies such as chemotherapy or targeted agents. However, in certain scenarios—particularly when lesions are deemed inoperable due to anatomical complexity, advanced disease, or multiple recurrences—percutaneous image-guided ablation may be considered. Although its role in achieving durable local control is limited by the often substantial tumor burden at diagnosis, ablation may offer clinical benefit in select patients. Given the aggressive nature of these malignancies, percutaneous intervention is frequently reserved for situations in which curative surgery is no longer feasible. In such cases, the therapeutic objective shifts toward palliation—aiming to reduce tumor volume, alleviate pain, preserve function, and improve quality of life. This palliative role is especially relevant in patients with poor performance status or limited life expectancy, where minimally invasive approaches can provide symptomatic relief with reduced procedural morbidity.
- Secondary Malignant Bone Tumors (Oligometastatic Disease): In select patients with a limited number of metastases (3–5 lesions, each <3 cm), cryoablation can be a targeted intervention. This is particularly relevant in cases where tumor progression risks compromising adjacent critical structures, such as spinal lesions [41].

Palliative Cryoablation

Cryoablation is increasingly employed as a palliative treatment for bone metastases, particularly in patients with advanced disease in whom conventional options such as pharmacologic analgesia, external beam radiotherapy, or surgical intervention are ineffective, contraindicated, or poorly tolerated. This minimally invasive technique offers a valuable alternative, capable of providing rapid and sustained pain relief, with the additional benefits of repeatability, low systemic toxicity, and minimal recovery time.

The pathophysiology of pain in bone metastases is multifactorial but is primarily related to tumor infiltration of the cortical bone and, critically, the periosteum—a highly innervated tissue whose stimulation is a major driver of nociceptive signaling. Periosteal involvement is often responsible for sharp, localized pain that is refractory to systemic treatments. Therefore, when performing cryoablation with palliative intent, it is essential that the entire lesion, including any portion infiltrating the periosteum, is encompassed within the ablation zone. Failure to include periosteal involvement may result in incomplete analgesia and persistent symptoms.

From a technical perspective, intraprocedural imaging—typically contrast-enhanced CT—is used to monitor iceball formation, ensuring that the ablation zone fully encompasses the lesion as well as the adjacent periosteal surface when infiltrated. In palliative settings, it is recommended that the nonperfused (ablated) volume at the end of the procedure also includes the periosteum, particularly in cases where pain is localized and correlates radiologically with cortical and periosteal involvement.

6.2.2 Contraindications

Absolute contraindications for ablation procedures are uncommon but include unsafe access, acute immunosuppression, active local or systemic infection, uncorrected coagulopathy, or lack of patient consent. Relative contraindications involve excessively large tumors or proximity to critical structures that cannot be adequately monitored or protected. In spinal procedures, the most common relative contraindications are unstable fractures and metastatic epidural spinal cord compression. Additionally, cryoablation can be impacted by the cold-sink effect, where nearby high-flow vascular structures dissipate the freezing temperature at the ablation site, potentially reducing its effectiveness [18].

6.3 Treatment of Benign Bone Lesions

6.3.1 Osteoid Osteoma

Osteoid osteoma is a frequent benign bone-forming tumor, accounting for approximately 12–14% of all primary bone neoplasms. It typically affects adolescents and young adults, most often during the second decade of life, with a marked male predominance reported in most series (male-to-female ratio ranging from 2:1–4:1) [68]. These lesions are usually small—less than 1.5 cm in diameter—and produce disproportionate pain, classically described as nocturnal and responsive to nonsteroidal anti-inflammatory drugs (NSAIDs), particularly acetylsalicylic acid. The pain is thought to result from high prostaglandin concentrations produced by the vascularized nidus [69, 70].

The most common location is the cortex of long bones, with over 50% of cases involving the femur or tibia [71, 72]. Nevertheless, 7–20% of osteoid osteomas arise in the spine, where they preferentially involve the posterior elements, especially in the lumbar region. Spinal involvement may lead to radicular symptoms or painful scoliosis in untreated cases, with reports indicating up to 70% of patients develop scoliosis if left untreated. Despite rare reports of spontaneous regression, most symptomatic cases warrant intervention [73, 74].

Histologically, the lesion is characterized by a small, highly vascular nidus composed of osteoid tissue and woven bone, surrounded by varying degrees of reactive sclerotic bone. Four morphological types have been described: intracortical, with dense sclerotic bone surrounding the nidus; periosteal, characterized by prominent periosteal reaction; spongiosal (medullary), which tends to induce less sclerosis; and subarticular, which may mimic arthritis due to associated synovial inflammation [75, 76]. At imaging, the nidus typically appears as a small, well-circumscribed lucency that may contain central mineralization, with surrounding cortical thickening and bone marrow or soft tissue edema. CT is the modality of choice for diagnosis, providing high-resolution visualization of the nidus and adjacent sclerosis, while MRI is sensitive in detecting associated reactive changes [77]. Technetium-99 m bone scintigraphy often shows a double-density sign, and early, intense contrast enhancement on gadolinium-enhanced MRI may further support the diagnosis [68].

Historically, osteoid osteomas were managed surgically through open excision of the nidus. However, the morbidity associated with surgery—including large incisions, blood loss, infection, neurovascular injury, spinal instability, and prolonged recovery—has led to the widespread adoption of image-guided percutaneous techniques [78]. Among these, radiofrequency ablation (RFA) has become the gold standard since the late 1990s, due to its high efficacy (reported success rates >90% after a single session) and low complication rates [79, 80].

More recently, percutaneous cryoablation has emerged as a compelling alternative to heat-based ablation techniques. Cryoablation offers several unique advantages that are particularly beneficial in the treatment of osteoid osteoma. The formation of the cryosphere can be visualized in real time during the procedure using intermittent noncontrast-enhanced CT scans, allowing precise control of the ablation margins. Unlike RFA, which relies on inductive heating, cryoablation induces a conductive freeze that can propagate more effectively through dense sclerotic bone, making it especially suitable for bone-forming tumors. This physical property also enables treatment of the nidus from an extraosseous position, potentially avoiding the need to directly penetrate the nidus with the cryoprobe.

In addition, cryoablation is typically better tolerated than heat-based ablation techniques. The anesthetic properties of cold allow many procedures to be performed under conscious sedation rather than general anesthesia, with patients often reporting less postprocedural pain. This makes cryoablation particularly attractive in the pediatric population or in lesions located in challenging anatomical regions such as the spine, where minimizing procedural discomfort and neurological risk is critical. The ablative volumes achievable with cryoablation may also be larger and more geometrically adaptable than those produced with RFA, which is particularly advantageous in eccentric or irregularly shaped lesions.

Given these characteristics, cryoablation represents a highly effective and safe option in the treatment arsenal for osteoid osteoma. It offers the precision of image guidance, the comfort of a less painful recovery, and the flexibility needed to manage lesions in difficult locations or in patients requiring a minimally invasive approach with optimal clinical outcomes.

In adult patients, procedures are typically performed under local anesthesia with or without intravenous analgesia or conscious sedation; general anesthesia is rarely necessary but may be used for deep or spinal lesions [64, 78, 81]. In pediatric populations, general anesthesia is commonly used to ensure immobility and comfort [82]. However, Pusceddu et al. demonstrated that percutaneous cryoablation can be safely and effectively performed under conscious sedation even in children, as their entire pediatric cohort underwent the procedure without general anesthesia [20].

Under CT or cone-beam CT guidance, access is gained using an 11–14G coaxial introducer, followed by the insertion of one or more cryoprobes. Probe positioning is determined based on lesion location and bone thickness—either intraosseous or adjacent to the nidus. Standard protocols typically include two freeze-thaw cycles, with 10 min of freezing followed by 8–10 min of passive or active thaw. In some pediatric protocols, a single freeze-thaw cycle (10 min freeze, 8 min passive thaw) has been shown to be equally effective while reducing sedation time and procedural complexity [20].

Thermal protection strategies are selectively employed when the lesion is located within 1 cm of sensitive structures such as nerves, cartilage, or skin.

In the prospective series by Michailidis et al., thermal insulation techniques were applied in 32% of cases. In the treatment of a humeral head lesion located near the axillary nerve, hydrodissection was performed to displace the nerve from the ablation zone, and a thermocouple was placed for real-time temperature monitoring throughout the freeze-thaw cycles. In another case involving a lumbar facet osteoid osteoma (L4–L5), an epidural hydrodissection technique was employed to insulate the adjacent nerve root, again guided by thermocouple monitoring. For superficially located lesions such as those in the medial malleolus, subcutaneous hydrodissection was used in combination with the application of a warm saline-filled surgical glove placed externally to protect the overlying skin from cryogenic injury [78].

Carbodissection was described in the series by Le Corroller et al., where CO_2 was injected using a spinal needle inserted into the intervertebral foramen to physically separate the dural sac and adjacent spinal nerve from the freezing zone. The same study emphasized the use of thermocouples placed near neural and cartilaginous structures to provide real-time feedback on tissue temperatures, enabling early interruption or modulation of cryoablation if thresholds were approached [64].

In the single-case report by Chan et al., which involved cryoablation of a glenoid osteoid osteoma, a warm saline glove was similarly used for cutaneous insulation, due to the superficial nature of the approach. This simple technique effectively prevented skin freezing and was accompanied by continuous CT monitoring of the iceball during both freezing phases, ensuring safe treatment margins without complications [81].

In pediatric cases reported in literature, although thermal protection was not routinely applied, trajectory planning and continuous imaging allowed safe treatment even in sensitive anatomical zones [20, 82, 83].

Clinical success—defined as complete pain relief and NSAID discontinuation—was consistently high across all series, with reported success rates ranging from 90.5% to 100% in both adult and pediatric populations [64, 78, 81, 82].

In literature, minor effects such as swelling or skin irritation are reported in <6% of adult cases [64, 78]. In pediatric cohorts, Whitmore et al. noted minor, self-limited complications in 21% of patients [82], whereas Pusceddu et al. reported no adverse events in those treated under conscious sedation [20].

6.3.2 Osteoblastoma

Osteoblastoma is a rare, benign bone-forming tumor, accounting for approximately 1% of all primary bone tumors [84]. It typically affects children and young adults, with a male predominance, and most commonly involves the posterior elements of the spine, long bones (such as the femur and tibia), and occasionally the craniofacial skeleton [85]. Histologically, it resembles osteoid osteoma but is generally larger in size (usually >1.5–2 cm), more expansile, and may show locally aggressive behavior, including cortical disruption and periosteal reaction. Pain is the most frequent symptom and may be persistent, intense, and less responsive to NSAIDs than in osteoid osteoma [85].

In imaging, osteoblastomas present as lytic or mixed lytic-sclerotic lesions with variable mineralization and may show bone expansion. They can mimic malignancy when aggressive features such as soft-tissue extension or rapid growth are present. Despite their benign histology, osteoblastomas require active treatment due to their symptomatic burden and potential for local recurrence [86].

Cryoablation represents a safe and effective option for the treatment of osteoblastoma, in both adult and pediatric patients, particularly in cases where surgery is contraindicated or anatomically challenging. Lesions located in the spine, lower limbs (e.g., femur, fibula, calcaneus), and small bones (e.g., metacarpals) have been successfully treated with percutaneous image-guided cryoablation [65, 87–89].

Access to the lesion is achieved using 10–14G bone trocars in pediatric cases [65]. Depending on the size and morphology of the lesion, cryoprobes are typically spaced 0.5–2 cm apart, with closer spacing (0.5–1.5 cm) preferred for small or compact lesions to ensure uniform iceball overlap, and wider spacing (1.5–2 cm) used in larger or irregularly shaped tumors to achieve a synergistic and confluent ablation volume [65, 87]. Osteoblastomas typically exceed 2 cm in diameter, with an average size of around 2.5 cm. Cryoablation has proven effective even for lesions up to

4 cm, as demonstrated in cases involving the ischium and proximal femur, where treatment was successfully performed using three cryoprobes to ensure complete and homogeneous coverage of the target volume [88, 89].

Cryoablation protocols varied between centers and were adapted to the lesion's characteristics and surrounding anatomy. In the series by Cazzato et al., freezing parameters included one or two probes, power settings from 40%–100%, and one or two freezing cycles, with a total freezing time ranging from 6–30 min, depending on tumor size and proximity to nontarget structures [87].

In contrast, the pediatric cohort reported by Serrano et al. followed a standardized protocol using two 10-min freezing cycles, separated by two thawing phases: in one center, a 10-min thaw (7 min passive, 3 min active), and in another, two 5-min active thaw cycles [65].

In two patients with sacral osteoblastomas previously unresponsive to thermal ablation, preablation embolization was performed during the same interventional session. This combined approach aimed to enhance the cryoablative effect by limiting lesion perfusion, thereby improving tissue freezing and minimizing the likelihood of further recurrence [87].

These variations reflect institutional preferences and the need to tailor the ablation strategy to the clinical scenario.

Due to the frequent proximity of osteoblastomas to critical anatomical structures—such as nerve roots, the spinal cord, joints, and skin—thermal protection strategies are a key component of procedural planning in cryoablation. These adjunctive measures are primarily indicated when the lesion lies less than 1 cm from at-risk structures, a scenario frequently encountered in spinal locations, including the cervical, thoracic, lumbar, and sacral segments, as well as in periarticular or subcutaneous regions. Thermocouples were the most consistently used measure, applied in 8 of 9 protected cases, and placed near the spinal canal or peripheral nerves to enable continuous temperature monitoring and reduce the risk of thermal injury. Hydrodissection was also employed in 5 cases, including treatments at the cervical spine, sacrum, and L5 level, to separate nerves or soft tissues from the ablation zone. Carbodissection was selectively used in one sacral lesion, in combination with hydrodissection and thermocouples, to increase safety margins in a location where soft tissue interfaces were complex and vascular.

Additionally, electrostimulation was used during needle positioning in at least two patients—both with sacral or lumbosacral involvement—where proximity to motor nerve roots required real-time functional monitoring. In contrast, only one case, involving a fibular lesion distant from any critical structure, was treated without the use of any protective technique [87].

In the mixed pediatric cohort reported by Serrano et al., which included both chondroblastoma and osteoblastoma, thermal protection was used in 5 out of 11 cases (45%). Focusing specifically on the four patients with osteoblastoma, three underwent insulation procedures: epidural pneumodissection and hydrodissection were performed for spinal lesions, and skin protection was used in one case involving the proximal humerus. The fourth osteoblastoma, located in the lumbar spine, was treated without insulation due to a safe probe trajectory [65].

In the series by Cazzato et al., two short-term complications were reported. One involved a 21-year-old male who developed a grade 3 neurological complication—characterized by motor and sensory impairment of the left upper limb—following cryoablation of an osteoblastoma at the left C5–C6 facet joint. While motor function recovered completely within 3 months, sensory symptoms persisted at the 12-month evaluation. The second case concerned a 21-year-old female who experienced a transient Horner syndrome (grade 2) after treatment of a T1 vertebral body lesion. The condition resolved fully within 48 h following the administration of high-dose corticosteroids.

Two patients experienced pain recurrence at the 12-month clinical follow-up. The first, a 6-year-old boy treated for a 20-mm L5 lamina osteoblastoma, had a 7-mm nodular recurrence detected on CE-MRI and was successfully retreated with percutaneous laser ablation. The second, a 21-year-old man with a sacral osteoblastoma (OB) previously treated with RFA and cryoablation, showed residual contrast enhancement at 6 months. Surgery was proposed but refused due to psychiatric comorbidity, and the patient was lost to follow-up [87].

In the case described by Poullain et al., involving a large osteoblastoma in the intertrochanteric region of the proximal femur, no immediate procedural complications were observed. However, the patient developed a cortical stress fracture at the periphery of the ablation zone approximately 6 weeks posttreatment. This event was attributed to premature mechanical loading during recovery and was managed conservatively, without resulting in long-term disability or instability [88].

In the pediatric cohort reported by Serrano et al., which included both chondroblastoma and osteoblastoma cases, only one short-term complication was observed among the four children treated specifically for osteoblastoma. This involved a transient radiculopathy affecting the right L2–L3 nerve roots following cryoablation of a thoracic lesion; symptoms gradually improved and resolved within 12 months [65].

6.3.3 Chondroblastoma

Chondroblastoma is a rare benign bone tumor, accounting for approximately 1–2% of all primary bone neoplasms and around 9% of benign bone tumors. It primarily affects adolescents and young adults, most commonly between the ages of 10 and 25, with a male predominance. The tumor typically arises in the epiphysis or apophysis of long bones—most frequently the proximal femur, distal femur, proximal tibia, and proximal humerus, although pelvic and vertebral locations have also been described. Despite its benign nature, the lesion may exhibit locally aggressive behavior and is typically associated with persistent joint-related pain, swelling, and decreased range of motion. On imaging, chondroblastomas appear as epiphyseal, lytic, eccentric lesions with a narrow zone of transition and often a sclerotic rim. MRI is particularly useful for identifying perilesional edema, which correlates with pain severity [90].

Given its location and proximity to articular cartilage, conventional **surgical curettage**, although effective, is associated with significant morbidity, risk of fracture, cartilage damage, and recurrence rates reported between 10% and 35% [90].

According to the literature, percutaneous cryoablation of chondroblastoma is consistently performed under general anesthesia, given the typical localization of these lesions in the epiphysis or near articular surfaces, and the need to ensure complete immobility during probe placement and ablation cycles [65, 91].

In the early experience reported by Thibaut et al., three adolescents with periarticular chondroblastomas underwent cryoablation using CT guidance. All lesions were smaller than 3.5 cm and located in proximity to the articular surface. Each procedure involved the coaxial placement of one or more 17G cryoprobes through 11G or 13G access cannulas, followed by two freeze-thaw cycles (10 min freeze, 6–10 min thaw). In superficial lesions, subcutaneous saline injection was used as a protective measure to avoid skin injury. One patient (33%) developed a local recurrence documented on MRI at 6 months, which was successfully managed with a second cryoablation session. All patients reported complete disappearance of pain (VAS = 0) within 48 h after the procedure. At 12-month follow-up, there was no evidence of recurrence, no cartilage or joint damage, and no immediate or delayed complications were observed [91].

These encouraging results were supported by the larger multicenter study by Serrano et al., which included seven pediatric patients with chondroblastoma, with lesions ranging from 8 mm–35 mm, most commonly in the proximal femur, distal femur, and acetabulum. In the series by Serrano et al., thermal protection was used in three of seven chondroblastoma cases, all involving periarticular lesions of the acetabulum and proximal femur, where joint hydrodissection was performed to protect adjacent structures. Among the seven patients treated, two moderate late complications were reported: one patient developed a trochanteric bursitis adjacent to the probe access path, and another experienced a tibial stress fracture. Neither event occurred within the ablation zone. Both were considered to be related to mechanical overuse following resolution of tumor-related pain, rather than direct effects of the cryoablation itself [65].

6.3.4 Aneurysmal Bone Cyst

Aneurysmal bone cysts (ABCs) are infrequent, benign bone lesions known for their locally destructive behavior. They consist of expansile, osteolytic cavities filled with blood and separated by fibrous septations of varying thickness. ABCs predominantly affect pediatric and adolescent populations, with the vast majority diagnosed before the age of 20, and tend to occur slightly more often in females [92]. Although these lesions typically originate in the metaphyseal regions of long bones, a substantial number—up to 30%—occur in the spinal column, especially involving the posterior elements and, in some cases, extending into the vertebral body [92, 93]. Patients usually present with localized pain, swelling, and reduced joint motion; when spinal involvement is present, neurologic deficits may also occur due to compression of adjacent neural structures. Imaging, particularly MRI, often reveals characteristic fluid–fluid levels, but histologic confirmation remains essential to exclude malignant mimics such as telangiectatic osteosarcoma [92, 94].

Historically, the standard treatment has been open surgical curettage, often supplemented with bone grafting or cementation. However, surgery can be invasive, especially in delicate or high-risk areas like the cervical spine, and recurrence remains a concern, with reported rates as high as 59% [95].

In light of these challenges, minimally invasive approaches have gained attention. Among them, image-guided percutaneous cryoablation has emerged as a valuable therapeutic option. This technique allows for controlled destruction of the lesion by applying cycles of freezing and thawing, which leads to cellular death and progressive ossification of the cyst cavity. Given its favorable safety profile and growing body of supporting evidence, cryoablation is increasingly being explored as a viable and effective treatment for ABCs, especially in pediatric patients and in locations where surgical access is risky or contraindicated.

This minimally invasive approach allows volumetric control of the ablation zone and offers the possibility of precise needle positioning, often under CT or, less frequently, MRI guidance. In pediatric patients, general anesthesia is typically required, and neuromonitoring is frequently adopted when lesions are near neurovascular structures.

In a prospective cohort of seven children, cryoablation was performed using coaxial cryoprobes under CT guidance. In cases of significant cortical thinning, direct probe insertion was used instead of a trocar. One case of premature physeal closure of the proximal femur was observed, resulting in coxa magna, while two other minor complications—transient paralytic ileus and an asymptomatic pathologic fracture—were also documented. Despite these, all patients showed clinical benefit, with a mean VAS score reduction from 1.9–0.3. Radiologically, one patient achieved a complete response, and the remaining showed a partial response with an average volume reduction of 81.9%. Two patients required repeat cryoablation due to persistent cystic activity, one undergoing three sessions in total [96].

MRI guidance has been explored as an alternative in children to avoid ionizing radiation. In a 5-year-old patient with a recurrent scapular lesion, MRI-guided cryoablation enabled precise visualization of the iceball and surrounding tissues. Pain resolution was immediate, with no complications or recurrence at 3-year follow-up. A single relapse in the coracoid process was successfully treated with a second procedure [97].

When treating spinal or sacral ABCs, specific precautions are needed. Advanced thermal protection methods such as epidural carbon dioxide dissection, foraminal warm saline infusion, and real-time thermocouple monitoring have been employed to avoid neurologic injury. In one reported case, cryoablation was combined with cementoplasty to stabilize a spinal segment. Despite a mild transient sensory deficit that resolved in two weeks, the patient returned to full athletic activity within six weeks, and a follow-up MRI at 18 months confirmed stable bone remodeling and no recurrence [66].

In cervicothoracic locations, where open surgery carries high morbidity, preprocedural embolization has been used to minimize bleeding risk during ablation. One such case involved NBCA embolization followed by cryoablation in a pediatric patient, with intraoperative neuromonitoring ensuring procedural safety. No complications or recurrence were observed at 16 months [61].

To promote early bone healing, cryoablation has also been combined with the injection of bone graft substitutes. In a series of six patients (ages 16–33), this combined approach was technically successful in all cases, with early remineralization observed—80% of cavity filling achieved at a median of 6 months, and one case achieving 100% at 3 months. No complications were recorded, and all patients experienced significant clinical improvement. The median follow-up was 31.5 months, and no recurrences were reported [98].

Cryoablation has also been evaluated in a larger pediatric series comparing it to other percutaneous options such as doxycycline sclerotherapy. In 21 patients undergoing 41 procedures, those treated with cryoablation required fewer sessions (mean 1.7) compared to sclerotherapy (mean 3), with similar clinical and radiological outcomes. Major complications were rare, occurring in 7.7% of procedures involving cryoablation or sclerotherapy. Follow-up imaging demonstrated cyst improvement in 85% of cases, while 93.8% of patients with pain or pathological fractures reported symptom resolution [99].

Taken together, these studies support the safety and efficacy of cryoablation for ABCs across a variety of anatomical sites and patient profiles. When needed, combined techniques such as embolization, cementoplasty, or grafting can be used to enhance treatment outcomes and reduce recurrence or mechanical complications. Cryoablation appears particularly valuable in cases where surgery has failed or is contraindicated due to location, age, or skeletal immaturity.

6.3.5 Chondromyxoid Fibroma

Chondromyxoid fibroma is a rare, benign bone tumor of cartilaginous lineage, most often seen in long bones. Curettage with grafting is standard, though recurrence can occur in up to 25% of cases [100].

Gowda et al. described a 17-year-old with multiple recurrences despite prior surgeries. A single cryotherapy probe was used to ablate the lesion. At 20-month follow-up, imaging showed mature bone formation and complete symptom resolution [67].

6.4 Treatment of Primary Malignant Bone Lesions

Primary malignant bone tumors—including osteosarcoma, Ewing's sarcoma, and chondrosarcoma—are rare entities, representing less than 1% of all newly diagnosed cancers annually. The cornerstone of treatment remains surgical resection, often combined with systemic chemotherapy or, in select cases, radiotherapy, depending on histologic subtype and staging.

Despite advancements in systemic therapies, many patients present with large-volume disease, limiting the feasibility of curative minimally invasive approaches. Nonetheless, percutaneous image-guided ablation techniques—such as cryoablation or radiofrequency ablation—may serve as valuable adjuncts within a multidisciplinary treatment framework, particularly in cases where tumors are located in anatomically complex, surgically inaccessible, or previously treated (recurrent) sites. These interventions may offer palliative benefit or local control in select patients deemed poor surgical candidates or when repeat resection carries excessive morbidity. However, the utility of ablative strategies remains constrained by tumor size and proximity to critical structures, often precluding complete tumor eradication at the time of diagnosis.

6.4.1 Osteosarcoma

Cryoablation has emerged as a valuable adjunctive and, in select cases, alternative strategy in the treatment of osteosarcoma—particularly in patients who are not ideal candidates for extensive surgical resection due to anatomical constraints, age, or advanced disease. Traditionally, osteosarcoma is managed with wide surgical resection and multi-agent chemotherapy. However, advances in ablative technologies have expanded the therapeutic arsenal for disease and symptom control.

In pediatric populations with unresectable or end-stage tumors, percutaneous cryoablation has been employed as a palliative option. In a multi-institutional retrospective study, Talbot et al. reported 89 ablative procedures—including 9 cryoablations—across 69 pediatric patients with various solid tumors, including 13 with osteosarcoma. Cryoablation was used primarily for symptom relief or local control in lesions inaccessible to surgery. Despite some grade $\geq$ 3 adverse events (e.g., postprocedural pain requiring IV medication), hospital stays were generally short, and the technique was well tolerated overall [101].

In patients with localized epiphyseal involvement, intraoperative cryoablation has enabled joint-preserving resections. Li et al. conducted a comparative study between cryo-assisted joint-sparing surgery and conventional endoprosthetic replacement in patients with osteosarcoma of the knee. Oncologic outcomes—including local recurrence, metastasis, and overall survival—were comparable. Although joint-sparing patients initially had reduced range of motion and lower MSTS (Musculoskeletal Tumor Society) scores at 1 year, outcomes equalized by year 3. Notably, joint-preserving surgery showed fewer long-term complications and better reconstruction durability [102].

Similarly, argon-based cryosurgery has been shown to safely sterilize juxta-articular osteosarcoma margins, allowing epiphyseal preservation. In a series of 12 patients, cryoablation enabled partial resection with no local recurrence in the preserved bone, and excellent functional recovery (mean MSTS score: 92.7%) [103].

Cryoablation also offers a reconstructive solution for very young patients, as described by Erwin and Cahyadi in a 5-year-old girl with proximal tibial osteosarcoma. After neoadjuvant chemotherapy, wide resection was combined with cryosurgical recycling of the tumor-bearing segment using liquid nitrogen. The segment was reimplanted and stabilized with dual plating and vascularized fibular grafting. No postoperative complications occurred, and radiographic union was achieved within one year. The patient demonstrated a good functional outcome, with an MSTS score of 76.6% [104].

In summary, cryoablation has shown promise in the management of osteosarcoma for:

- Local tumor control in anatomically challenging or functionally critical sites
- Pain palliation in advanced, unresectable cases
- Joint preservation, particularly in juxta-articular tumors
- Biological reconstruction, especially in pediatric patients

However, case selection is key. Complications such as infection, fracture, or local recurrence may occur, underscoring the need for careful planning and follow-up. Further prospective studies are needed to validate long-term oncological safety and functional benefits.

6.4.2 Ewing's Sarcoma

Ewing sarcoma is a highly aggressive malignant small round cell tumor, most commonly affecting children and young adults. While first-line treatment involves a combination of systemic chemotherapy, radiotherapy, and surgical resection, management becomes significantly more complex in cases of recurrence, metastasis, or anatomically inoperable disease. In such contexts, cryoablation has emerged as a promising palliative modality for local control and symptom relief.

A multi-institutional retrospective study conducted across five pediatric oncology centers examined the use of site-directed ablative therapies in children and young adults with advanced solid tumors, including 15 patients diagnosed with Ewing sarcoma. Although stereotactic body radiation therapy (SBRT) was the primary modality for pain palliation in this cohort, cryoablation demonstrated feasibility and safety, particularly in the context of tumor burden reduction and local control [101].

A particularly illustrative case was detailed by Lessard et al., involving a 9-year-old girl with multiply recurrent pelvic Ewing sarcoma who had received cumulative high-dose chemotherapy and radiation. The tumor, located in the sacrum with epidural extension, caused progressive pain and threatened neurologic compromise. Given prior maximum radiation to the pelvis and proximity to the sacral plexus, CT-guided percutaneous cryoablation was selected as a targeted modality for pain palliation and tumor cytoreduction. To minimize the risk of neural injury—particularly to the S1 nerve root—intraoperative neurophysiological monitoring with somatosensory-evoked potentials (SSEPs) was employed throughout the procedure. Five percutaneous cryoprobes with 3 cm active tips were positioned to surround the tumor, followed by two freeze-thaw cycles (10 min each, with 8-min thaw). Continuous SSEP recordings allowed real-time assessment of neural function, which remained stable during ablation. The patient achieved complete pain relief within 24 h, and imaging confirmed effective tumor necrosis without enhancement on contrast MRI. However, given the unavoidable proximity of the iceball to the S2–S3 roots, the patient developed neurogenic bladder and bowel incontinence—highlighting the balance between efficacy and risk in high-stakes anatomical regions [105].

6.4.3 Chondrosarcoma

Chondrosarcomas are malignant cartilage-forming tumors known for their resistance to chemotherapy and radiotherapy. For low-grade (Grade I) tumors, especially when they are confined to bone without soft tissue extension, minimally invasive approaches such as intralesional curettage combined with cryoablation are increasingly favored over wide surgical resection, due to favorable functional and oncologic outcomes.

The primary indication for cryoablation in chondrosarcoma is a radiologically and clinically diagnosed low-grade tumor with features of aggressiveness (e.g., endosteal scalloping >2/3 of cortical thickness, pain, or progressive enlargement) but without extraosseous soft tissue extension. Differentiating low-grade chondrosarcoma from enchondroma remains a diagnostic challenge; thus, many authors recommend a combined evaluation using clinical history, imaging, and, when needed, histological review by musculoskeletal pathology experts [106, 107].

Multiple studies report excellent oncologic control using curettage with cryoablation. Meftah et al. documented a 90.7% recurrence-free survival at 10 years in 42 patients with low-grade chondrosarcoma treated with this technique. Importantly, all local recurrences occurred in lesions with initial soft tissue extension, and no metastases were observed [106]. Mohler et al. confirmed these findings in a cohort of 46 grade I chondrosarcoma patients, with only two local recurrences and no significant complications, suggesting that this approach is highly effective in properly selected patients [107].

A similar study by Souna et al. on 15 patients showed no recurrence at a mean of 8 years, reinforcing the reliability of this method for grade I chondrosarcomas without cortical breakthrough [108].

The effectiveness of cryoablation in the treatment of chondrosarcoma strongly depends on the accuracy of tumor grading prior to intervention. In clinical practice, however, discrepancies between biopsy-based grading and the final histological diagnosis are not uncommon, particularly due to intratumoral heterogeneity—a well-known limitation in cartilaginous tumors.

In a reported series, five patients underwent curettage and cryoablation under the assumption of having atypical cartilaginous tumors (ACT) or low-grade (grade 1) chondrosarcoma based on biopsy. However, postoperative pathology revealed all five cases were in fact grade 2 chondrosarcomas, as preoperative MRI had initially suggested. This grading mismatch highlights a critical limitation of core needle biopsy, which may fail to capture more aggressive tumor regions due to sampling error. Oncologic outcomes for the misclassified grade 2 cases treated with intralesional cryosurgery were suboptimal: only 60% achieved recurrence-free survival. However, none of the patients developed distant metastases, and all remained alive and disease-free at follow-up, indicating that local recurrence in grade 2 disease—while concerning—may not always carry systemic implications [109].

Recent proteomic analyses have revealed that cryoablation modulates several oncogenic pathways in chondrosarcoma tissue, including PI3K-Akt and mitogen-activated protein kinase (MAPK) signaling. Madda et al. demonstrated that postcryoablation specimens exhibited downregulation of fibronectin and annexin-1, molecules involved in tumor progression, suggesting a potential biological benefit beyond local cytotoxicity [110].

6.4.4 Sacral Chordoma

Sacral chordoma is a rare malignant tumor often difficult to manage surgically due to its size, deep location, and proximity to critical neural and vascular structures. While wide resection remains the gold standard, it can lead to significant morbidity. In this context, cryoablation offers a minimally invasive alternative, especially in inoperable patients or those refusing surgery. In a retrospective study by Li et al., nine patients with sacral chordoma were treated using CT-guided percutaneous cryoablation. All patients achieved complete response (CR): 66.7% after one session, and the remainder after two sessions. No major complications were reported. The treatment led to a significant reduction in pain (VAS from 7.3 to 4.2) and improvement in functional status (score from 3.2 to 1.4). Two patients (22.2%) experienced local recurrence, successfully managed with repeat ablation or embolization. No distant metastases occurred, and the median progression-free survival was 36.8 months [111].

However, findings from Cherix et al. present a more cautious perspective. In their long-term follow-up study of four patients treated with image-guided percutaneous cryoablation for unresectable sacrococcygeal chordoma, technical feasibility was confirmed in all cases, but complete freezing of tumor volume was achieved in only 60% of procedures. Notably, 90% of treated lesions recurred after a mean of 8.1 months, with a 5-year survival rate of 50%. The high recurrence rate was attributed to the anatomical complexity of the sacral region, which often limited the extent of ablation due to proximity to critical structures like sacral nerve roots and the rectum. Only one patient remained disease-free, and this was due to subsequent carbon-ion radiotherapy. Furthermore, one case of major neurological complication (permanent perianal anesthesia) was reported, highlighting potential procedural risks [112].

Cryoablation (CA) should be considered a valuable option in multidisciplinary treatment plans, particularly when surgery is contraindicated, but its use in curative settings warrants careful patient selection and should ideally be complemented by adjunctive therapies such as advanced radiation modalities.

6.5 Treatment of Bone Metastatic Disease

Bone is the third most frequent location for metastatic spread of carcinomas, following the lungs and liver [113]. Although surgical resection is seldom feasible due to the typically poor prognosis of these patients, bone metastases often result in serious complications such as spinal cord compression, pathological fractures, and persistent, debilitating pain, all of which have a profound impact on quality of life [114–116].

In this context, cryoablation has gained increasing recognition within the field of thermal ablation for skeletal metastases. Its ability to conform to irregular tumor contours and its real-time monitoring capabilities have made it particularly advantageous. Compared to thermal techniques based on heat energy—such as radiofrequency or microwave ablation—cryoablation is generally associated with reduced procedure-related pain [117].

Although curative intent is rarely achievable, the literature emphasizes the value of cryoablation in achieving local disease control and symptom palliation, making it a valuable option within the multidisciplinary strategy for managing metastatic bone disease.

6.5.1 Curative Treatment

The Cardiovascular and Interventional Radiological Society of Europe defines curative intent in the treatment of bone metastases as the complete and definitive destruction of the tumor through ablation techniques [19]. This approach is primarily indicated in oligometastatic patients, typically those presenting with fewer than three lesions, each measuring less than 3 cm [18]. Ideal candidates are individuals with favorable prognostic indicators—including younger age, preserved cortical bone architecture, absence of metastases beyond the bone, good functional status, and a slowly progressing primary disease. However, such a profile is relatively uncommon among the general population of oncology patients.

6.5.1.1 Local Tumor Control

Multiple studies demonstrate that cryoablation offers effective and durable local tumor control (LTC) in oligometastatic patients. In a cohort of 40 patients with 50 bone metastases from renal cell carcinoma, LTC was achieved in 82% of lesions, with control rates reaching 96% in patients who had five or fewer metastases [118]. A significant predictor of success was the extent of the ablative margin: lesions where the iceball extended ≥1 cm beyond the tumor edge had a substantially lower recurrence risk (mean margin 2.2 cm in controlled lesions vs. 1.35 cm in recurrent cases, $p = 0.005$).

Similar efficacy was reported in a multicenter study of patients undergoing image-guided thermal ablation (mainly cryoablation) for oligometastatic bone disease. At 1–2 years, local progression-free survival (LPFS) rates were 76.8% and 71.7%, respectively [119]. These outcomes were associated with smaller lesion size (<2–3 cm), preserved cortical architecture, and absence of adjacent neural structures, emphasizing the importance of precise anatomical assessment.

Another prospective study evaluating cryoablation in 52 patients with 122 bone lesions demonstrated a 67% complete response rate at 1-year follow-up [120]. Predictive factors for success included the absence of cortical bone erosion and the presence of metachronous rather than synchronous metastases, suggesting more indolent disease biology and better response to localized therapy.

6.5.1.2 Pain Control

Cryoablation not only serves an oncologic role but also provides robust and sustained pain relief—even in patients treated with curative intent. The mechanism involves destruction of sensory nerve fibers, tumor devascularization, and reduction of local inflammatory cytokines.

In a retrospective series involving 28 cryoablation procedures, patients experienced a statistically significant reduction in pain scores from a pretreatment mean of 6.9–3.5 at three months ($p < 0.0001$), even in curative-intent cohorts [121]. These results confirm that local tumor ablation directly translates to early and substantial symptom improvement.

A larger study evaluating thermal ablation in 72 patients found that 74% of lesions treated for pain showed meaningful reduction in VAS scores, especially when procedures were augmented with cementoplasty for structural reinforcement in weight-bearing bones [122].

Additional evidence from patients with osseous metastases from non-small cell lung cancer demonstrated similar benefits, with pain scores decreasing from 7.5 to 3.7 at four weeks postprocedure ($p < 0.00001$) [123].

6.5.1.3 Progression-Free Survival and Systemic Delay

An important benefit of cryoablation in oligometastatic disease is its potential to delay systemic therapy and prolong progression-free intervals, especially relevant in hormone-sensitive malignancies.

In a cohort of prostate cancer patients undergoing cryoablation for limited bone metastases, the median progression-free survival (PFS) was 21 months, and in patients who had not yet initiated androgen deprivation therapy (ADT), systemic therapy could be deferred by a median of 29 months [124]. These findings suggest that local ablation not only controls visible disease but may extend systemic stability, allowing for therapeutic deintensification.

Such benefits are especially impactful in younger patients or those with significant concerns about the side effects of long-term systemic treatments.

6.5.1.4 Safety and Complications

Cryoablation is generally well tolerated, with a low rate of major complications, particularly when standard protective measures are applied. Across studies, the rate of grade ≥ 3 complications ranges from 2.6% to 5% [120, 122].

Documented serious adverse events include:

- Femoral nerve injury (due to the close proximity of the iceball to neurovascular bundles)
- Hemothorax (typically related to lesions near the ribs or pleura)
- Epidural hematoma (in spinal procedures)
- Infection following cementoplasty (requiring antibiotics or surgical drainage) [120, 122, 125].

Most major complications occurred in anatomically sensitive locations like the sacrum, spine, and pelvis. For this reason, technical precautions such as real-time thermocouple monitoring, hydrodissection to separate adjacent organs, and saline insulation around nerves are essential for safe ablation, especially in curative settings.

Minor complications—such as transient postablation pain flares, soft tissue edema, or low-grade fevers—are more common but usually self-limiting and managed conservatively.

6.5.1.5 Technical and Prognostic Considerations

Successful curative cryoablation depends on a combination of technical precision and appropriate patient selection. Key factors that correlate with improved outcomes include:

- Oligometastatic Status: Patients with ≤5 lesions showed significantly better LTC rates (96%) than those with more extensive disease (53.3%, $p = 0.001$) [118].
- Small Tumor Volume: Lesions <2–3 cm in diameter are more easily encompassed by effective iceball margins, improving ablation completeness.
- Favorable Anatomic Location: Lesions distant from the spinal cord or major nerve roots reduce procedural risk. Conversely, pelvic or vertebral metastases require meticulous planning, including probe angulation and protective maneuvers.
- Iceball Coverage: Achieving a ≥ 1 cm ablative margin beyond all visible tumor edges is critical to minimize recurrence.

6.5.2 Palliative Treatment

For patients experiencing significant pain from bone metastases (typically ≥6 on the VAS scale), palliative interventions are a key component of care. The primary objective is not curative, but rather symptom control through tumor debulking, prevention of pathological fractures, and decompression in cases of spinal involvement. Among available techniques, cryoablation has gained prominence as a minimally invasive option, particularly when standard therapies such as analgesics, radiotherapy, or surgery are ineffective or poorly tolerated. It offers several advantages, including rapid onset of pain relief, repeatability, minimal systemic effects, and short recovery times. The pain associated with bone metastases is often linked to tumor extension into the cortical bone and periosteum—the latter being a richly innervated structure critical in pain generation. Effective cryoablation must therefore encompass not only the tumor mass but also any periosteal infiltration. Incomplete coverage may result in suboptimal pain control.

6.5.2.1 Pain Control

Pain palliation remains the primary indication for cryoablation in the metastatic bone setting. In a multicenter prospective trial, Callstrom et al. demonstrated that cryoablation reduced worst pain scores from a baseline of 7.1–1.4 over 24 weeks, with 75% of patients reporting a clinically significant pain decrease by the first week of follow-up [126]. An earlier interim analysis by the same group showed consistent findings, with a reduction in pain from 6.7 to3.8 by week 4 and improved ability to perform daily activities [127].

Prologo et al. retrospectively analyzed 50 cryoablation procedures and found a rapid median pain reduction from 8 to 3 within 24 h, sustained at 3 months, along with a 70% decrease in opioid consumption [128]. Similarly, Motta et al. reported a significant drop in VAS scores from 7.6 to 2.1 within two weeks postprocedure, highlighting the utility of cryoablation in quick symptom relief [129].

In the MOTION trial, Jennings et al. demonstrated that 70% of patients achieved a ≥ 2-point reduction in BPI pain scores at 8 weeks, with a median duration of pain control of 6.3 months and no significant pain flares [130]. Yang et al. further confirmed these analgesic benefits in a cohort of patients with osteolytic metastases, noting a reduction in mean pain scores from 7.1 to 1.8 at six months, even in patients previously unresponsive to radiotherapy [131]. In a smaller series focusing on sternal lesions, Hegg et al. showed a mean pain score decrease from 7.0 to 1.8, with sustained relief in the majority of patients [132].

6.5.2.2 Local Tumor Control

While the main aim of cryoablation in this setting is symptom relief, local tumor control has been frequently observed. Jennings et al. reported a 74% local control rate at 12 months, especially in tumors less than 3 cm in size and without cortical breach [130]. In a similar experience, Motta et al. observed lesion stability or regression in 87.5% of cases, particularly when cryoablation was combined with cementoplasty in weight-bearing regions [129].

Hegg et al. also demonstrated local shrinkage of sternal metastases in 68% of patients, with repeat ablation proving effective in cases of partial response [132]. Wallace et al., in a larger cohort of musculoskeletal metastases, reported stable or decreasing tumor size in 80% of cases three months posttreatment, reinforcing the potential of cryoablation to delay disease progression [133].

6.5.2.3 Functional Status and Prognosis

Beyond pain relief, cryoablation positively influences patient functionality and independence. Yang et al. showed that nearly half of the treated patients improved their ECOG performance status, with 30% regaining ambulation after treatment [131]. Prologo et al. similarly reported that 76% of patients achieved improved physical autonomy, with reduced opioid use and better tolerance of daily activities [128]. Thacker et al. found that patients treated with cryo had faster functional recovery, earlier return to mobility, and fewer postprocedural limitations, compared to patients treated with radiofrequency ablation [51].

6.5.2.4 Safety and Complications

Cryoablation has demonstrated a favorable safety profile across multiple studies. In Callstrom's 2013 multicenter study, only one major complication—osteomyelitis—was observed among 61 patients, corresponding to a 1.6% rate [126]. The MOTION trial reported 4.4% of patients experiencing common terminology criteria for adverse events (CTCAE) grade ≥ 3 events, with transient nerve injury and bleeding being the most serious, all of which were managed conservatively [130].

Prologo et al. reported an 11% overall complication rate, mostly consisting of mild frostbite, hematomas, or transient neuropathy, none of which required surgical intervention [128]. Similarly, Motta et al. noted no major complications in their cohort, emphasizing the use of thermocouples and hydrodissection techniques to enhance safety [129]. Auloge et al., in a large retrospective review, reported a major complication rate of 2.5%: fractures represented 50% [17].

6.5.2.5 Technical Considerations

- Ablation Margins: It is recommended a double freeze-thaw cycle with at least a 5 mm iceball margin beyond the tumor edge to ensure complete ablation and reduce recurrence risk [127].
- Protection of Critical Structures: Advised hydrodissection and thermocouple monitoring, particularly in the spine and pelvis [130].
- Mechanical Stability: Cryocementoplasty and balloon separation to reinforce load-bearing bones and prevent fractures postablation [128].
- Anesthesia Management: Motta et al. showed that cryotherapy under local anesthesia is feasible in patients with poor functional reserve (ASA III). This allows safe intervention without the risks associated with general anesthesia, especially in elderly or comorbid patients [129].
- Probe Strategy: Auloge et al. found that using >3 cryoprobes increased complication risk, especially in long bones and elderly patients, highlighting the need for optimized probe planning [17, 134].

6.6 Cryoablation vs. Other Treatments

6.6.1 Cryoablation vs. RFA: Analysis of Literature

Thermal ablation represents a cornerstone in the multidisciplinary management of bone metastases, especially for pain palliation and local tumor control. Among the most established techniques are cryoablation (CA) and radiofrequency ablation (RFA). While both achieve tissue necrosis through thermal energy, they differ significantly in mechanism, procedural characteristics, safety, and clinical outcomes.

6.6.1.1 Pain Control

Pain palliation is a primary goal in the treatment of bone metastases, especially in patients with advanced disease. Multiple studies have demonstrated that both cryoablation (CA) and radiofrequency ablation (RFA) are effective modalities in achieving pain relief. However, CA appears to offer superior outcomes in immediate pain control and reduced postprocedural analgesic needs.

Thacker et al. showed that patients treated with CA experienced a median *decrease* in morphine-equivalent analgesic use within 24 h of the procedure, whereas those who underwent RFA had a *median increase* in opioid consumption. This difference was statistically significant ($p = 0.03$), and CA was also associated with shorter hospital stays (median 2.5 days vs. 5 days, $p = 0.003$) [51]. Similarly, a retrospective study comparing 274 patients reported significantly fewer cases of postprocedural pain in the CA group (2.3%) than in the RFA group (30.3%, $p < 0.001$) [135].

Vaswani et al. further supported these findings, demonstrating a reduction in median pain scores from 8 to 3 after thermal ablation ($p < 0.001$), with comparable efficacy between RFA and CA for sarcoma metastases [122].

In a retrospective propensity-matched study of 50 patients with solitary osteolytic painful bone metastases, Zugaro et al. demonstrated that CA led to a higher complete response (CR) rate at 12 weeks (32%) compared to RFA (20%), with statistical significance only seen in the CA group. Partial responses were also recorded in both arms (CA 36%, RFA 44%). Notably, only CA significantly reduced opioid use from baseline (36% of patients were opioid-free at 12 weeks, vs. 20% in RFA). Both techniques improved self-reported quality of life (QoL), but CA showed a greater increase in QoL scores (from 3.9 to 6.1) versus RFA (from 3.6 to 5.6), confirming its superior efficacy in pain relief and patient-centered outcomes [135].

6.6.1.2 Local Tumor Control

Local tumor control (LTC) is increasingly relevant in the management of oligometastatic patients, where curative intent may be pursued. Studies have shown that both CA and RFA can achieve substantial rates of LTC, though cryoablation might be advantageous in specific contexts.

Deschamps et al. found that in curative-intent treatments, cryoablation was selected more frequently for larger or complex lesions due to better real-time monitoring with CT and the ability to place multiple probes. This technical flexibility may translate into more precise treatment margins [120]. In oligometastatic cohorts, Cazzato et al. reported a 1-year local progression-free survival (LPFS) of 76.8% and a 2-year LPFS of 71.7%, with BM size >2 cm being the only predictor of progression [119].

Notably, Erie et al. specifically evaluated patients with oligometastatic prostate cancer treated with percutaneous image-guided ablation (predominantly cryoablation, 89%) and found an LTC rate of 83% at a median follow-up of 27 months. Importantly, in the androgen-deprivation therapy (ADT)-naïve subgroup, local control was achieved in 100% of metastases, with a median ADT-free survival of 29 months. This suggests that ablative therapy can meaningfully delay systemic therapy in well-selected patients [124].

In a population of metastatic sarcomas, Vaswani et al. reported a 1-year LTC of 70% overall, but 100% in the subset with oligometastatic disease [122]. These findings suggest that when well-selected, patients undergoing CA may derive robust local control outcomes.

Although the Zugaro et al. study did not primarily assess long-term local tumor control (LTC), a recurrence rate was reported in 12% of CA cases and 8% of RFA cases, suggesting similar efficacy between the two modalities over short-term follow-up [135].

6.6.1.3 Functional Status and Prognosis

While both modalities aim at pain relief and local tumor suppression, CA may offer additional advantages by preserving adjacent neural and structural integrity due to the visualizability of the iceball during treatment. This technical characteristic of CA supports safer interventions near sensitive anatomical regions and may facilitate faster recovery, ultimately impacting quality of life and functional status positively [120].

Cazzato et al. observed that in sacral metastases treated with curative intent, patients undergoing CA had prolonged pain relief with minimal impact on neurologic function [125].

Beyond pain control, Zugaro et al. reported significant improvements in functional well-being and QoL. Using the McGill Quality of Life questionnaire, CA patients showed a greater improvement in QoL scores at 12 weeks compared to those treated with RFA [135].

6.6.1.4 Safety and Complications

Both techniques demonstrate a favorable safety profile, but CA appears to be associated with fewer minor complications. A large retrospective propensity-matched study by De Marini et al. reported no significant difference in major complications (RFA 1.5% vs. CA 2.7%, $p = 1$), but significantly more minor complications with RFA (33.3% vs. 6.0%, $p < 0.001$), largely due to postprocedural pain [136].

Additionally, the improved visualization during CA may contribute to fewer inadvertent injuries to adjacent structures. Deschamps et al. emphasized that the ability to monitor the ice ball under CT allows better control of the ablation zone, reducing the likelihood of thermal damage to nearby nerves or organs [120].

Zugaro et al. documented an excellent safety profile for both procedures, with only one transient nerve injury per group (RFA and CA), both resolving within 10 days with steroid treatment. No major complications or extended hospitalizations were reported. These results underscore the minimally invasive nature of both techniques, with comparable complication rates (~4%). However, the better post-procedural analgesia in CA patients also suggests a more favorable safety/tolerability profile in terms of overall recovery [135].

6.6.1.5 Technical Considerations

From a technical standpoint, RFA and CA differ significantly in mechanism and application. RFA uses high-frequency alternating current to induce coagulative necrosis, with optimal effectiveness in smaller, more contained lesions. Conversely, CA employs argon gas to induce cellular apoptosis via freezing, allowing simultaneous use of multiple probes and better adaptation to irregular lesion shapes.

CT-guided visualization of the iceball in CA provides real-time feedback and spatial control, making it particularly useful for complex anatomical locations, including near critical neural structures or within the pelvis and spine [120, 122].

CA is also associated with a potentially longer procedural time due to freeze-thaw cycles, yet this is offset by improved tolerance and lower analgesic needs postintervention.

Both cryoablation and radiofrequency ablation represent powerful tools in the interventional management of bone metastases, offering meaningful pain relief and tumor control. Cryoablation appears to provide better periprocedural pain control, reduced hospital stay, and lower minor complication rates, making it the preferred modality in many scenarios, especially for complex or larger lesions, and in oligometastatic settings where local control is paramount.

While both techniques are efficacious, the selection should be individualized based on lesion characteristics, anatomic location, and patient goals, with cryoablation gaining increasing favor in modern practice due to its enhanced safety and precision.

6.6.2 Cryoablation vs. Radiation Therapy: Analysis of Literature

Bone metastases are among the most frequent and debilitating complications in advanced cancer patients, often associated with intense pain and reduced quality of life. External beam radiation therapy (EBRT) has long been the mainstay for palliation, providing symptom relief in a majority of patients. However, with the evolution of image-guided minimally invasive procedures, CA has emerged as an effective alternative, offering advantages such as rapid onset of pain relief and the possibility of local tumor control. The comparative evaluation of CA and RT is essential to guide personalized care strategies, especially in patients with limited disease burden or those experiencing refractory pain.

6.6.2.1 Pain Control and Quality of Life

Radiotherapy is effective in reducing pain in approximately 60% of patients, with single-fraction RT (SFRT) and multiple-fraction RT (MFRT) offering comparable pain control but differing in duration of effect and retreatment rates [137]. However, pain relief may take 4–12 weeks to manifest fully after RT, potentially limiting its utility in cases where rapid symptom control is needed.

Cryoablation, by contrast, provides more immediate pain relief. Di Staso et al. compared CA, RT, and their sequential combination in a propensity-matched study involving 175 patients with solitary painful bone metastases. Complete response (CR) rates were significantly higher in the CA (32%) and CA + RT (72%) groups compared to RT alone (11.2%) ($p < 0.0001$). Moreover, the use of CA alone or in combination resulted in significantly reduced need for narcotics and improved self-rated quality of life scores compared to RT [138].

6.6.2.2 Clinical Outcomes and Cost-Effectiveness

Although RT is generally more accessible and cost-effective, its efficacy may decline with repeated use due to cumulative toxicity. Cryoablation, while more expensive initially, is valuable in retreatment scenarios, particularly after RT failure. Chang et al. used a Markov model to assess cost-effectiveness, finding that combining RT followed by CA (RT-ablation) was cost-effective, especially in patients with longer survival (>19 months). In contrast, upfront CA strategies were not economically favorable [137].

6.6.2.3 Combined Modality Therapy

Evidence from Di Staso et al. suggests a synergistic benefit when CA is followed by RT. The rationale for this sequence lies in the differing mechanisms of action and oxygen dependency: CA effectively ablates the hypoxic tumor core, while RT can target the more oxygenated tumor periphery. The combination may also exploit tumor microenvironment changes induced by ablation, enhancing RT sensitivity [138].

This sequential approach yielded superior pain control and reduction in opioid use, although long-term oncologic outcomes remain to be defined. No major complications were reported, and the treatment was well tolerated, with most adverse events being transient neuropathies or mild infections.

Nevertheless, growing evidence supports a role for CA, particularly in the following scenarios:

- Patients with refractory pain after RT
- Solitary metastases amenable to percutaneous access
- Longer life expectancy where durable control is desired
- Contraindications to further RT

From a procedural standpoint, clinical decision-making must also integrate technical and anatomical factors—particularly in the spine. The cardiovascular and interventional radiological society of europe (CIRSE) recommends several practical guidelines:

- In cases of vertebral metastases with epiduritis and neurologic symptoms, **radiotherapy should precede vertebroplasty**.
- When stereotactic body radiotherapy (SBRT) is intended with a curative aim, **SBRT should be performed before vertebroplasty**, to minimize the theoretical risk of cement-driven tumor cell embolization.
- Following SBRT for small vertebral lesions, **vertebroplasty may be performed secondarily** to reduce fracture risk due to SBRT-induced osteonecrosis [18].

Finally, future research should investigate the role of CA in immunomodulation, its combination with systemic therapies, and its potential use in enhancing local tumor control in oligometastatic disease.

6.7 Conclusions

Cryoablation represents a transformative advance in the interventional management of bone lesions, combining oncologic efficacy with favorable safety and tolerability. Its ability to achieve cytotoxic temperatures with high spatial precision—while preserving nearby neurovascular and structural integrity—makes it uniquely suited for treating lesions in challenging anatomical locations. Clinical evidence supports its effectiveness in both benign and malignant conditions, including osteoid osteoma, osteoblastoma, chondroblastoma, aneurysmal bone cysts, oligometastatic bone disease, and select primary malignancies. The procedure's anesthetic effect, real-time imaging visibility, and compatibility with adjunctive therapies such as cementoplasty and embolization further enhance its clinical utility. While complications remain rare and manageable, careful planning, advanced thermal protection techniques, and multidisciplinary collaboration are essential to optimize outcomes. As research continues to explore its immunologic potential and integration with systemic therapies, cryoablation is poised to play an increasingly central role in the personalized, image-guided treatment of musculoskeletal tumors.

References

1. Arnott J. Practical illustrations of the remedial efficacy of a very low or anesthetic temperature in cancer. Lancet. 1850;2:257–9.
2. Sabel MS. Cryo-immunology: a review of the literature and proposed mechanisms for stimulatory versus suppressive immune responses. Cryobiology. 2009;58(1):1–11.
3. O'Rourke AP, Haemmerich D, Prakash P, Converse MC, Mahvi DM, Webster JG. Current status of liver tumor ablation devices. Expert Rev Med Devices. 2007;4:523–37.
4. Erinjeri JP, Clark TW. Cryoablation: mechanism of action and devices. J Vasc Interv Radiol. 2010;21(8 Suppl):S187–91.

5. Hoffmann NE, Bischof JC. The cryobiology of cryosurgical injury. Urology. 2002 Aug;60(2 Suppl 1):40–9.
6. Theodorescu D. Cancer cryotherapy: evolution and biology. Rev Urol. 2004;6(Suppl 4):S9–S19.
7. Chu KF, Dupuy DE. Thermal ablation of tumours: biological mechanisms and advances in therapy. Nat Rev Cancer. 2014;14(3):199–208.
8. Jansen MC, van Hillegersberg R, Schoots IG, Levi M, Beek JF, Crezee H, van Gulik TM. Cryoablation induces greater inflammatory and coagulative responses than radiofrequency ablation or laser induced thermotherapy in a rat liver model. Surgery. 2010;147(5):686–95.
9. Erinjeri JP, Thomas CT, Samoilia A, Fleisher M, Gonen M, Sofocleous CT, Thornton RH, Siegelbaum RH, Covey AM, Brody LA, Alago W Jr, Maybody M, Brown KT, Getrajdman GI, Solomon SB. Image-guided thermal ablation of tumors increases the plasma level of interleukin-6 and interleukin-10. J Vasc Interv Radiol. 2013;24(8):1105–12.
10. Ahmad F, Gravante G, Bhardwaj N, Strickland A, Basit R, West K, Sorge R, Dennison AR, Lloyd DM. Changes in interleukin-1β and 6 after hepatic microwave tissue ablation compared with radiofrequency, cryotherapy and surgical resections. Am J Surg. 2010;200(4):500–6.
11. Gravante G, Sconocchia G, Ong SL, Dennison AR, Lloyd DM. Immunoregulatory effects of liver ablation therapies for the treatment of primary and metastatic liver malignancies. Liver Int. 2009;29(1):18–24.
12. Chen Z, Meng L, Zhang J, Zhang X. Progress in the cryoablation and cryoimmunotherapy for tumor. Front Immunol. 2023;25:14.
13. Wing MG, Rogers K, Jacob G, Rees RC. Characterisation of suppressor cells generated following cryosurgery of an HSV-2-induced fibrosarcoma. Cancer Immunol Immunother. 1988;26(2):169–75.
14. Yamashita T, Hayakawa K, Hosokawa M, Kodama T, Inoue N, Tomita K, Kobayashi H. Enhanced tumor metastases in rats following cryosurgery of primary tumor. Gan. 1982;73(2):222–8.
15. Kammoun T, Prévot E, Serrand C, et al. Feasibility and safety of single-probe cryoablation with liquid nitrogen: an initial experience in 24 various tumor lesions. Cancers (Basel) 2022;14(21).
16. Nomori H, Yamazaki I, Adachi T. Cryoablation using liquid nitrogen for metastatic lung cancers. Clin Oncol. 2022;7:1932.
17. Auloge P, Cazzato RL, Rousseau C, et al. Complications of percutaneous bone tumor cryoablation: a 10-year experience. Radiology. 2019;291(2):521–8.
18. Ryan A, Byrne C, Pusceddu C, Buy X, Tsoumakidou G, Filippiadis D. CIRSE standards of practice on thermal ablation of bone Tumours. Cardiovasc Intervent Radiol. 2022;45(5):591–605.
19. Gangi A, Tsoumakidou G, Buy X, Quoix E. Quality improvement guidelines for bone tumour management. Cardiovasc Intervent Radiol. 2010;33(4):706–13.
20. Pusceddu C, Vergantino E, Santucci D, Marsico S, Cappucci M, Vaccarino F, Beomonte Zobel B, Grasso RF, Faiella E. Percutaneous Cryoablation under conscious sedation: a safe, effective and painless option for the treatment of pediatric osteoid Osteoma. J Clin Med. 2023;12(21):6889.
21. Kelekis A, Cornelis F, Tutton S, Filippiadis D. Metastatic osseous pain control: bone ablation and cementoplasty. Semin Interv Radiol. 2017;34(04):328–36.
22. Tomasian A, Jennings JW. Percutaneous minimally invasive thermal ablation for management of osseous metastases: recent advances. Int J Hyperth. 2019;36(2):3–12.
23. Tomasian A, Dehdashti F, Jennings JW. Percutaneous minimally invasive thermal ablation of musculoskeletal lesions: usefulness of PET-computed tomography. PET Clin. 2018;13(4):579–85.
24. Pellerin O, Medioni J, Vulser C, Déan C, Oudard S, Sapoval M. Management of painful pelvic bone metastasis of renal cell car- cinoma using embolization, radio-frequency ablation,

and cementoplasty: a prospective evaluation of efficacy and safety. Cardiovasc Interv Radiol. 2013;37(3):730–6.
25. Gennaro N, Sconfienza LM, Ambrogi F, Boveri S, Lanza E. Thermal ablation to relieve pain from metastatic bone disease: a systematic review. Skeletal Radiol. 2019;48(8):1161–9.
26. Napoli A, Anzidei M, Marincola BC, Brachetti G, Ciolina F, Cartocci G, Marsecano C, Zaccagna F, Marchetti L, Cortesi E, Catalano C. Primary pain palliation and local tumor control in bone metastases treated with magnetic resonance-guided focused ultrasound. Investig Radiol. 2013;48(6):351–8.
27. Grasso RF, Faiella E, Luppi G, Schena E, Giurazza F, Del Vescovo R, D'Agostino F, Cazzato RL, Beomonte Zobel B. Percutaneous lung biopsy: comparison between an augmented reality CT navigation system and standard CT-guided technique. Int J Comput Assist Radiol Surg. 2013;8:837–48.
28. Chehab MA, Brinjikji W, Copelan A, Venkatesan AM. Navigational tools for interventional radiology and interventional oncology applications. Semin Interv Radiol. 2015;32:416–27.
29. Wood BJ, Zhang H, Durrani A, Glossop N, Ranjan S, Lindisch D, Levy E, Banovac F, Borgert J, Krueger S, et al. Navigation with electromagnetic tracking for interventional radiology procedures: a feasibility study. J Vasc Interv Radiol JVIR. 2005;16:493–505.
30. Appelbaum L, Sosna J, Nissenbaum Y, Benshtein A, Goldberg SN. Electromagnetic navigation system for CT-guided biopsy of small lesions. AJR Am J Roentgenol. 2011;196:1194–200.
31. Bruners P, Penzkofer T, Nagel M, Elfring R, Gronloh N, Schmitz-Rode T, Günther RW, Mahnken AH. Electromagnetic tracking for CT-guided spine interventions: phantom, ex-vivo and in-vivo results. Eur Radiol. 2009;19:990–4.
32. Meier-Meitinger M, Nagel M, Kalender W, Bautz WA, Baum U. Computer-assisted navigation system for interventional CT-guided procedures: results of phantom and clinical studies. ROFO Fortschr Geb Rontgenstr Nuklearmed. 2008;180:310–7.
33. Aghayev E, Ebert LC, Christe A, Jackowski C, Rudolph T, Kowal J, Vock P, Thali MJ. CT data-based navigation for post-mortem biopsy—a feasibility study. J Forensic Leg Med. 2008;15:382–7.
34. Khan MF, Dogan S, Maataoui A, Gurung J, Schiemann M, Ackermann H, Wesarg S, Sakas G, Vogl TJ. Accuracy of biopsy needle navigation using the Medarpa system–computed tomography reality superimposed on the site of intervention. Eur Radiol. 2005;15:2366–74.
35. Zhang Z, Shao G, Zheng J, Wen S, Zeng H, Hao W, Luo J, Guo L. Electromagnetic navigation to assist with computed tomography-guided thermal ablation of liver tumors. Minim Invasive Ther Allied Technol MITAT Off J Soc Minim Invasive Ther. 2020;29:275–82.
36. Liu J-F, Jiao D-C, Ren J-Z, Zhang W-G, Han X-W. Percutaneous bone biopsy using a flat-panel cone beam computed tomography virtual navigation system. Saudi Med J. 2018;39:519–23.
37. Faiella E, Castiello G, Bernetti C, Pacella G, Altomare C, Andresciani F, Beomonte Zobel B, Grasso RF. Impact of an augmented reality navigation system (SIRIO) on bone percutaneous procedures: a comparative analysis with standard CT-guided technique. Curr Oncol. 2021;28:1751–60.
38. Faiella E, Casati R, Pileri M, Pacella G, Altomare C, Vergantino E, Bruno A, Beomonte Zobel B, Grasso RF. Augmented reality navigation system (SIRIO) for neuroprotection in vertebral Tumoral ablation. Curr Oncol. 2024;31(9):5088–97.
39. Gage AA, Guest K, Montes M, et al. Effect of varying freezing and thawing rates in experimental cryosurgery. Cryobiology. 1985;22:175–82.
40. Kurup AN, Schmit GD, Morris JM, Atwell TD, Schmitz JJ, Weisbrod AJ, Woodrum DA, Eiken PW, Callstrom MR. Avoiding complications in bone and soft tissue ablation. Cardiovasc Intervent Radiol. 2017;40(2):166–76.
41. McMenomy BP, Kurup AN, Johnson GB, et al. Percutaneous cryoablation of musculoskeletal oligometastatic disease for complete remission. J Vasc Interv Radiol. 2013;24:207–13.
42. Orsi F, Hamiddin AS, Sattin C, Pizzi C, Varano GM, Della Vigna P, Mauri G, Maiettini D, Bonomo G. Liquid nitrogen-based cryoablation: complication rates for lung, bone, and soft tissue tumors cryoablation. Br J Radiol. 2024;97(1163):1863–9.

43. Bageacu S, Kaczmarek D, Lacroix M, Dubois J, Forest J, Porcheron J. Cryosurgery for resectable and unresectable hepatic metastases from colorectal cancer. Eur J Surg Oncol. 2007;33(5):590–6.
44. Gage AA, Baust J. Mechanisms of tissue injury in cryosurgery. Cryobiology. 1998;37(3):171–86.
45. Jia J, Pollock M. The pathogenesis of non-freezing cold nerve injury: observations in the rat. Brain. 1997;120(pt 4):631–46.
46. Littrup PJ, Jallad B, Vorugu V, et al. Lethal isotherms of cryoablation in a phantom study: effects of heat load, probe size, and number. J Vasc Interv Radiol. 2009;20(10):1343–51.
47. Rutkove SB. Effects of temperature on neuromus- cular electrophysiology. Muscle Nerve. 2001;24(7):867–82.
48. Haveman J, Van Der Zee J, Wondergem J, Hoogeveen JF, Hulshof MC. Effects of hyperthermia on the peripheral nervous system: a review. Int J Hyperth. 2004;20(4):371–91.
49. Xu D, Pollock M. Experimental nerve thermal injury. Brain. 1994;117(pt 2):375–84.
50. Chosy SG, Nakada SY, Lee FT Jr, Warner TF. Monitoring renal cryosurgery: predictors of tissue necrosis in swine. J Urol. 1998;159(4):1370–4.
51. Thacker PG, Callstrom MR, Curry TB, et al. Palliation of painful metastatic disease involving bone with imaging-guided treatment: comparison of patients' immediate response to radiofrequency Ablation and cryoablation. AJR Am J Roentgenol. 2011;197(2):510–5.
52. Haveman J, Wondergem J, van Dam WM, van der Kracht AH. Irradiation of the rat sciatic nerve leads to delayed recovery from function loss after heat treatment or mechanical damage. Neurosci Res Commun. 1994;14(1):1–7.
53. Kurup AN, Morris JM, Schmit GD, Atwell TD, Weisbrod AJ, Murthy NS, Callstrom MR. Neuroanatomic considerations in percutaneous tumor ablation. Radiographics. 2013;33(4):1195–215.
54. Kurup AN, Morris JM, Boon AJ, et al. Motor evoked potential monitoring during cryoablation of musculoskeletal tumors. J Vasc Interv Radiol. 2014;25(11):1657–64.
55. Yoon JT, Nesbitt J, Raynor BL, Roth M, Zertan CC, Jennings JW. Utility of motor and somatosensory evoked potentials for neural Thermoprotection in ablations of musculoskeletal tumors. J Vasc Interv Radiol. 2020;31(6):903–11.
56. Tsoumakidou G, Garnon J, Ramamurthy N, Buy X, Gangi A. Interest of electrostimulation of peripheral motor nerves during percutaneous thermal ablation. Cardiovasc Intervent Radiol. 2013;36(6):1624–8.
57. Autrusseau PA, Garnon J, Auloge P, Weiss J, Dalili D, Caudrelier J, Cazzato RL, Koch G, Gangi A. Hydrodissection of the retro-sternal space to protect the pericardium during sternal Cryoablation. Cardiovasc Intervent Radiol. 2020;43(9):1371–7.
58. Garnon J, Cazzato RL, Caudrelier J, Nouri-Neuville M, Rao P, Boatta E, Ramamurthy N, Koch G, Gangi A. Adjunctive Thermoprotection during percutaneous thermal ablation procedures: review of current techniques. Cardiovasc Intervent Radiol. 2019;42(3):344–57.
59. Khan MA, Deib G, Deldar B, Patel AM, Barr JS. Efficacy and safety of percutaneous microwave ablation and cementoplasty in the treatment of painful spinal metastases and myeloma. AJNR Am J Neuroradiol. 2018;39(7):1376–83.
60. Deschamps F, de Baere T. Cementoplasty of bone metastases. Diagn Interv Imaging. 2012;93(9):685–9. https://doi.org/10.1016/j.diii.2012.06.009. Epub 2012 Aug 11
61. Griauzde J, Gemmete JJ, Farley F. Successful treatment of a musculoskeletal tumor society grade 3 aneurysmal bone cyst with N-butyl cyanoacrylate embolization and percutaneous cryoablation. J Vasc Interv Radiol. 2015;26(6):905–9.
62. Lee JH, Stein M, Roychowdhury S. Percutaneous treatment of a sacral metastasis with combined embolization, cryoablation, alcohol ablation and sacroplasty for local tumor and pain control. Interv Neuroradiol. 2013;19(2):250–3.
63. Sundararajan SH, Calamita S, Girgis P, Ngo G, Ranganathan S, Giglio M, Gendel V, Goyal S, Nosher J, Roychowdhury S. Sequential interventional Management of Osseous Neoplasms via embolization, Cryoablation, and Osteoplasty. J Oncol. 2019;14:2019.

64. Le Corroller T, Vives T, Mattei JC, Pauly V, Guenoun D, Rochwerger A, Champsaur P. Osteoid Osteoma: percutaneous CT-guided Cryoablation is a safe, effective, and durable treatment option in adults. Radiology. 2022;302(2):392–9.
65. Serrano E, Zarco F, Gill AE, Hawkins CM, Macías N, Inarejos Clemente EJ, Torner F, Barber I, Corominas D, González EL, López-Rueda A, Gómez FM. Percutaneous cryoablation of chondroblastoma and osteoblastoma in pediatric patients. Insights Imaging. 2021;12(1):106.
66. Tsoumakidou G, Too CW, Garnon J, et al. Treatment of a spinal aneurysmal bone cyst using combined image-guided cryoablation and cementoplasty. Skeletal Radiol. 2015;44:285–9.
67. Gowda PC, Dunlap RH, Ahlawat S, Gross JM, Morris CD, Lyons GR. Recurrent chondromyxoid fibroma of the distal femur treated with percutaneous cryoablation. Skeletal Radiol. 2023;52(12):2497–501.
68. Kransdorf MJ, Stull MA, Gilkey FW, Moser RP Jr. Osteoid osteoma. Radiographics. 1991;11(4):671–96.
69. Huang AJ. Radiofrequency ablation of osteoid osteoma: difficult-to-reach places. Semin Musculoskelet Radiol. 2016;20(5):486–95.
70. Yalcinkaya U, Doganavsargil B, Sezak M, et al. Clinical and morphological characteristics of osteoid osteoma and osteoblastoma: a retrospective single- center analysis of 204 patients. Ann Diagn Pathol. 2014;18(6):319–25.
71. Rosenthal D, Callstrom MR. Critical review and state of the art in interventional oncology: benign and metastatic disease involving bone. Radiology. 2012;262(3):765–80.
72. Tsoumakidou G, Thénint MA, Garnon J, Buy X, Steib JP, Gangi A. Percutaneous image-guided laser photocoagulation of spinal osteoid osteoma: a single-institution series. Radiology. 2016;278(3):936–43.
73. Rybak LD, Gangi A, Buy X, et al. Thermal ablation of spinal osteoid osteomas close to neural elements: technical considerations. Multicenter Stud. 2010;195:W293–8.
74. Haibach H, Farrell C, Gaines RW. Osteoid osteoma of the spine: surgically correctable cause of painful scoliosis. CMAJ. 1986;135:895–9. Medline
75. Hakim DN, Pelly T, Kulendran M, Caris JA. Benign tumours of the bone: a review. J Bone Oncol. 2015;4(02):37–41.
76. Klein MH, Shankman S. Osteoid osteoma: radiologic and pathologic correlation. Skeletal Radiol. 1992;21(01):23–31.
77. Chai JW, Hong SH, Choi JY, Koh YH, Lee JW, Choi JA, Kang HS. Radiologic diagnosis of osteoid osteoma: from simple to challenging findings. Radiographics. 2010;30:737–49.
78. Michailidis A, Panos A, Samoladas E, Dimou G, Mingou G, Kosmoliaptsis P, Arvaniti M, Giankoulof C, Petsatodis E. Cryoablation of osteoid osteomas: is it a valid treatment option? World J Radiol. 2024;16(9):389–97.
79. Rosenthal DI, Hornicek FJ, Wolfe MW, Jennings LC, Gebhardt MC, Mankin HJ. Percutaneous radiofrequency coagulation of osteoid osteoma compared with operative treatment. J Bone Joint Surg Am. 1998;80(6):815–21.
80. Rosenthal DI, Hornicek FJ, Torriani M, Gebhardt MC, Mankin HJ. Osteoid osteoma: percutaneous treatment with radiofrequency energy. Radiology. 2003;229(1):171–5.
81. Chan LHD, Chien PYC, Chan THF. A rare cause of shoulder pain: osteoid osteoma of the scapular glenoid treated with cryoablation. Radiol Case Rep. 2023;19(1):136–40.
82. Whitmore MJ, Hawkins CM, Prologo JD, Marshall KW, Fabregas JA, Yim DB, Monson D, Oskouei SV, Fletcher ND, Williams RS. Cryoablation of osteoid Osteoma in the pediatric and adolescent population. J Vasc Interv Radiol. 2016;27(2):232–7.
83. Thurlow PC, Azhideh A, Ho CK, Stratchko LM, Pooyan A, Alipour E, Hosseini N, Chalian M. Thermal protection techniques for image-guided musculoskeletal ablation. Radiographics. 2025;45(4).
84. Lucas DR. Osteoblastoma. Arch Pathol Lab Med. 2010;134:1460–6.
85. Arrigoni F, Barile A, Zugaro L, Fascetti E, Zappia M, Brunese L, Masciocchi C. CT-guided radiofrequency ablation of spinal osteoblastoma: treatment and long-term follow-up. Int J Hyperth. 2018;34:321–7.

86. Izzo A, Zugaro L, Fascetti E, Bruno F, Zoccali C, Arrigoni F. Management of Osteoblastoma and Giant Osteoid Osteoma with percutaneous Thermoablation techniques. J Clin Med. 2021;10:5717.
87. Cazzato RL, Auloge P, Dalili D, De Marini P, Garnon J, Koch G, et al. Percutaneous image-guided Cryoablation of Osteoblastoma. AJR Am J Roentgenol. 2019;213(5):1157–62.
88. Poullain F, Mattei JC, Rochwerger A, Souteyrand P, Larousserie F, Jacopin T, et al. Percutaneous cryoablation of osteoblastoma in the proximal femur. Skeletal Radiol. 2020;49(9):1467–71.
89. Kumasaka S, et al. CT-guided percutaneous cryoablation of an aggressive osteoblastoma: a case report. J Vascul Interv Radiol. 26(11):1746–8.
90. Xu H, Nugent D, Monforte HL, Binitie OT, Ding Y, Letson GD, et al. Chondroblastoma of bone in the extremities: a multicenter retrospective study. J Bone Joint Surg Am. 2015;97(11):925–31.
91. Thibaut A, Bouhamama A, Boespflug A, Vaz G, Cuinet M, Kalenderian AC, Menassel B, Ricoeur A, Mastier C, Pilleul F. Percutaneous cryotherapy for treatment of Chondroblastoma: early experience. Cardiovasc Intervent Radiol. 2019;42(2):304–7.
92. Papagelopoulos PJ, Currier BL, Shaughnessy WJ, et al. Aneurysmal bone cyst of the spine. Management and outcome. Spine (PhilaPa 1976). 1998;23:621–8.
93. Hay MC, Paterson D, Talor TK. Aneurysmal bone cysts of the spine. J Bone Joint Surg (Br). 1978;60-B:406–11.
94. Restrepo R, Zahrah D, Pelaez L, Temple HT, Murakami JW. Update on aneurysmal bone cyst: pathophysiology, histology, imaging and treatment. Pediatr Radiol. 2022;52:1601–14.
95. Cottalorda J, Bourelle S. Current treatments of primary aneurysmal bone cysts. J Pediatr Orthop B. 2006;15:155–67.
96. Schlickewei CW, et al. Cryoablation of aneurysmal bone cysts in children: a prospective multicenter study. J Vasc Interv Radiol. 2024;
97. Fritz J, et al. MRI-guided percutaneous Cryoablation of a recurrent ABC in a child. Skeletal Radiol. 2018;47(6):833–8.
98. Alkuhaimi TS, et al. Feasibility of percutaneous combined Cryoablation and bone graft substitute for symptomatic bone cysts. Cardiovasc Intervent Radiol. 2023;46(4):512–8.
99. Arleo TL, et al. Percutaneous image-guided treatment of ABCs: a retrospective comparative series. Pediatr Radiol. 2022;52(7):1215–24.
100. Schajowicz F, Gallardo H. Chondromyxoid fibroma (fibromyxoid chondroma) of bone. A clinico-pathological study of thirty-two cases. J Bone Joint Surg Br. 1971;53(2):198–216.
101. Talbot LJ, Schechter A, Mothi SS, Ragan M, Aldrink JH, Brungardt J, Dasgupta R, Lautz TB, Rajeswaran S, Moya-Mendez ME, Tracy ET, Temple M, Davidoff AM. Use of palliative site-directed ablation in pediatric oncology: a retrospective study from the pediatric surgical oncology research collaborative. Pediatr Blood Cancer. 2025;72(2).
102. Li J, Lu Y, Chen G, Li M, Xiao X, Ji C, Wang Z, Guo Z. Cryoablation-aided joint retention surgery for epiphysis involvement in osteosarcoma compared with endoprosthetic replacement. Bone Joint J. 2021;103:1421.
103. Li J, Guo Z, Yang Q, Ji C, Wang Z. Adjuvant argon-based cryoablation for joint-preserving tumor resection in patients with juxta-articular osteosarcoma around the knee. Cryobiology. 2015;71(2):236–43.
104. Erwin US, Cahyadi SD. Cryosurgery and vascularized fibular graft reconstruction in proximal tibia osteosarcoma in young children: a case report. Int J Surg Case Rep. 2021;89:106568.
105. Lessard AM, Gilchrist J, Schaefer L, Dupuy DE. Palliation of recurrent Ewing sarcoma of the pelvis with cryoablation and somatosensory-evoked potentials. J Pediatr Hematol Oncol. 2009;31(1):18–21.
106. Meftah M, Schult P, Henshaw RM. Long-term results of intralesional curettage and cryosurgery for treatment of low-grade chondrosarcoma. J Bone Joint Surg Am. 2013;95(15):1358.
107. Mohler DG, Chiu R, McCall DA, Avedian RS. Curettage and cryosurgery for low-grade cartilage tumors is associated with low recurrence and high function. Clin Orthop Relat Res. 2010;468(10):2765.

108. Souna BS, Belot N, Duval H, Langlais F, Thomazeau H. No recurrences in selected patients after curettage with cryotherapy for grade I chondrosarcomas. Clin Orthop Relat Res. 2010;468(7):1956–62.
109. Deckers C, de Leijer EM, Flucke U, de Rooy JWJ, Schreuder HWB, Dierselhuis EF, van der Geest ICM. Curettage and cryosurgery for enchondroma and atypical cartilaginous tumors of the long bones: oncological results of a large series. J Surg Oncol. 2021;123(8):1821–7.
110. Madda R, Chen CM, Chen CF, Wang JY, Wu PK, Chen WM. Effect of Cryoablation treatment on the protein expression profile of low-grade central chondrosarcoma identified by LC-ESI-MS/MS. J Am Soc Mass Spectrom. 2021;32(6):1469–89.
111. Li L, Jiang XF, Sun LJ, Fu YF, Zhang W. Computed tomography-guided argon-helium cryoablation for sacrum chordoma. Medicine (Baltimore). 2020;99(42):e22604.
112. Cherix S, Traverso A, Bazan AA, Gallusser N, Heutschi-Ozturk H, Abou-Khalil S, Goetti P, Letovanec I, Montemurro M, Bize P. Image-guided percutaneous cryoablation of unresectable sacrococcygeal chordoma: feasibility and outcome in a selected group of patients with long term follow-up. J Surg Oncol. 2021;123(2):497–504.
113. Errani C, Bazzocchi A, Spinnato P, Facchini G, Campanacci L, Rossi G, Mavrogenis AF. What's new in management of bone metastases? Eur J Orthop Surg Traumatol. 2019;29:1367–75.
114. Papalexis N, Parmeggiani A, Peta G, Spinnato P, Miceli M, Facchini G. Minimally invasive interventional procedures for metastatic bone disease: a comprehensive review. Curr Oncol. 2022;29:4155–77.
115. Hong S, Youk T, Lee SJ, Kim KM, Vajdic CM. Bone metastasis and skeletal-related events in patients with solid cancer: a Korean nationwide health insurance database study. PLoS One. 2020;15:*e0234927.*
116. Cazzato RL, Auloge P, De Marini P, Boatta E, Koch G, Dalili D, Rao PP, Garnon J, Gangi A. Spinal tumor ablation: indications, techniques, and clinical management. Tech Vasc Interv Radiol. 2020;23:100677.
117. Munk PL, Murphy KJ, Gangi A, Liu DM. Fire and ice: percutaneous ablative therapies and cement injection in Management of Metastatic Disease of the spine. Semin Musculoskelet Radiol. 2011;15:125–34.
118. Gardner CS, Ensor JE, Ahrar K, Huang SY, Sabir SH, Tannir NM, Lewis VO, Tam AL. Cryoablation of bone metastases from renal cell carcinoma for local tumor control. J Bone Joint Surg Am. 2017;99(22):1916–26.
119. Luigi Cazzato R, Auloge P, De Marini P, Rousseau C, Chiang JB, Koch G, Caudrelier J, Rao P, Garnon J, Gangi A. Percutaneous image-guided ablation of bone metastases: local tumor control in oligometastatic patients. Int J Hyperth. 2018;35(1):493–9.
120. Deschamps F, Farouil G, Ternes N, Gaudin A, Hakime A, Tselikas L, Teriitehau C, Baudin E, Auperin A, de Baere T. Thermal ablation techniques: a curative treatment of bone metastases in selected patients? Eur Radiol. 2014;24(8):1971–80.
121. Arrigoni F, Bianchi G, Formiconi F, Palumbo P, Zugaro L, Gravina GL, Barile A, Masciocchi C. CT-guided cryoablation for management of bone metastases: a single center experience and review of the literature. Radiol Med. 2022;127(2):199–205.
122. Vaswani D, Wallace AN, Eiswirth PS, Madaelil TP, Chang RO, Tomasian A, Jennings JW. Radiographic local tumor control and pain palliation of sarcoma metastases within the musculoskeletal system with percutaneous thermal ablation. Cardiovasc Intervent Radiol. 2018;41(8):1223–32.
123. Ma Y, Wallace AN, Waqar SN, Morgensztern D, Madaelil TP, Tomasian A, Jennings JW. Percutaneous image-guided ablation in the treatment of osseous metastases from non-small cell lung cancer. Cardiovasc Intervent Radiol. 2018;41(5):726–33.
124. Erie AJ, Morris JM, Welch BT, Kurup AN, Weisbrod AJ, Atwell TD, Schmit GD, Kwon ED, Callstrom MR. Retrospective review of percutaneous image-guided ablation of Oligometastatic prostate cancer: a single-institution experience. J Vasc Interv Radiol. 2017;28(7):987–92.

125. Cazzato RL, De Marini P, Leonard-Lorant I, Dalili D, Koch G, Autrusseau PA, Mayer T, Weiss J, Auloge P, Garnon J, Gangi A. Percutaneous thermal ablation of sacral metastases: assessment of pain relief and local tumor control. Diagn Interv Imaging. 2021;102(6):355–61.
126. Callstrom MR, Dupuy DE, Solomon SB, Beres RA, Littrup PJ, Davis KW, Paz-Fumagalli R, Hoffman C, Atwell TD, Charboneau JW, Schmit GD, Goetz MP, Rubin J, Brown KJ, Novotny PJ, Sloan JA. Percutaneous image-guided cryoablation of painful metastases involving bone: multicenter trial. Cancer. 2013;119(5):1033–41.
127. Callstrom MR, Atwell TD, Charboneau JW, Farrell MA, Goetz MP, Rubin J, Sloan JA, Novotny PJ, Welch TJ, Maus TP, Wong GY, Brown KJ. Painful metastases involving bone: percutaneous image-guided cryoablation--prospective trial interim analysis. Radiology. 2006;241(2):572–80.
128. Prologo JD, Passalacqua M, Patel I, Bohnert N, Corn DJ. Image-guided cryoablation for the treatment of painful musculoskeletal metastatic disease: a single-center experience. Skeletal Radiol. 2014;43(11):1551–9.
129. Motta A, Caltabiano G, Palmucci S, Failla G, Basile A. Feasibility of percutaneous cryoablation of vertebral metastases under local anaesthesia in ASAIII patients. Eur J Radiol. 2017;95:13–7.
130. Jennings JW, Prologo JD, Garnon J, Gangi A, Buy X, Palussière J, Kurup AN, Callstrom M, Genshaft S, Abtin F, Huang AJ, Iannuccilli J, Pilleul F, Mastier C, Littrup PJ, de Baère T, Deschamps F. Cryoablation for palliation of painful bone metastases: the MOTION multicenter study. Radiol Imag Cancer 2021;3(2).
131. Yang Y, Li Y, Wu Y, Qiu S, Liu C, Wang Q, Hong Y, Lyu J, Zhang Y, Du D. Retrospective analysis of CT-guided percutaneous cryoablation for treatment of painful osteolytic bone metastasis. Cryobiology. 2020;92:203–7.
132. Hegg RM, Kurup AN, Schmit GD, Weisbrod AJ, Atwell TD, Olivier KR, Moynihan TJ, Callstrom MR. Cryoablation of sternal metastases for pain palliation and local tumor control. J Vasc Interv Radiol. 2014;25(11):1665–70.
133. Wallace AN, McWilliams SR, Connolly SE, Symanski JS, Vaswani D, Tomasian A, Vyhmeister R, Lee AM, Madaelil TP, Hillen TJ, Jennings JW. Percutaneous image-guided Cryoablation of musculoskeletal metastases: pain palliation and local tumor control. J Vasc Interv Radiol. 2016;27(12):1788–96.
134. Torabi S, Ahmadzade M, Ghorani H, Sarvari M, Rouientan H, Trinh K, Manzari Tavakoli G, Afsharzadeh M, Uppot RN, Ghasemi-Rad M. Image-guided cryoablation for palliation of painful bone metastases: a systematic review and meta-analysis. Skeletal Radiol. 2025;54:1715.
135. Zugaro L, DI Staso M, Gravina GL, Bonfili P, Gregori L, Franzese P, Marampon F, Tombolini V, Di Cesare E, Masciocchi C. Treatment of osteolytic solitary painful osseous metastases with radiofrequency ablation or cryoablation: a retrospective study by propensity analysis. Oncol Lett. 2016;11(3):1948–54.
136. De Marini P, Cazzato RL, Auloge P, Koch G, Dalili D, Garnon J, Gangi A. Percutaneous image-guided thermal ablation of bone metastases: a retrospective propensity study comparing the safety profile of radio-frequency ablation and cryo-ablation. Int J Hyperth. 2020;37(1):1386–94.
137. Chang EM, Shaverdian N, Capiro N, Steinberg ML, Raldow AC. Cost effectiveness of external beam radiation therapy versus percutaneous image-guided Cryoablation for palliation of uncomplicated bone metastases. J Vasc Interv Radiol. 2020;31(8):1221–32.
138. Di Staso M, Gravina GL, Zugaro L, Bonfili P, Gregori L, Franzese P, Marampon F, Vittorini F, Moro R, Tombolini V, Di Cesare E, Masciocchi C. Treatment of solitary painful osseous metastases with radiotherapy, Cryoablation or combined therapy: propensity matching analysis in 175 patients. PLoS One. 2015;10(6):e0129021.

High-Intensity Focused Ultrasound (HIFU)

7

Franco Orsi and Gianluca Maria Varano

Abbreviations

HIFU	High-Intensity Focused Ultrasound
MR-HIFU	Magnetic Resonance-Guided High-Intensity Focused Ultrasound
US-HIFU	Ultrasound-Guided High-Intensity Focused Ultrasound
EBRT	External Beam Radiation Therapy
PRFS	Proton Resonance Frequency Shift
QoL	Quality of Life
CTCAE	Common Terminology Criteria for Adverse Events
PET-CT	Positron Emission Tomography–Computed Tomography
SUV	Standardized Uptake Value
BPI	Brief Pain Inventory
EORTC	European Organisation for Research and Treatment of Cancer
SREs	Skeletal-Related Events
MEDD	Morphine Equivalent Daily Dose
MRI	Magnetic Resonance Imaging
CT	Computed Tomography

7.1 Introduction

Bone represents one of the most common sites for metastatic spread in cancer patients. With approximately 280,000 new cases of bone metastases annually in the United States alone, this clinical scenario presents a significant healthcare challenge

F. Orsi (✉) · G. M. Varano
Interventional Radiology, IRCCS Istituto Europeo di Oncologia, Milan, Italy
e-mail: franco.orsi@ieo.com

C. Pusceddu, S. Marsico (eds.), *Malignant Bone Lesions and Beyond*,
https://doi.org/10.1007/978-3-032-00018-7_7

[8]. As advances in cancer treatment continue to improve overall survival rates, the number of patients living with bone metastases is expected to increase further [9]. These lesions significantly impact quality of life by causing severe pain, pathological fractures, spinal cord or nerve root compression, and hypercalcemia—conditions collectively known as skeletal-related events (SREs).

The management of bone metastases traditionally involves a multidisciplinary approach. External beam radiation therapy (EBRT) has long represented the standard of care for palliative treatment of cancer-induced bone pain. However, limitations exist with this approach, as approximately 40% of patients undergoing EBRT do not experience substantial pain improvement [4]. Moreover, radiation therapy poses challenges, including limitations on retreatment due to cumulative dose constraints, delayed onset of pain relief (taking up to 4 weeks), and potential side effects that can adversely affect patient comfort and quality of life [3].

In this therapeutic landscape, High-Intensity Focused Ultrasound (HIFU) has emerged as a promising noninvasive treatment option for bone metastases. This technology utilizes focused ultrasound energy to induce precise thermal ablation at a targeted focal point, resulting in coagulative necrosis and denervation of pain-transmitting nerve fibers in the periosteum without damaging surrounding tissues [5]. With the introduction of guidance systems using either magnetic resonance imaging (MR-HIFU) or ultrasound (US-HIFU), this modality has gained significant attention for both the palliative treatment of painful bone metastases and local tumor control.

This chapter aims to provide interventional radiologists with a comprehensive understanding of HIFU principles, mechanisms of action, technical aspects, clinical applications, efficacy, safety, and future perspectives specifically for the treatment of malignant bone lesions.

7.2 Basic Principles of HIFU

7.2.1 Physical Principles and Mechanisms of Action (Fig. 7.1)

High-intensity focused ultrasound represents a sophisticated technological application of acoustic energy to induce biological effects in precisely targeted tissues. Modern HIFU systems generate ultrasound waves within a frequency range of 0.2–4 MHz, with peak compression pressures reaching up to 70 MPa and peak rarefaction pressures of up to 20 MPa. The acoustic intensity typically ranges from 100 to 10,000 W/cm^2 [7]. These high-energy ultrasound waves converge on a small target volume where several mechanisms produce therapeutic effects.

The primary mechanism of HIFU therapy involves thermal effects. When ultrasound waves propagate through tissues, they cause molecular vibration, which results in frictional heating. At the focal point where energy concentrates, temperatures can rapidly rise above 56 °C, a threshold that, when maintained for at least one second, induces coagulative necrosis. This thermal mechanism constitutes the

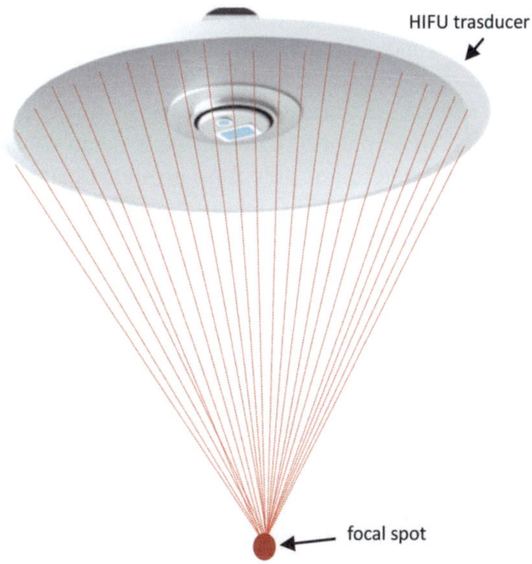

Fig. 7.1 A general schematic illustrating how the transducer focuses acoustic waves on a single focal spot, where the delivered energy is concentrated and interacts with the targeted tissue, leading to a rapid temperature increase

predominant mode of action for therapeutic ablation in HIFU treatments of bone lesions [10].

Beyond thermal effects, HIFU can also generate mechanical effects at high acoustic intensities. These include acoustic cavitation (the formation, oscillation, and collapse of gas-filled microbubbles), radiation force, and acoustic streaming. While these mechanical effects are generally avoided in clinical HIFU for bone lesions due to their less predictable nature, they form the basis of histotripsy, an emerging HIFU technique with potential applications in oncology [11].

HIFU also produces significant vascular effects. Through thermal coagulation of blood vessels, HIFU can cause thrombosis and tumor ischemia, further contributing to tumor cell death. The comprehensive nature of these effects makes HIFU a multifaceted approach to treating bone lesions, though current clinical applications primarily rely on the thermal mechanism, which remains the only mechanism with regulatory approval for commercial use [12] in the USA.

7.2.2 Tissue-Ultrasound Interaction in Bone

The interaction between ultrasound energy and bone tissue differs significantly from that observed in soft tissues, creating unique considerations for HIFU treatment of bone lesions. Bone possesses an acoustic absorption coefficient approximately 50 times greater than soft tissue [13].

When ultrasound waves encounter bone, approximately 70% of the acoustic energy is reflected at the bone-soft tissue interface. A substantial portion of the remaining energy is absorbed within the first few millimeters of the bone surface, with only minimal energy penetrating deeper into the bone structure. This high absorption and reflection initially appeared to limit HIFU applications to superficial bone lesions. However, researchers later recognized that this property actually provides advantages in treating bone pain.

The preferential heating of the periosteum—the most richly innervated structure of mature bone responsible for pain signal conduction—leads to thermal denervation and rapid pain relief. This understanding has informed the development of two primary approaches for HIFU treatment of bone lesions. The wide-beam approach is utilized when cortical bone remains intact; here, the focused ultrasound beam is positioned at the bone surface or slightly behind it, with energy absorbed by the cortical surface leading to periosteal denervation. Alternatively, the direct approach is employed when bone metastases feature transcortical growth (osteolytic lesions). In this scenario, the ultrasound beam is focused directly on the tumor component, allowing for tumor ablation in addition to pain relief [5].

7.3 HIFU Technology and Image Guidance

7.3.1 HIFU Systems

Modern HIFU technology consists of sophisticated devices comprising a generator and a transducer working in concert. The generator produces ultrasound energy, which the transducer focuses onto a well-defined target at a given distance within the body. Contemporary systems use phased array transducers containing multiple piezoelectric elements that can be individually adjusted in amplitude and phase by specific software. This advanced design allows for precise focal spot steering without requiring physical movement of either the transducer or the patient, significantly enhancing treatment flexibility and precision.

HIFU systems are generally categorized according to their configuration and clinical application. Extracorporeal transducers represent the most versatile category, available in compact flat, curved, and helmet-like designs (dedicated to neuro applications). These systems allow targeting of both superficial and deep structures accessible through the skin, making them particularly suitable for bone lesions. Notable examples include the Exablate 2000/2100 (InSightec Ltd., Haifa, Israel), Sonalleve (Profound Medical, Mississauga, Canada), and the JC HIFU system (Chongqing Haifu Medical Technology Co., Ltd., Chongqing, China). These systems have been extensively studied and validated for bone metastasis treatment.

For bone lesions, extracorporeal systems predominate in clinical practice. These systems enable sequential sonications, with each sonication covering a focal volume of 0.2–5 mm^3 and lasting only a few seconds. Multiple sonications can be performed in a precise pattern to cover larger treatment volumes, allowing for customization of the treatment approach based on the specific characteristics of the bone lesion.

7.3.2 Image Guidance Systems

The safe and effective delivery of HIFU therapy requires dedicated image guidance for planning, targeting, and monitoring of treatment. Two primary modalities have emerged as the mainstays of HIFU guidance: magnetic resonance imaging and ultrasound.

MR-guided HIFU (MR-HIFU or MRgFUS) offers several distinct advantages that have made it the preferred approach in many clinical settings, particularly for bone lesions. Its superior soft tissue contrast enables precise target delineation, allowing clinicians to clearly distinguish between tumor tissue, healthy bone, and adjacent critical structures. Perhaps most importantly, MR guidance provides real-time temperature monitoring using proton resonance frequency shift (PRFS) thermometry, offering quantitative feedback on treatment progress and safety. This capability allows immediate assessment of therapeutic response and facilitates multi-planar imaging for comprehensive treatment planning.

Typical MR-HIFU systems integrate the HIFU transducer within the MRI table of 1.5 T or 3.0 T scanners. During treatment, the MRI provides both anatomical information for precise targeting and thermal mapping to ensure both safety and efficacy. As described by Scipione et al. [12], PRFS thermometry allows quantitative temperature measurements with an accuracy of 1 °C, spatial resolution of 1 mm, and temporal resolution of 3 s—parameters that enable exquisite control over the ablation process.

For bone treatments specifically, there are limitations to direct temperature measurements within cortical bone or bone marrow. This is due to the lack of mobile protons in cortical bone and the inability to apply PRFS thermometry in fat tissues. However, temperature monitoring in adjacent soft tissues provides sufficient feedback to ensure treatment efficacy while maintaining safety parameters.

Ultrasound-guided HIFU (US-HIFU or USgFUS) presents an alternative approach with distinct advantages in certain clinical scenarios. US guidance offers real-time imaging capability with rapid frame rates, lower cost, and greater accessibility than MRI, and no contraindications related to MRI compatibility. Treatment sessions generally require less time than MR-guided procedures. In US-HIFU systems, both imaging and therapeutic elements are incorporated in a stereotactically controlled or handheld device. Tissue-change monitoring is based on alterations in echogenicity rather than direct temperature measurement, which can limit quantitative treatment assessment, especially in deeper tissues.

While both guidance methods have proven effective for bone lesions, MR-HIFU generally predominates in developed countries due to its superior target visualization and temperature monitoring capabilities, particularly for non-flat bones and deep-seated lesions. The choice between guidance systems ultimately depends on lesion characteristics, institutional resources, and specific clinical scenarios.

7.4 Patient Selection and Clinical Workflow

7.4.1 Patient Selection Criteria

The success of HIFU treatment for malignant bone lesions begins with appropriate patient selection. A careful evaluation of potential candidates must consider multiple factors that influence both technical feasibility and clinical outcomes. Optimal candidates typically present with confirmed bone metastases causing moderate to severe pain (generally scoring 4 or higher on a 0–10 pain scale). These lesions should be located in non-spinal regions, with the exception of posterior elements below the level of the conus medullaris, and should not involve the skull due to technical limitations of ultrasound transmission through the skull.

For treatment feasibility, the target lesions must be clearly identifiable on MRI, CT, or ultrasound imaging. They should maintain a distance of at least 1 cm from the skin surface and major nerve bundles to prevent inadvertent thermal damage to these structures. The risk of pathological fracture must be carefully evaluated, with the MIRELS scoring system commonly employed to assess stability [14]; patients with scores of 7 or lower are generally considered suitable candidates, while those with higher scores may require surgical stabilization before or instead of HIFU treatment.

Clinical eligibility also considers previous treatments and prognosis. HIFU has shown particular value for patients who have not responded adequately to standard radiation therapy, those unsuitable for radiation due to previous exposure or comorbidities, or those who decline radiation therapy. Given the palliative nature of the procedure and the resources involved, patients should have a life expectancy of at least 3 months to derive meaningful benefit from the intervention.

Several conditions may preclude HIFU treatment. Patients with contraindications to MRI cannot undergo MR-HIFU procedures, though US-HIFU may remain an option in some cases. Technical contraindications include lesions with a high risk of fracture, those located too close to the skin surface or major nerve bundles, and the presence of metallic implants in the acoustic beam path. Patient factors such as inability to maintain the required position for treatment, extensive scarring in the acoustic beam path, or the proximity of bowel or lung in the acoustic pathway may also render HIFU unsuitable [3].

7.4.2 Pre-treatment Assessment

Comprehensive pre-treatment assessment forms the foundation of successful HIFU therapy for bone lesions. This process begins with a thorough clinical evaluation to characterize the patient's pain experience using standardized tools such as the Visual Analog Scale or Numerical Rating Scale. Clinicians should document current analgesic medication use, including type, frequency, and dosage, to establish a baseline for assessing treatment response. Quality of life assessments using validated questionnaires such as the Brief Pain Inventory Quality of Life, EORTC QLQ-BM22, or

EORTC QLQ-C30 provide important baseline metrics for evaluating the impact of treatment on patient well-being.

Imaging assessment plays a crucial role in treatment planning and patient selection. Unenhanced CT scans provide essential information for characterizing lesions as osteoblastic, osteolytic, or mixed, and for assessing cortical integrity—factors that influence the technical approach to HIFU treatment. MRI offers detailed delineation of metastatic lesions, their extent, and their relationship to surrounding structures, information vital for precise treatment planning. For patients with suspected widespread metastatic disease, bone scintigraphy or PET-CT may help determine the extent of disease and guide treatment prioritization. Conventional radiography retains value for assessing fracture risk and skeletal stability, particularly for lesions in weight-bearing bones.

The imaging evaluation serves multiple purposes beyond diagnosis. It plays a critical role in treatment planning, helping establish the optimal acoustic window and beam path configuration as well as patient position during the treatment. Key parameters evaluated include target lesion size, location, extent, accessibility to ultrasound, and the presence of any acoustic obstacles that might interfere with treatment delivery, as highlighted by Scipione et al. [12] in their clinical review of HIFU applications.

7.4.3 Clinical Workflow

The clinical workflow for HIFU treatment of bone metastases follows a systematic approach designed to maximize safety and efficacy. The process begins with careful patient preparation, including anesthesia planning based on the treatment location and individual patient factors. General anesthesia is typically preferred for treating upper trunk lesions such as those in the proximal humerus, scapula, sternum, or clavicle, where patient movement must be minimized. For lesions in the lower trunk, spine, or extremities, spinal anesthesia or regional nerve blocks often provide adequate pain control while reducing systemic risks. In select cases involving peripheral extremity treatments, conscious sedation may be enough.

Patient positioning represents a critical step in the procedure, as it directly impacts the quality of the acoustic window. The target lesion must be positioned directly over the HIFU transducer to achieve the optimal treatment approach. Ideal positioning aims to create the shortest possible beam path with minimal anatomical obstacles, enhancing energy delivery to the target while reducing the risk of complications.

Pre-treatment imaging and planning then establish the foundation for precise therapy. After acquiring planning images via MRI or ultrasound, clinicians define the target volume and identify critical structures to avoid. The treatment region, skin surface, bone cortex, and adjacent tissues are carefully segmented, with "no-pass" regions designated to protect sensitive structures. Anatomical fiducials are established to compensate for potential patient movement during treatment, ensuring maintained targeting accuracy.

The treatment planning phase involves selecting appropriate parameters such as sonication locations, number of sonications, energy levels, and cooling durations based on lesion characteristics. For intact cortical bone, the focal spot is typically positioned behind the cortical bone (wide-beam approach) or directly on the surface. For lesions with cortical erosion, the focus spot targets both tumor tissue and the bone-tumor interface. Before proceeding to therapeutic sonications, low-energy test sonications verify system calibration and patient positioning.

During treatment delivery, sequential therapeutic sonications target the designated treatment volume. With MR-HIFU, real-time temperature monitoring guides energy deposition, while US-HIFU relies on echogenicity changes to assess treatment progress. Treatment parameters vary based on lesion characteristics; intact cortical bone typically requires lower energy levels (1500–3000 J), while osteolytic lesions with cortical erosion may need higher energy levels (2500–6500 J) to achieve therapeutic effects.

Posttreatment assessment includes immediate imaging, typically contrast-enhanced MRI for MR-HIFU procedures, to evaluate the treated area. The skin is carefully examined for potential burns, vital signs are monitored, and pain assessment establishes early response to treatment. For patients undergoing procedures with regional anesthesia, same-day discharge is often possible, while those receiving general anesthesia typically require 24-h observation before discharge.

Follow-up evaluations occur at regular intervals, commonly scheduled at 1 day, 1 week, 1 month, and 3 months posttreatment. These assessments track pain scores, medication use, quality-of-life metrics, and imaging findings to document treatment response over time. This structured approach ensures comprehensive care throughout the patient journey from initial consultation through long-term follow-up.

7.5 Clinical Applications and Efficacy

7.5.1 Pain Palliation in Bone Metastases (Figs. 7.2 and 7.3)

The primary application of HIFU for malignant bone lesions centers on pain palliation. The mechanism underlying this effect involves thermal ablation of the highly innervated periosteum, leading to denervation and interruption of pain signal transmission. This approach has demonstrated remarkable efficacy across numerous clinical studies, establishing HIFU as a valuable tool in the multimodal management of painful bone metastases.

The landmark FDA-approved Phase III trial provided compelling evidence for HIFU's efficacy [1]. This randomized, placebo-controlled study of 147 patients (112 receiving MR-HIFU, 35 receiving placebo treatment) demonstrated a response rate at 3 months of 64.3% in the MR-HIFU group compared to 20% in the placebo group ($p < 0.001$). Complete response, defined as complete pain relief without

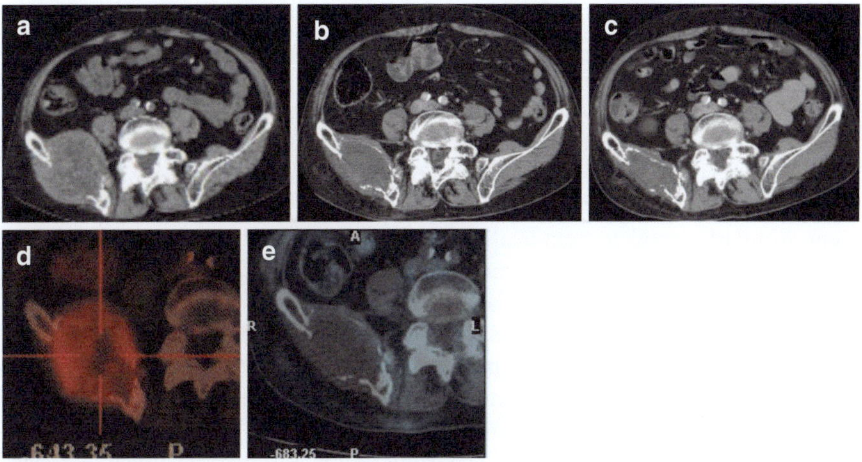

Fig. 7.2 A 69-year-old male with a large, painful iliac bone metastasis from a bladder carcinoma, recurrent after prior radiotherapy. (**a**) Axial CT image demonstrates the extensive osteolytic lesion; (**d**) corresponding FDG-PET image shows intense metabolic activity. Three months after treatment with ultrasound-guided HIFU (USg-HIFU); (**b**) follow-up CT reveals marked tumor shrinkage, with complete resolution of FDG uptake on PET; (**e**) At 6 months post-HIFU, the lesion shows further reduction in size and early signs of peripheral bone remineralization

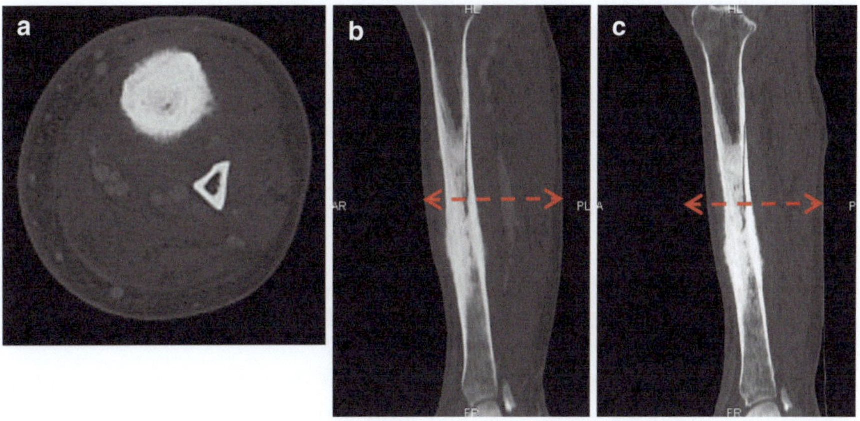

Fig. 7.3 (**a**) CT scan shows a sclerotic bone metastasis from prostate cancer involving the left tibia, causing severe pain with a Visual Analogue Scale (VAS) score of 9/10 despite prior radiotherapy. The lesion extends over 6 cm in the cranio-caudal direction, as illustrated in the Multiplanar Reconstruction (MPR) image. (**b**) Following HIFU treatment performed for palliative purposes, the patient reported a significant reduction in pain (VAS 1/10), and the circumference of the leg decreased, reflecting a reduction in the inflammatory process, as shown in (**c**)

increased analgesic usage, was achieved in 23.2% of MR-HIFU patients versus 5.7% of placebo patients. Perhaps most tellingly, the mean pain score reduction reached 3.6 points in the MR-HIFU group compared to just 0.7 points in the placebo group, representing a clinically significant improvement in patient comfort.

Meta-analyses have further confirmed these findings across broader patient populations. A systematic review examined 26 studies encompassing 799 patients [4]. Their analysis revealed overall pain response rates of 79% at 3 months posttreatment. Similarly, another meta-analysis of 15 studies with 362 patients showed a significant reduction in the pain score from an average of 6.74 at baseline to 2.28 at 5–14 weeks following HIFU treatment [15].

When compared to conventional radiation therapy, HIFU demonstrates distinct advantages in certain aspects of pain management. A matched-pair study comparing MR-HIFU to radiation therapy found significantly faster pain relief with MR-HIFU (evident at 1–2 weeks) with comparable long-term efficacy at 1–3 months [2]. This rapid onset of pain relief, typically occurring within 1–7 days posttreatment, contrasts favorably with radiation therapy's slower response timeline, which can extend to 3–4 weeks.

The durability of HIFU's analgesic effect has also been documented in longer-term studies. A study following patients for 12 months posttreatment demonstrated sustained pain reduction that, while showing some attenuation over time, remained significantly improved from baseline at the one-year mark (10.9% reduction, $p < 0.01$) [16]. This lasting benefit translates to meaningful improvements in patient function and quality of life throughout the palliative care journey.

Beyond pain reduction, HIFU treatment frequently enables reductions in pain medication requirements. Across studies, approximately 55.8% of patients were able to discontinue pain medication entirely following HIFU treatment, while an additional 33% achieved significant dose reductions. This medication-sparing effect carries substantial quality of life benefits by reducing opioid-related side effects such as constipation, sedation, and cognitive impairment that often complicate cancer pain management.

7.6 Tumor Control and Bone Quality Improvement

While pain palliation represents the primary goal of HIFU therapy for bone metastases, growing evidence suggests significant benefits for local tumor control and bone quality improvement as well. Several studies have documented objective tumor responses following HIFU treatment, extending its potential utility beyond symptom management.

Studies have assessed tumor response at 3 months posttreatment. Findings demonstrated complete response in 11.1% of patients, partial response in 22.2%, stable disease in 55.6%, and progressive disease in only 11.1% of cases [6]. These results suggest that HIFU not only alleviates pain but also exerts meaningful effects on tumor burden in a substantial proportion of patients.

Metabolic imaging has provided additional evidence of HIFU's tumor-controlling effects. PET/CT with 18F-Fluorodeoxyglucose (**18F-FDG**) has been used to assess metabolic response, documenting significant reduction or complete resolution of metabolic activity in treated lesions [17]. The observed decrease in SUV values by 25–35% in responsive lesions reflects a meaningful reduction in tumor metabolic activity following HIFU intervention.

Volumetric analysis revealed an average decrease in enhancing tumor volume by 50.2% at 1 month and a further 44% reduction at 3 months compared to baseline measurements [18]. This progressive volume reduction demonstrates HIFU's ongoing effect on tumor burden beyond the immediate treatment period.

Perhaps most remarkably, HIFU treatment has demonstrated the potential to improve bone quality through remineralization—a unique advantage not commonly seen with other ablative approaches. Studies have reported that 27.7% of patients with osteolytic lesions showed increased bone density with restoration of cortical bone following HIFU treatment. Conversely, 16.7% of patients with sclerotic lesions experienced decreased bone density, potentially reflecting normalization of bone architecture, while 55.6% showed no significant bone density changes [6].

CT evidence of increased bone density in 44% of treated lesions has been documented [18], supporting the concept that HIFU may induce beneficial structural changes in affected bone. These improvements in bone quality likely result from a combination of thermal ablation of tumor cells, reduced osteoclast activity, and potential promotion of osteoblastic activity after treatment, though the precise mechanisms continue to be investigated.

7.7 HIFU for Primary Malignant Bone Tumors

While HIFU applications for bone metastases have received the most extensive clinical evaluation, emerging evidence suggests promising results for primary malignant bone tumors as well. Though studied less extensively, available data indicate potential benefits for local tumor control in appropriately selected cases.

A study reported outcomes in 80 patients with primary bone malignancies, including 62 osteosarcomas, three Ewing sarcomas, ten chondrosarcomas, and five tumors of other histologies. They achieved complete tumor ablation (100%) in 69 patients and partial ablation (> 50%) in the remaining 11 patients. Remarkably, local tumor progression occurred in only 5 of the 69 completely ablated tumors at a mean follow-up of 36.8 months, with the study reporting a 5-year overall survival rate of 50.5% [19].

In a smaller series, seven patients with extremity osteosarcomas were treated using HIFU, achieving complete response in 42.9% and partial response in 42.9% of cases, with a 5-year survival rate of 71.4% [20]. These findings, while preliminary, suggest potential applications for HIFU in selected cases of primary bone malignancies.

Perhaps most compelling is a randomized study comparing chemotherapy plus HIFU ($n = 36$) versus chemotherapy alone ($n = 36$) for osteosarcoma treatment. This investigation demonstrated significantly higher overall response (88.9% vs. 66.7%) and disease control rates (94.4% vs. 75.0%) in the combined therapy group. More impressively, improved 2-year (69.4% vs. 52.8%) and 3-year survival rates (38.9% vs. 22.2%) were observed in patients receiving the combined approach [21], suggesting potential survival benefits when HIFU is integrated with conventional treatment modalities.

These studies collectively indicate that HIFU may offer meaningful contributions to local tumor control in primary bone malignancies, particularly when combined with standard treatments such as chemotherapy. While further research is needed to define optimal patient selection criteria and treatment protocols, these preliminary findings open promising avenues for HIFU applications beyond metastatic disease.

7.8 Impact on Quality of Life and Analgesic Use

The ultimate measure of any palliative intervention lies in its impact on patients' quality of life and functional status. HIFU treatment has demonstrated positive effects on these critical outcomes, extending its benefits beyond pain control alone.

In the landmark study, patients receiving MR-HIFU showed a 2.4-point better BPI-QoL score compared to the placebo group at 3 months posttreatment [1]. This difference represents a clinically meaningful improvement in quality-of-life metrics that directly reflect patients' ability to engage in daily activities and maintain functional independence.

Studies have documented improvement in QLQ-C15-PAL overall quality-of-life scores from 49.99 at baseline to 56.07 at 90 days following HIFU intervention [22]. Particularly notable were improvements in physical and emotional function subscales, reflecting enhanced mobility and psychological well-being after treatment.

Research has found significant improvements in both functional interference and psychosocial aspect scores throughout a 12-month follow-up period. While some attenuation of benefit was observed in later months, scores remained significantly improved from baseline at the one-year mark [16], demonstrating HIFU's durable impact on quality of life.

The reduction in analgesic requirements following HIFU represents another crucial benefit for patients in palliative settings. Meta-analyses have documented average morphine equivalent daily dose (MEDD) reductions of 15.11 mg at 2 weeks, 10.87 mg at 1 month, and 5.53 mg at 3 months posttreatment [4]. Studies have reported that 63.6% of patients were able to discontinue pain medication entirely, while the remaining 36.4% achieved dosage reductions of 50% or greater [18].

Research has similarly found that 72.2% of patients discontinued medication completely, 16.7% maintained stable dosage, and only 11.1% required reintroduction of pain medications during the follow-up period [6]. These medication-sparing effects carry profound implications for patients' comfort and function, as reduced analgesic requirements mean fewer medication-related side effects and improved cognitive function and alertness during a critical period in patients' lives.

7.9 Safety Profile and Complications

One of HIFU's most compelling advantages for treating bone lesions lies in its excellent safety profile. The noninvasive nature of the procedure contributes to minimal complications compared to surgical or other percutaneous interventions, making it particularly suitable for fragile patients with limited treatment options.

The most commonly reported adverse events are minor and typically resolve spontaneously within days to weeks. Treatment-related pain represents the most frequent complaint, manifesting as sonication pain during the procedure, positioning discomfort related to maintaining the required treatment position, or post-procedural pain that typically resolves within 72 h. These experiences can generally be managed with temporary analgesic adjustments without requiring significant intervention.

Skin effects occur in a minority of patients, with first-degree burns reported in approximately 5%–10% of treatments. These superficial thermal injuries typically resolve without sequelae within 1–2 weeks. More significant second-degree burns occur less frequently (1–2% of cases) and generally resolve within 2–4 weeks with appropriate wound care. Other minor effects include local edema and swelling, transient numbness or paresthesia, and occasional fatigue or low-grade fever—all of which typically resolve spontaneously with supportive care.

Serious adverse events are rare in HIFU treatment of bone lesions. A comprehensive meta-analysis examining 799 patients from 26 studies reported that only 0.9% of patients experienced major adverse events (CTCAE grade ≥ 3), while 5.9% experienced minor complications (CTCAE grade ≤ 2) [4]. Third-degree skin burns occur extremely rarely and typically result from protocol deviations or noncompliance with treatment guidelines rather than the inherent risk of properly performed procedures.

Fractures have been reported in approximately 1–2% of cases, though establishing causality remains challenging, as pathological fractures commonly occur as a natural consequence of metastatic bone disease itself. Nerve injuries remain rare when proper safety margins (≥ 1 cm from major nerve bundles) are maintained during treatment planning and delivery.

7.10 Technical Considerations and Challenges

Despite its significant therapeutic potential, HIFU treatment of bone lesions presents several technical challenges that require careful consideration for optimal outcomes. Successfully navigating these challenges demands a thorough understanding of acoustic principles, detailed pre-treatment planning, and ongoing technical innovations.

Acoustic access and beam path planning represent fundamental considerations for any HIFU procedure, particularly for bone lesions. Several obstacles can impede effective acoustic access, including nontarget bone in the beam path that can absorb and reflect ultrasound energy, air-filled organs such as bowel or lung that cause reflection and scattering, and surgical scars or implants that can distort the beam path. An adequate acoustic coupling between the transducer and the skin is also essential to prevent complications such as skin burns and to improve treatment efficiency by reducing energy absorption in the superficial skin layers. Careful selection of the acoustic window helps overcome these challenges by optimizing transducer position relative to the target, minimizing the distance between transducer and target tissue, and avoiding critical structures in the beam path. However, certain anatomical locations remain difficult to access due to positioning limitations, while prolonged positioning requirements can cause patient discomfort and compromise treatment delivery.

Bone tissue presents specific technical challenges for HIFU treatment. One significant limitation involves temperature monitoring capabilities. Direct temperature measurement in bone remains impossible with current MR thermometry techniques, necessitating reliance on monitoring temperature in adjacent soft tissues as a surrogate measure. This indirect approach makes it challenging to assess treatment completeness in real-time, potentially affecting treatment precision. The heterogeneous acoustic properties of bone further complicate treatment delivery. Variations in bone density substantially affect ultrasound absorption and heating patterns, while different responses in osteolytic versus osteoblastic lesions necessitate tailored treatment approaches. The transition zones between tumor and healthy bone present particularly variable acoustic properties, requiring careful planning to ensure adequate treatment throughout the target volume.

Determining optimal energy requirements and dosimetry for bone HIFU represents another challenge. Finding the appropriate acoustic power for different bone densities requires balancing treatment efficacy with safety considerations. Similarly, adapting treatment parameters for lesions with cortical destruction versus intact cortex demands a nuanced understanding of ultrasound-tissue interactions in different pathological states.

Several approaches have emerged to address these challenges. Treatment planning strategies have evolved to include the wide-beam approach for intact cortical bone (positioning the focus behind the bone) and the direct approach for osteolytic lesions with cortical erosion (focusing on tumor tissue). Multi-angle approaches have been developed for complex anatomical locations where direct access is limited. Technical adaptations include adjustment of ultrasound parameters based on lesion characteristics, use of phased array transducers for electronic steering of the focal spot, and implementation of motion compensation techniques to account for patient movement during treatment.

Imaging enhancements have also contributed to improved HIFU delivery for bone lesions. Fusion of pre-treatment CT with real-time MR provides improved bone visualization during treatment planning and execution. Ongoing development of alternative temperature monitoring techniques aims to overcome the limitations of conventional thermometry in bone tissues. The use of contrast-enhanced imaging for immediate posttreatment assessment helps verify treatment adequacy and identify any areas requiring additional attention.

7.11 Comparison with Other Treatment Modalities

Understanding HIFU's place in the therapeutic armamentarium requires a thorough comparison with other established treatment approaches for bone metastases. Each modality offers distinct advantages and limitations that inform optimal treatment selection for individual patients.

Radiation therapy remains the standard of care for painful bone metastases, but HIFU provides several distinct advantages in specific clinical scenarios. The timeline for pain relief represents one of the most significant differences between these approaches. HIFU typically produces pain improvement within 1–7 days, while radiation therapy requires 2–4 weeks for maximal effect. This rapid onset can prove valuable for patients with severe pain requiring urgent intervention. Response rates vary between modalities, with HIFU demonstrating rates of 60–100% across studies compared to 50–70% for single-fraction radiation treatment. Perhaps most importantly, HIFU faces no dose limitations and can be repeated as needed, while radiation therapy encounters cumulative dose constraints that may limit retreatment options, particularly in previously irradiated areas.

The matched-pair study comparing MR-HIFU to radiation therapy confirmed these different response patterns, showing significantly faster pain relief with HIFU at 1–2 weeks, with comparable efficacy emerging at 1–3 months [2]. This temporal difference may prove critical for patients with severe pain or limited life expectancy, where rapid symptom control significantly impacts quality of life.

Compared to other ablation methods such as radiofrequency, microwave, and cryoablation, HIFU offers unique advantages stemming from its completely noninvasive nature. While these other techniques require percutaneous needle insertion—with attendant risks of bleeding, infection, and tumor seeding—HIFU eliminates these concerns entirely. This distinction proves particularly valuable for patients who have coagulopathies, are immunocompromised, or have prior complications from invasive procedures. Moreover, the extracorporeal nature of the energy source used in HIFU allows for precise modulation of both the shape and size of the treatment area, adapting to the extent and geometry of the target lesion. This represents a fundamental difference from percutaneous techniques, where the ablation zone has a fixed shape and volume, typically forming concentrically around the applicator.

The guidance systems employed also differ substantially between modalities. MR-HIFU offers real-time thermal mapping that provides quantitative feedback during treatment—a capability lacking in most conventional ablation approaches. This feedback allows precise energy titration to achieve therapeutic temperatures while minimizing collateral damage. However, HIFU's accessibility remains limited by acoustic access requirements, whereas other ablation techniques can reach most lesions, including those in the spine, that might be inaccessible to ultrasound energy.

For appropriate cases, HIFU may offer an alternative to surgical intervention, particularly for patients with high operative risk or those declining surgery. The outpatient nature of most HIFU procedures, minimal recovery time, and low complication rate contrast favorably with the inpatient admission, significant recovery period, and higher complication risks associated with surgical management. However, surgery maintains essential advantages for mechanical stabilization and fracture prevention/treatment in weight-bearing bones—functions that HIFU cannot provide. Consequently, HIFU remains primarily indicated for non-weight-bearing bones or lesions with low fracture risk when considered as an alternative to surgical approaches.

7.12 Combined Treatment Approaches

Emerging evidence suggests substantial benefits may derive from combining HIFU with other treatment modalities, leveraging complementary mechanisms of action to enhance overall therapeutic effects. These integrated approaches may offer synergistic benefits that exceed those of individual treatment modalities used sequentially or in isolation.

The combination of HIFU and radiation therapy represents one of the most promising integrative strategies. The complementary mechanisms suggest potential synergistic effects: HIFU provides rapid pain relief through periosteal denervation, while radiation therapy contributes sustained tumor control through different cytotoxic pathways. Beyond sequential benefits, HIFU-induced hyperthermia may enhance radiation effectiveness through several mechanisms, including increased tumor oxygenation, inhibition of DNA repair, and enhanced immune recognition of tumor cells. This radiosensitizing effect potentially enables dose reduction in radiation therapy when combined with HIFU, limiting cumulative radiation exposure.

Initial clinical evidence supporting this combined approach has emerged from several studies. A feasibility study evaluated combined MR-HIFU and radiation therapy in six patients with painful bone metastases [23]. Their findings demonstrated both safety and promising efficacy, with 83% of patients experiencing significant pain response at 7 days and 60% maintaining response at 4 weeks posttreatment. No treatment-related severe adverse events were observed, supporting the feasibility of this combined approach.

The ongoing FURTHER trial (Focused Ultrasound and RadioTHERapy for non-invasive palliative pain treatment in patients with bone metastasis) represents a critical step in evaluating this integrated strategy. This European Union-funded multicenter three-arm randomized trial compares MR-HIFU alone, radiation therapy alone, and combined treatment for first-line management of painful bone metastases. Results from this landmark study will provide valuable insights into the relative efficacy and optimal sequencing of these complementary treatment modalities.

Combining HIFU with systemic therapies presents another promising avenue for enhanced management of bone lesions. The integration of HIFU with chemotherapy has shown particularly encouraging results in primary bone tumors. Wang's randomized study of osteosarcoma treatment demonstrated significantly improved response and survival rates when HIFU was added to conventional chemotherapy [21]. This synergy likely results from multiple mechanisms: HIFU provides local tumor control while chemotherapy addresses micrometastatic disease, HIFU-induced hyperthermia may enhance drug delivery to the tumor site, and thermal ablation potentially reduces tumor burden to improve chemotherapy efficacy against remaining viable cells.

For patients receiving targeted therapies, HIFU offers complementary local tumor debulking while maintaining systemic treatment. This approach may reduce the burden on systemic therapy, potentially delaying resistance development or allowing dose modifications to manage side effects while maintaining disease control. Emerging evidence also suggests HIFU may induce immunomodulatory effects that could enhance immunotherapy efficacy. Studies have documented increases in TNF-α, IL-2, and IL-8 following HIFU treatment, changes that may favorably condition the tumor microenvironment for enhanced checkpoint inhibitor activity, though clinical validation of these effects requires further investigation.

The combination of bone-targeted agents such as bisphosphonates or denosumab with HIFU represents another logical integration of complementary mechanisms. While HIFU provides rapid pain control and local tumor ablation, bone-targeted agents offer systemic prevention of skeletal-related events through inhibition of osteoclast activity. This comprehensive approach addresses both symptomatic lesions and prevention of new skeletal complications, potentially offering more complete management of metastatic bone disease. However, formal studies of this combined approach remain limited, highlighting an area for future clinical investigation.

7.13 Future Perspectives and Emerging Applications

The evolution of HIFU technology continues to expand its potential applications for malignant bone lesions, with several technological developments poised to overcome current limitations and extend treatment capabilities. Advanced imaging integration stands at the forefront of these innovations, with the fusion of multiple imaging modalities enhancing planning precision and treatment guidance. Development of alternative temperature monitoring techniques specifically adapted for bone tissue may overcome current thermometry limitations, while real-time tumor response assessment tools could enable dynamic treatment adaptation based on observed biological effects.

Treatment planning algorithms continue to advance, with automated segmentation and planning systems reducing operator dependence and improving consistency. Simulation-based optimization of treatment parameters using acoustic and thermal modeling promises more precise energy delivery tailored to individual lesion characteristics. Perhaps most importantly, patient-specific treatment planning based on bone density and tumor characteristics will allow truly personalized approaches that maximize therapeutic benefit while minimizing complications.

Hardware innovations further expand HIFU's potential applications. More flexible transducer designs enable better anatomical access to previously challenging locations, while higher power systems facilitate faster treatments, reducing procedure duration and improving patient tolerance. Smaller, more portable systems increase accessibility of this technology, potentially extending its benefits to broader patient populations, including those in resource-limited settings.

Several emerging applications may substantially expand HIFU's role in managing malignant bone lesions. Histotripsy—a non-thermal mechanical ablation technique using focused ultrasound—offers potential advantages for sclerotic lesions that respond less favorably to conventional thermal ablation. By mechanically fractionating tissue through controlled cavitation, histotripsy may overcome the limitations of thermal approaches in certain lesion types. Initial preclinical results in canine osteosarcoma models have shown promise [24], suggesting potential clinical applications in the future.

Drug delivery enhancement using HIFU represents another frontier with significant potential. Techniques originally developed for HIFU-induced blood-brain barrier opening have been adapted for enhancing therapeutic delivery to bone tumors. By transiently increasing vascular and cellular permeability through mechanical effects, HIFU may enhance the delivery of chemotherapeutic agents, immunotherapies, or radiopharmaceuticals to bone lesions. This approach potentially allows reduced systemic dosing while maintaining or improving local efficacy, limiting side effects while preserving therapeutic benefit.

The immunomodulatory effects of HIFU have gained increasing attention as potential mechanisms for enhancing systemic tumor control. Emerging evidence suggests HIFU may enhance tumor antigen presentation through the release of damage-associated molecular patterns and tumor-specific antigens following thermal ablation. This immunogenic cell death potentially enhances recognition by the immune system, creating opportunities for synergy with immunotherapeutic approaches. Initial evidence of cytokine modulation following HIFU treatment supports this concept, though further research is needed to optimize protocols for maximizing immunogenic effects.

Current research suggests potential expansion of HIFU indications beyond current applications. Advancements in spine applications represent a particularly significant frontier, with the development of techniques for safe treatment of vertebral metastases potentially opening treatment options for patients with this common and challenging disease manifestation. Preliminary studies on posterior elements have demonstrated feasibility, while ongoing refinement of planning techniques to avoid spinal cord injury continues to improve safety profiles for these applications.

Perhaps most ambitiously, the application of HIFU with curative intent in carefully selected cases of oligometastatic disease has been proposed. Through complete ablation of solitary metastases in conjunction with effective systemic therapy, this approach aims to achieve durable disease control or even cure in highly selected patients. Integration of HIFU into multimodal treatment approaches for definitive management of oligometastatic disease represents an evolving paradigm that may fundamentally change treatment goals from palliation to cure for specific patient subgroups.

7.14 Conclusion

High-intensity focused ultrasound has emerged as a valuable therapeutic option for the management of malignant bone lesions. Its noninvasive nature, excellent safety profile, and demonstrated efficacy for pain palliation position it as an important addition to the interventional radiologist's armamentarium. The rapid onset of pain relief—typically within days rather than the weeks required for radiation therapy—offers particular advantages for patients with severe symptoms or limited life expectancy.

Beyond pain palliation, growing evidence supports HIFU's efficacy for local tumor control and improvement in bone quality through remineralization. These effects extend its potential applications from purely palliative interventions to tumor-directed therapy with potential impact on disease progression. The integration of HIFU with other treatment modalities, including radiation therapy, systemic treatments, and bone-targeted agents, offers promising avenues for enhanced therapeutic effects through complementary mechanisms of action.

Technological advancements continue to expand HIFU capabilities and overcome current limitations. Improvements in imaging integration, treatment planning algorithms, and hardware design enhance treatment precision and accessibility. Emerging applications such as histotripsy, drug delivery enhancement, and immunomodulation further broaden the potential clinical impact of this technology.

While challenges remain—particularly regarding acoustic access limitations, temperature monitoring in bone tissue, and optimal patient selection criteria—ongoing research and clinical experience continue to refine approaches to these issues. The favorable risk-benefit profile of HIFU treatment supports its integration into comprehensive management strategies for malignant bone lesions.

References

1. Hurwitz MD, Ghanouni P, Kanaev SV, et al. Magnetic resonance-guided focused ultrasound for patients with painful bone metastases: phase III trial results. J Natl Cancer Inst. 2014;106(5)
2. Lee HL, Kuo CC, Tsai JT, Chen CY, Wu MH, Chiou JF. Magnetic resonance-guided focused ultrasound versus conventional radiation therapy for painful bone metastasis: a matched-pair study. J Bone Joint Surg Am. 2017;99(18):1572–8.
3. Huisman M, Ter Haar G, Napoli A, et al. International consensus on use of focused ultrasound for painful bone metastases: current status and future directions. Int J Hyperth. 2015;31(3):251–9.
4. Baal JD, Chen WC, Baal U, Wagle S, Baal JH, Link TM, Bucknor MD. Efficacy and safety of magnetic resonance-guided focused ultrasound for the treatment of painful bone metastases: a systematic review and meta-analysis. Skeletal Radiol. 2021;50(12):2459–69.
5. Napoli A, Anzidei M, Marincola BC, et al. MR Imaging-guided focused ultrasound for treatment of bone metastasis. Radiographics. 2013;33(6):1555–68.
6. Napoli A, Anzidei M, Marincola BC, et al. Primary pain palliation and local tumor control in bone metastases treated with magnetic resonance-guided focused ultrasound. Investig Radiol. 2013;48(6):351–8.

7. De Maio A, Alfieri G, Mattone M, Ghanouni P, Napoli A. High-intensity focused ultrasound surgery for tumor ablation: a review of current applications. Radiology: Imaging. Cancer. 2024;6(1)
8. Li S, Peng Y, Weinhandl ED, et al. Estimated number of prevalent cases of metastatic bone disease in the US adult population. Clin Epidemiol. 2012;4:87–93.
9. Tsukamoto S, Kido A, Tanaka Y, et al. Current overview of treatment for metastatic bone disease. Curr Oncol. 2021;28(5):3347–72.
10. Siedek F, Yeo SY, Heijman E, et al. Magnetic resonance-guided high-intensity focused ultrasound (mr-hifu): technical background and overview of current clinical applications (Part 1). Rofo. 2019;191(6):522–30.
11. Khokhlova VA, Fowlkes JB, Roberts WW, et al. Histotripsy methods in mechanical disintegration of tissue: towards clinical applications. Int J Hyperth. 2015;31(2):145–62.
12. Scipione R, Anzidei M, Bazzocchi A, Gagliardo C, Catalano C, Napoli A. HIFU for bone metastases and other musculoskeletal applications. Semin Intervent Radiol. 2018;35(4):261–7.
13. Yeo SY, Bratke G, Grüll H. High intensity focused ultrasound for treatment of bone malignancies – 20 years of history. Cancer. 2023;15(1):108.
14. Mirels H. Metastatic disease in long bones. A proposed scoring system for diagnosing impending pathologic fractures. Clin Orthop Relat Res. 1989;249:256–64.
15. Han X, Huang R, Meng T, Yin H, Song D. The roles of magnetic resonance-guided focused ultrasound in pain relief in patients with bone metastases: a systemic review and meta-analysis. Front Oncol. 2021;11:712230.
16. Chen ZQ, Wang CR, Ma XJ, et al. Evaluation of quality of life using EORTC QLQ-BM22 in patients with bone metastases after treatment with magnetic resonance guided focused ultrasound. Orthop Surg. 2018;10(3):264–71.
17. Wang Y, Wang W, Tang J. Primary malignant tumours of the bony pelvis: US-guided high intensity focused ultrasound ablation. Int J Hyperth. 2013;29(7):683–7.
18. Gianfelice D, Gupta C, Kucharczyk W, Bret P, Havill D, Clemons M. Palliative treatment of painful bone metastases with MR imaging-guided focused ultrasound. Radiology. 2008;249(1):355–63.
19. Chen W, Zhu H, Zhang L, et al. Primary bone malignancy: effective treatment with high-intensity focused ultrasound ablation. Radiology. 2010;255(3):967–78.
20. Li C, Wu P, Zhang L, Fan W, Huang J, Zhang F. Osteosarcoma: limb salvaging treatment by ultrasonographically guided high-intensity focused ultrasound. Cancer Biol Ther. 2009;8(12):1102–8.
21. Wang C. Therapeutic Effects of adriamycin combined with high-intensity focused ultrasound on osteosarcoma. J Balk Union Oncol. 2019;24(2):826–31.
22. Harding D, Giles SL, Brown MRD, et al. Evaluation of quality of life outcomes following palliative treatment of bone metastases with magnetic resonance-guided high intensity focused ultrasound: an international multicentre study. Clin Oncol. 2018;30(4):233–42.
23. Bartels MMTJ, Verpalen IM, Ferrer CJ, et al. Combining radiotherapy and focused ultrasound for pain palliation of cancer induced bone pain; a stage I/IIa study according to the IDEAL framework. Clin Transl Radiat Oncol. 2021;27:57–63.
24. Arnold L, Hendricks-Wenger A, Coutermarsh-Ott S, et al. Histotripsy ablation of bone tumors: feasibility study in excised canine osteosarcoma tumors. Ultrasound Med Biol. 2021;47(12):3435–46.

Irreversible Electroporation

8

Claudio Pusceddu, Claudio Cau, and Salvatore Marsico

8.1 Introduction

Irreversible electroporation (IRE) is a method of nonthermal ablation that uses high voltage electrical pulses to change the permeability of the cell membrane, leading to cell death. The nonthermal mechanism of action is a motivating factor behind using IRE for the ablation of lesions. Current clinical applications include treating lesions in the prostate, liver, and pancreas as well as sarcomas and desmoid tumors. Given the body of evidence supporting its safety and efficacy for various clinical uses, IRE is considered well-studied, especially in the field of urology. The use of IRE in humans was first published in 2010 and reported the use of IRE for prostate cancer [1]. The procedure was well tolerated by the 16 patients under study with no reported complications. Postoperative biopsies performed three weeks post-procedure confirmed no residual cancer in the treated area. A specific device for the IRE procedure, the NanoKnife System (AngioDynamics, Latham, NY, USA), received 510 k clearance by the US Food and Drug Administration (FDA) in 2008 for surgical ablation of soft tissue. While the technology has been in use since 2008, it has been updated and refined over time.

Additionally, the amount of evidence supporting the safety and efficacy of IRE for the treatment of prostate cancer has increased dramatically since the first

C. Pusceddu (✉)
Department of Radiology, Mater Olbia Hospital, Olbia, Cagliari, Italy

Interventional Oncology Institute, Barcelona, Spain

C. Cau
Department of Radiology, Mater Olbia Hospital, Olbia, Italy

S. Marsico
Department of Radiology, Hospital del Mar, Barcelona, Spain

Interventional Oncology Institute, Barcelona, Spain

C. Pusceddu, S. Marsico (eds.), *Malignant Bone Lesions and Beyond*,
https://doi.org/10.1007/978-3-032-00018-7_8

in-human studies. As a result, the United Kingdom National Institute for Health and Care Excellence (NICE) published a guidance specifically about IRE for prostate cancer in 2023, concluding that the procedure works and there are no major safety concerns in the short- and medium term [2]. IRE was also included as an investigational treatment option in the EAU–EANM–ESTRO–ESUR–ISUP–SIOG Guidelines on Prostate Cancer. In addition to prostate cancer, the literature supports the use of IRE in other surgical applications. For example, in recognition of the unique mechanism of action of IRE and given the evidence supporting its use, the NanoKnife System received an FDA Breakthrough Device Designation for the treatment of pancreatic cancer in 2018. Multiple studies have demonstrated the safety of IRE for tumor ablation near critical structures, including vascular, biliary, nervous, and urinary structures, better than conventional thermal ablative techniques [3–5] When treating lesions in the liver, thermal ablation risks damaging large vessels, bile ducts, gall bladder, hepatic capsule, and other organs [6]. IRE is a viable treatment option for both primary liver cancer and colorectal liver metastases [7] when these lesions are not good candidates for surgical resection and thermal ablative techniques. For prostate cancer, the use of IRE can reduce treatment side effects common with radical treatments, such as urinary incontinence, erectile dysfunction, and bowel problems, by preserving vital structures [3–5]. In some cases, IRE can be used for lesions treated unsuccessfully by thermal ablation or previously viewed as unresectable [8]. For pancreatic cancer, tumors are often unresectable due to their location near vital structures. IRE provides a treatment option for patients with advanced disease whose tumors are not amenable to surgical resection and has also been shown to prolong overall survival [9]. [10] IRE can also be used for margin accentuation for resectable tumors to achieve a microscopic negative margin. With its nonthermal mechanism of action, the IRE ablation zone is not subject to the heat-sink effect and can preserve adjacent vital structures, making it an attractive option for unresectable tumors. Thus far, the clinical evidence supports the safety and efficacy of IRE in the short- and medium term.

8.2 Mechanism of Action

The cell membrane is selectively permeable to ions and organic molecules and controls the movement of substances in and out of cells. Certain electrical fields, when applied across a cell, can permeabilize the cell membrane through a process that was named electroporation [11].

Electroporation can be simply described as the process of creating nanopores on the cell membrane using an electrical field (Fig. 8.1).

The image illustrates three major types of molecular transport across the cell membrane. **Simple diffusion** allows small nonpolar molecules to move directly through the lipid bilayer without the need for transport proteins. **Facilitated diffusion** involves specific membrane transporter proteins that enable the passive movement of polar or larger molecules along their concentration gradient. **Primary active transport** requires energy from ATP hydrolysis to move molecules against

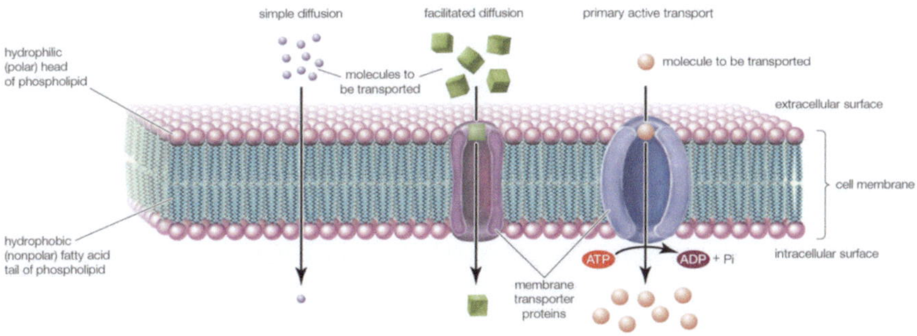

Fig. 8.1 Mechanisms of membrane transport across the lipid bilayer

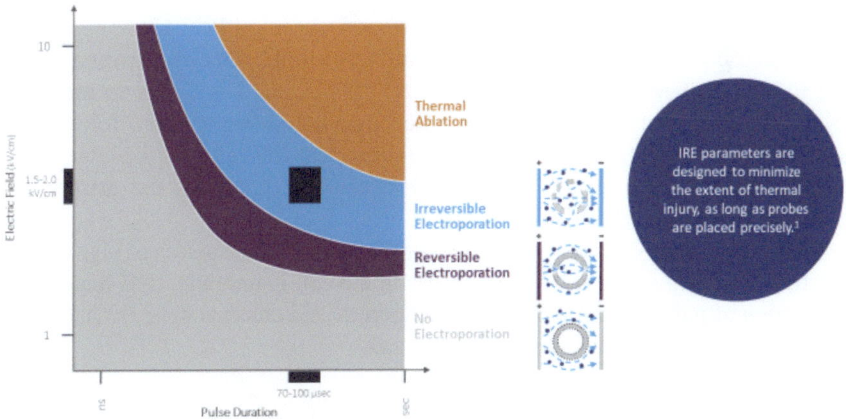

Fig. 8.2 Electroporation-based tissue response as a function of electric field and pulse duration

their concentration gradient through membrane-bound ATPase transporters. The lipid bilayer is composed of **phospholipids**, with hydrophilic (polar) heads facing the aqueous environments and hydrophobic (nonpolar) fatty acid tails oriented inward.

As a function of field amplitude and duration, permeabilization can be either reversible or irreversible [12]. In the case of IRE, after delivering high-voltage pulses above a sufficient threshold, the cells within the electrical field are irreversibly damaged (Fig. 8.2).

The diagram illustrates the relationship between electric field strength (y-axis) and pulse duration (x-axis) in determining the biological effects of electroporation. At lower field intensities and shorter durations, no electroporation occurs (gray area). **Reversible electroporation** (purple) enables temporary membrane permeability, typically used for drug or gene delivery. **Irreversible electroporation (IRE)** (blue) induces permanent membrane disruption, leading to cell death while preserving extracellular matrix structure, and is the therapeutic target in IRE-based ablation. At higher energy levels and prolonged pulse durations, **thermal ablation** (orange) dominates, leading to coagulative necrosis. The schematic on the right highlights the zones of tissue response based on electrode placement, and emphasizes that appropriate IRE parameters are designed to minimize collateral thermal injury.

The electric field changes the electrochemical potential across the cell membrane and induces instabilities in the polarized cell membrane lipid bilayer. The unstable membrane then alters its shape, forming aqueous pathways that possibly are nanoscale pores through the membrane. Electroporation is commonly used in medicine and biotechnology to introduce nonpermeable chemical species across the cell membrane, ranging from small molecules such as fluorescent dyes, drugs, and radioactive tracers to high molecular weight molecules such as antibodies, enzymes, nucleic acids, and DNA (Fig. 8.3) [13].

The image illustrates the sequence of events induced by IRE. Upon application of an electric field (E), targeted cells undergo **irreversible electroporation**, resulting in the permanent disruption of the cell membrane. This leads to **apoptosis** (within hours), characterized by controlled membrane degradation, followed by **phagocytosis** (over days), where immune cells clear the resulting cellular debris. Unlike thermal ablation, this nonthermal mechanism preserves the extracellular matrix and avoids coagulative necrosis.

IRE uses a direct current (DC) generator that creates short pulses of high-voltage electric current to create irreversible pores in the cell membrane. IRE requires the generation of pulses of up to 3000 V of amplitude and currents up to 50 A [14].

The electrical pulse parameters for IRE are:

- Number of pulses: 20 + 70/80 (90–100 in total)
- Length: 70–90 μs
- Electric Field amplitude: 1500 V/cm

The number of probes that are used during an IRE procedure is dependent on the size and the shape of the desired zone of tissue ablation. Also, because the

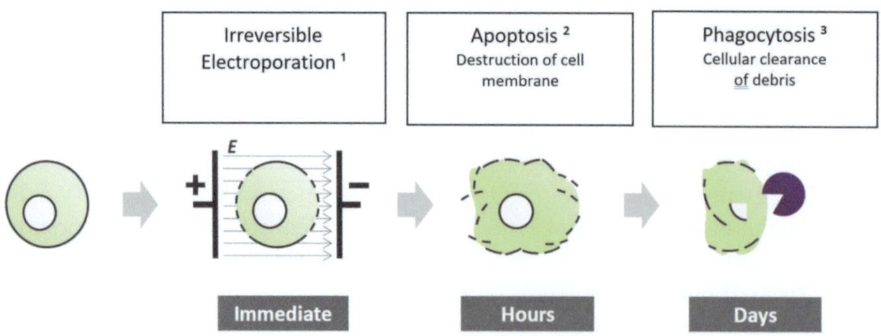

Fig. 8.3 Cellular response timeline following irreversible electroporation (IRE)

amplitude and the gradient of the field depend on the applied voltage as well as on the distance between the electrodes, the treatment parameter for voltage is dependent on the distance between probes within the targeted tissue [15]. A dedicated ECG needs to be used to synchronize IRE pulses with the refractory period of the cardiac rhythm in order to minimize the risk of arrhythmias.

Additionally, conventional thermal ablation techniques may result in the "heat-sink effect," in which perivascular tissues are not completely ablated, leading to incomplete tumor ablation. As a nonthermal ablation technique, IRE is not limited by this phenomenon [16]. IRE lesions show a sharp demarcation between ablated and nonablated tissues, while thermal ablation techniques show a transitional zone of partially damaged tissue where insufficient temperatures were reached [17].

Lastly, treatment with IRE may be faster than other techniques as ablation occurs in seconds rather than minutes due to the use of high-speed electrical currents rather than heat or cold as used in other ablative techniques. Therefore, the time needed to complete the procedure is largely determined by the time it takes to place the ablation probes rather than the ablation itself [18]. A typical IRE procedure for a solid tumor, with a size of approximately 3 cm in diameter, uses 90 pulses with an ultra-short pulse length of 100 microseconds. A single pair of electrode probes takes approximately two minutes, depending on the patient's heart rate. Therefore, even with a pullback ablation technique, total IRE treatment is approximately 6–12 minutes. This is possible due to the utilization of extremely high-speed electric currents as a means of creating cell death, whereas other ablation techniques use hot or cold temperatures.

8.3 Clinical Use of IRE in Liver

Hepatocellular carcinoma (HCC) is one of the most frequently occurring solid tumors worldwide [19]. While surgical resection and liver transplantation are often curative treatment options, the vast majority of patients are not eligible due to factors including comorbidities, liver function reserve, tumor stage, and location and size of tumors. Percutaneous ablation was established as a treatment approach for hepatic tumors that are unresectable [20].

Common techniques such as radiofrequency ablation (RFA) and microwave ablation (MWA) are based on heat-induced damage, which are limited by the heat-sink effect when treating lesions near major vessels and the potential for damaging the tissue of other nearby structures. For lesions located near critical structures, IRE is an appealing alternative due to its nonthermal mechanism of action. IRE is included in the National Comprehensive Cancer Network (NCCN) Clinical Practice Guidelines for HCC due to these advantages over RFA [21].

An initial ablate-and-resect study (COLDFIRE-1) in ten patients with colorectal cancer liver metastases (CRLM) demonstrated that IRE applied two hours prior to resection was associated with cell death and necrosis of the metastases [22]. A phase II study (COLDFIRE-2) showed that in 51 patients with CRLM $\leq$5.0 cm, at 12 months, 68% were alive without local recurrence, and the local control rate after retreatment was 74% [23]. Such data show that IRE may be an effective treatment for CRLM unsuitable for resection or thermal ablation. Other studies including patients with both primary and secondary liver cancer suggest differences in key outcomes like overall survival between these patient populations.

Niessen et al. conducted a long-term survival analysis of 71 patients with inoperable malignant hepatic tumors with a median follow-up time of 35.7 months [24]. Approximately half of the patients had primary liver tumors (HCC and cholangiocellular carcinoma), and the other half had secondary liver cancer (CRLM or other liver metastases). The median overall survival of patients with primary liver cancer and secondary liver cancer was 26.8 months and 19.9 months, respectively, though this difference was not statistically significant. An average survival time of 24.3 months was reported for CRLM, which is more favorable than previously reported survival times ranging from 18 to 21.7 months for patients with CRLM receiving palliative chemotherapy [25]. [26]

In one of the largest multicenter studies to date, Fruhling et al. reported on 149 patients in Sweden with HCC or CRLM with a median follow-up time of 58 months [27]. Median overall survival was 35.0 months and 27.0 months, for HCC and CRLM, respectively. Local ablation success, defined as no evidence of residual or recurrent tumor within 10 mm from the ablated tumor, at 6 and 12 months, was 58.3% and 40.3% for HCC, and 37.7% and 25.4% for CRLM. Less than one-fifth of patients in the study had a complication. While Overall Survival (OS) and ablation success were lower than previous reports for RFA and MWA, this finding is likely explained by the severity of the disease in patients treated with IRE. The authors concluded that this study further demonstrated that IRE is a safe ablation modality for patients with liver tumors that are not suitable for surgery or thermal ablation.

Gupta et al. conducted a meta-analysis of the safety and efficacy of IRE for liver malignancies, including 25 studies ($n = 776$) [28]. The pooled overall survival at 6, 12, 24, and 36 months was 93.28%, 81.29%, 61.47%, and 40.88%, respectively, with better overall survival at 12 and 36 months for HCC. The overall complication rate was 23.7% with major complications occurring in 6.9% of patients. Pooled overall survival estimates were lower than what was previously reported for RFA and MWA, which is explained by the fact that patients are generally selected for IRE when thermal ablation is contraindicated. As the literature on IRE for the treatment of hepatic lesions continues to evolve, formal comparisons to other ablative techniques are warranted. While the current evidence supports potential benefit for patients, the clinical use of IRE continues to develop as more patients are treated.

8.4 Clinical Use of IRE in Pancreas

Pancreatic cancer is the third leading cause of cancer death in the United States with a 5-year survival rate of 12.5% [29]. While the 5-year survival rate is higher following resection of the tumor, only about 15–20% of pancreatic cancers are resectable [29]. [30] Treatment is complex for patients with locally advanced pancreatic cancer (LAPC), defined by involvement of nearby vessels without metastases.

Historically, unresectable LAPC had a poor median overall survival ranging from 9 to 16 months depending on the treatment regimen [31]. [32] IRE is a viable treatment option for patients with LAPC due to its nonthermal mechanism of action, which allows for the ablation of tumors while preserving surrounding vital structures and avoiding the heat-sink effect. There are currently two uses of IRE: in situ IRE for the ablation of unresectable lesions and margin accentuation, which is used when resection is feasible, but there is concern for positive margins.

Martin et al. conducted a prospective registry study of 200 patients with LAPC, with 150 patients undergoing IRE alone and 50 with pancreatic resection plus IRE for margin accentuation using the open approach [33]. The median overall survival from diagnosis was 24.9 months, which doubled previous reports of overall survival for patients treated with chemotherapy or radiation therapy alone. Results from this study were confirmed by the American Hepato-Pancreato-Biliary Association (AHPBA) and the Pancreatic Registry study, a prospective, multinational study of patients with LAPC treated with IRE using the open approach [34]. Patients received induction chemotherapy and/or external beam radiation therapy per institutional protocol followed by in situ IRE or IRE with resection. A total of 152 patients were treated with a median overall survival from diagnosis of 30.7 months.

PANFIRE-2, a prospective, phase II trial, studied the safety and efficacy of percutaneous IRE for LAPC (n = 40) and locally recurring pancreatic cancer (n = 10) [35]. Median overall survival was 17 months from the diagnosis of LAPC and 16 months from the diagnosis of recurrence, which exceeded the target median OS for patients receiving no induction chemotherapy or gemcitabine-based induction chemotherapy (11.6 months) and for those receiving induction 5-fluorouracil, leucovorin, irinotecan, and oxaliplatin (FOLFIRINOX) (14.9 months), suggesting a survival benefit over standard of care.

In 2024, a multidisciplinary panel with IRE experts, surgeons, and interventional radiologists provided a guideline for IRE treatment in pancreas using a three-step modified Delphi Consensus [36]. Regardless of the relatively small panel, consensus was reached on 147/158 items (93%), which indicates unanimity on the recommendations regarding the number of preoperative cycle FOLFIRINOX (preferably four cycles), patient selection, contraindication, IRE procedure, and follow-up.

While registry studies and single-arm trials support the effectiveness of IRE for the treatment of LAPC, especially in combination with induction chemotherapy, and FOLFIRINOX in particular, comparative studies and ideally randomized controlled trials are needed to validate results. Two ongoing randomized controlled trials, the PAL-PIE study in the United Kingdom and the DIRECT study in the United States, will assess the efficacy of IRE plus chemotherapy vs. chemotherapy alone. Future research may also compare IRE performed through the open vs. percutaneous approach. As more patients are treated, IRE device(s) and the science behind them will continue to evolve and develop.

8.5 IRE in Musculoskeletal (MSK) and for Other Clinical Uses

IRE is an emerging treatment option for the ablation of musculoskeletal and soft tissue tumors in cases where surgery is not indicated (Figs. 4–8). An initial experiment using rabbit femurs was conducted to determine the ablation threshold of cortical bone and evaluate the ablated bone segment [37]. The results showed that IRE ablation preserved the structural integrity of the bone cortex, and the ablated area regenerated quickly, with revascularization appearing 4 weeks post-IRE and osteogenic activity peaking 8 weeks after IRE. Furthermore, the negative effects on bone mechanics resolved within 8 weeks. Currently, the literature on IRE for the treatment of bone tumors in humans is limited to case reports. In one case report, IRE was used as a curative treatment for Ewing's sarcoma in a 9-year-old girl [38]. While the results from animal models and case reports are promising, larger clinical studies are needed to establish the safety and efficacy of IRE for treating these conditions.

Another potential use of IRE is for the treatment of aggressive fibromatosis, or desmoid tumors. A small retrospective study of six patients with aggressive fibromatosis was treated with IRE. A total of eight tumors were treated, and 100% of the tumors achieved Choi partial response, though none met the criteria for Response Evaluation Criteria In Solid Tumors (RECIST) 1.1 partial response [39]. Five out of eight tumors met the RECIST criteria for progressive disease. Overall, this small study demonstrated that IRE may provide local control of aggressive fibromatosis, though recurrence is expected. Additional research is needed to understand the role of IRE for the treatment of desmoid tumors. Despite the limited data, IRE is included as a potential ablation technique in the NCCN Clinical Practice Guidelines for Soft Tissue Sarcoma, which covers desmoid tumors. As with any treatment option, the IRE device(s) have and will continue to evolve iteratively, and the science has and will continue to develop as more patients are treated.

8.6 Initial Clinical Applications of Irreversible Electroporation for Bone Metastases (Figs. 8.4, 8.5, 8.6, 8.7, and 8.8)

The patient was referred for percutaneous ablation and, after the interdisciplinary tumor board discussion, was selected for CT-guided IRE as a nonthermal, structurally preserving approach. Written informed consent was obtained for both the procedure and publication of data.

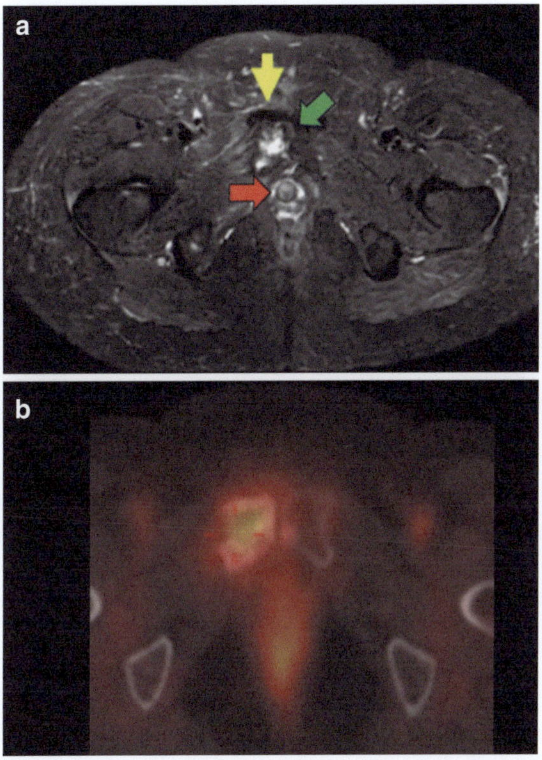

Fig. 8.4 A 55-year-old woman with a history of hormone receptor-positive, HER2-negative breast cancer, diagnosed in 2013, was initially managed with radical mastectomy, axillary dissection, adjuvant chemotherapy, radiotherapy, and long-term endocrine therapy. She later developed widespread osseous metastatic disease, managed palliatively with capecitabine. (**a**) Axial fat-suppressed T2-weighted (DP-FS) MR image of the pelvis demonstrating a hyperintense osteolytic lesion (yellow arrow) involving the **right pubic bone**. This anatomical relationship to adjacent critical structures, including the urethra (red arrow) and pubic symphysis (green arrow), was a key factor in selecting a nonthermal ablation approach (IRE). (**b**) Axial fused PET/CT image of the pelvis showing intense Fluorodeoxyglucose (FDG) uptake in a **lytic lesion of the** right pubic bone, consistent with metabolically active bone metastasis

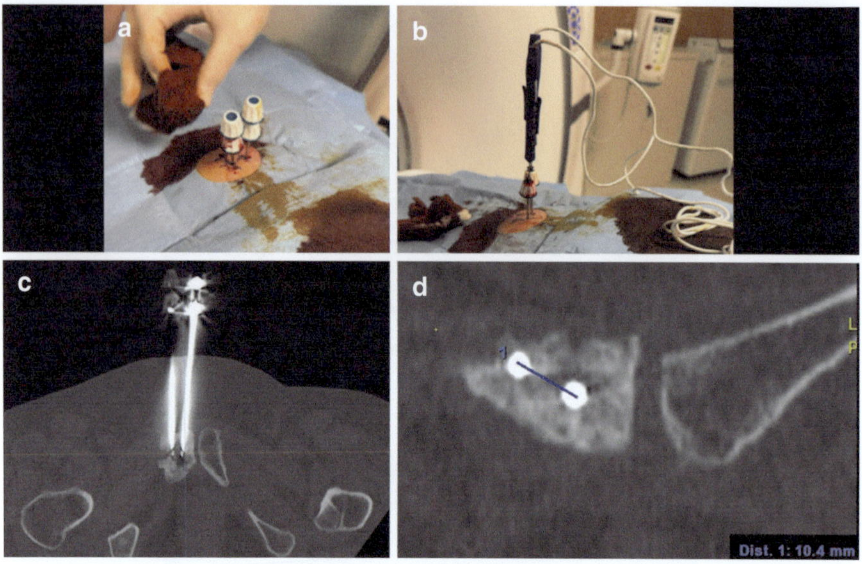

Fig. 8.5 (**a**) Intraoperative view of the sterile setup showing the insertion of two 12-gauge coaxial bone access cannulae for transosseous approach to the right pubic bone under CT guidance. (**b**) Intraoperative view showing coaxial insertion of the 19-gauge Nanoknife® IRE electrodes (AngioDynamics®) through the bone access cannulae. (**c**) Axial Maximum Intensity Projection (MIP) reconstruction showing aligned placement of the right-sided 19-gauge IRE electrode targeting the osteolytic metastasis. (**d**) Coronal CT reconstruction demonstrating that the two IRE electrodes are positioned at an appropriate distance from each other, ensuring correct inter-electrode spacing for optimal electric field distribution

Fig. 8.6 Axial fused PET/CT image obtained **3 months after IRE treatment** showing **complete metabolic response** of the previously treated pubic bone metastasis. No residual FDG uptake is observed at the ablation site, consistent with successful local tumor control

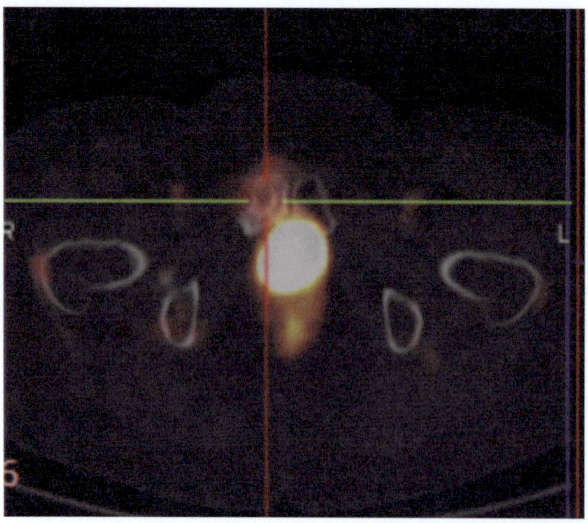

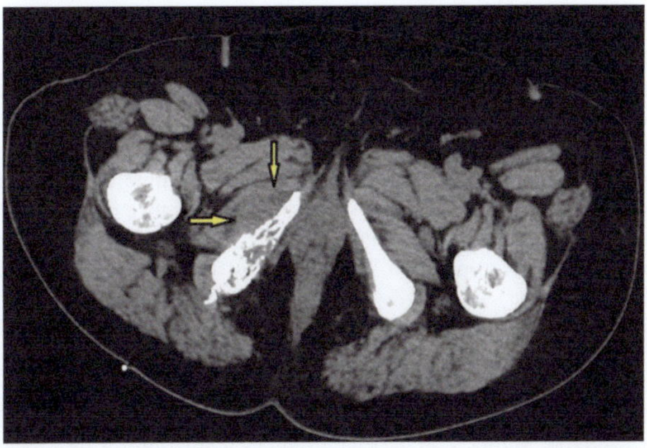

Fig. 8.7 A 62-year-old man with a history of prostate cancer was treated with radiotherapy. He developed a right ischial bone metastasis previously irradiated and was also treated with thermal ablation and cementoplasty, which initially provided pain relief. Recently, a painful and functionally limiting extraosseous component appeared (yellow arrows), leading to severe debilitation and inability to stand

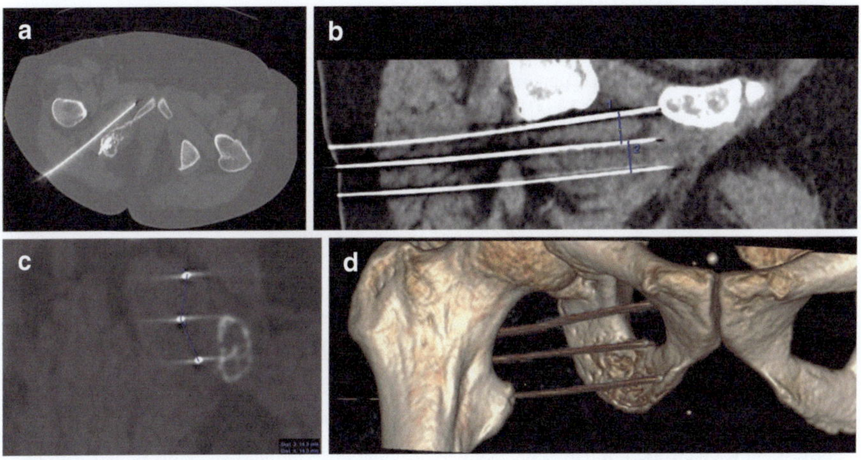

Fig. 8.8 CT-guided procedural images. (**a**) Axial CT image showing the correct positioning of a percutaneous needle within the ischiatic lesion. (**b**) Coronal reformation depicting the accurate placement of three irreversible electroporation (IRE) electrodes, well-spaced and aligned across the target lesion. (**c**) Sagittal MIP reconstruction confirming the optimal inter-electrode distances for effective IRE delivery. (**d**) Volume-rendered 3D reconstruction illustrating the final electrode configuration and spatial relationship with the periischiatic metastatic lesion

References

1. Onik G, Rubinsky B. Irreversible electroporation: first patient experience focal therapy of prostate cancer. In: Rubinsky B, editor. Irreversible electroporation, series in biomedical engineering. Berlin: Springer; 2010. p. 235–47.
2. National Institute for Health and Care Excellence. Irreversible electroporation for treating prostate cancer 2023.(NICEguideline IPG768). https://www.nice.org.uk/guidance/ipg768.
3. Lee EW, Chen C, Prieto VE, et al. Advanced hepatic ablation technique for creating complete cell death: irreversible electroporation. Radiology. 2010;255:426–33. https://doi.org/10.1148/radiol.10090337.
4. Maor E, et al. The effect of irreversible electroporation on blood vessels. Technol Cancer Res Treat. 2007;6(4):307–12. https://doi.org/10.1177/153303460700600407.
5. Narayanan G, Bhatia S, Echenique A, et al. Vessel patency post irreversible electroporation. Cardiovasc Intervent Radiol. 2014;37(6):1523–9. https://doi.org/10.1007/s00270-014-0988-9.
6. Teratani T, Yoshida H, Shiina S, et al. Radiofrequency ablation for hepatocellular carcinoma in so-called high-risk locations. Hepatology. 2006;43(5):1101–8. https://doi.org/10.1002/hep.21164.
7. Meijerink MR, Ruarus AH, Vroomen LGPH, et al. Irreversible electroporation to treat Unresectable colorectal liver metastases (COLDFIRE-2): a phase II, two-center, Single-arm clinical trial. Radiology. 2021;299(2):470–80. https://doi.org/10.1148/radiol.2021203089.
8. Rubinsky B, Onik G, Mikus P. Irreversible electroporation: a new ablation modality–clinical implications. Technol Cancer Res Treat. 2007;6:37–48. https://doi.org/10.1177/153303460700600106.
9. Holland MM, Bhutiani N, Kruse EJ, et al. A prospective, multi-institution assessment of irreversible electroporation for treatment of locally advanced pancreatic adenocarcinoma: initial outcomes from the AHPBA pancreatic registry. HPB (Oxford). 2019;21(8):1024–31. https://doi.org/10.1016/j.hpb.2018.12.004.
10. Martin RC 2nd, Kwon D, Chalikonda S, et al. Treatment of 200 locally advanced (stage III) pancreatic adenocarcinoma patients with irreversible electroporation: safety and efficacy. Ann Surg. 2015;262(3):486–94. https://doi.org/10.1097/SLA.0000000000001441.
11. Davalos, et al. Tissue ablation with irreversible electroporation. Ann Biomed Eng. 2005;33(2):223–31. https://doi.org/10.1007/s10439-005-8981-8.
12. Davalos, et al. Ann Biomed Eng. 2005;33(2):223–31.
13. Bertacchini C, Margotti PM, Bergamini E, Lodi A, Ronchetti M, Cadossi R. Design of an irreversible electroporation.
14. Pech M, Janitzky A, Wendler JJ, Strang C, Blaschke S, Dudeck O, et al. Irreversible electroporation of renal cell carcinoma: a first-in-man phase I clinical study. Cardiovasc Intervent Radiol. 2011;34:132.
15. Deodhar A, Dickfeld T, Single GW, Hamilton WC Jr, Thornton RH, Sofocleous CT, et al. Irreversible electroporation near the heart: ventricular arrhythmias can be prevented with ECG synchronization. AJR Am J Roentgenol. 2011;196:W330–5.
16. Onik, et al. Irreversible electroporation: implications for prostate ablation. Techn Cancer Res. 2007;6(4):1–6. https://doi.org/10.1177/153303460700600405. System for clinical use. Technol Cancer Res Treat. 2007;6:313–20.
17. Wagstaff PG, Buijs M, van den Bos W, et al. Irreversible electroporation: state of the art. Onco Targets Ther. 2016;9:2437–46. https://doi.org/10.2147/OTT.S88086.
18. Onik, et al. Irreversible electroporation: implications for prostate ablation. Techn Cancer Res. 2007;6(4):1–6. https://doi.org/10.1177/153303460700600405.
19. Siegel, et al. Cancer statistics, 2024. CA Cancer J Clin. 2024;2024(74):12–49. https://doi.org/10.3322/caac.21820.
20. Shiina et al. Percutaneous ablation for hepatocellular carcinoma: comparison of various ablation techniques and surgery. 2018. https://doi.org/10.1155/2018/4756147.

21. Benson et al. Hepatocellular Carcinoma, Version 2.2023, NCCN Clinical Practice Guidelines in Oncology. 2023. https://www.nccn.org/guidelines/guidelinesdetail?category=1&id=1514.
22. Scheffer et al. Ablation of colorectal liver metastases by irreversible electroporation: results of the COLDFIRE-I ablate-and-resect study. 2014. https://doi.org/10.1007/s00330-014-3259-x.
23. Meijerink, et al. Irreversible electroporation to treat Unresectable colorectal liver metastases (COLDFIRE-2): a phase II, two-center. Single-Arm Clinical Trial. 2021; https://doi.org/10.1148/radiol.2021203089.
24. Niessen et al. Percutaneous Irreversible Electroporation: Long-term survival analysis of 71 patients with inoperable malignant hepatic tumors, 2017. https://doi.org/10.1038/srep43687.
25. de Gramont A, et al. Leucovorin and fluorouracil with or without oxaliplatin as first-line treatment in advanced colorectal cancer. J Clin Oncol. 2000;18:2938–47. https://doi.org/10.1200/JCO.2000.18.16.2938.
26. Giacchetti S, et al. Phase III multicenter randomized trial of oxaliplatin added to chronomodulated fluorouracilleucovorin as first- line treatment of metastatic colorectal cancer. J Clin Oncol. 2000;18:136–47. https://doi.org/10.1200/JCO.2000.18.1.136.
27. Fruhling et al. Irreversible electroporation of hepatocellular carcinoma and colorectal cancer liver metastases: a nationwide multicenter study with short- and long-term follow up. 2023. https://doi.org/10.1016/j.ejso.2023.107046.
28. Gupta et al. Efficacy and safety of irreversible electroporation for malignant liver tumors: a systematic review and meta-analysis. 2021. https://doi.org/10.1007/s00330-021-07742-y.
29. Habermehl D, Brecht IC, Bergmann F, et al. Chemoradiation in patients with isolated recurrent pancreatic cancer-therapeutical efficacy and probability of re-resection. Radiat Oncol. 2013;31(8):27. https://doi.org/10.1186/1748-717X-8-27.
30. Varadhachary GR, Tamm EP, Abbruzzese JL, et al. Borderline resectable pancreatic cancer: definitions, management, and role of preoperative therapy. Ann Surg Oncol. 2006;13(8):1035–46. https://doi.org/10.1245/ASO.2006.08.011.
31. Loehrer PJ Sr, Feng Y, Cardenes H, et al. Gemcitabine alone versus gemcitabine plus radiotherapy in patients with locally advanced pancreatic cancer: an eastern cooperative oncology group trial. J Clin Oncol. 2011;29(31):4105–12. https://doi.org/10.1200/JCO.2011.34.8904.
32. Rombouts SJ, Walma MS, Vogel JA, et al. Systematic review of resection rates and clinical outcomes after FOLFIRINOX-based treatment in patients with locally advanced pancreatic cancer. Ann Surg Oncol. 2016;23(13):4352–60. https://doi.org/10.1245/s10434-016-5373-2.
33. Martin, et al. Treatment of 200 locally advanced (stage III) pancreatic adenocarcinoma patients with irreversible electroporation. Safety Efficacy. 2015; https://doi.org/10.1097/SLA.0000000000001441.
34. Holland et al. A prospective, multi-institution assessment of irreversible electroporation for treatment of locally advanced pancreatic adenocarcinoma: initial outcomes from the AHPBA pancreatic registry. 2019. https://doi.org/10.1016/j.hpb.2018.12.004.
35. Ruarus, et al. Percutaneous irreversible electroporation in locally advanced and recurrent pancreatic cancer (PANFIRE-2): a multicenter, prospective, Single-arm. Phase II Study. 2020; https://doi.org/10.1148/radiol.2019191109.
36. Vos, et al. Consensus guidelines of irreversible electroporation for pancreatic tumors: protocol standardization using the modified Delphi technique. Semin Intervent Radiol. 2024; https://doi.org/10.1055/s-0044-1787164.
37. Song et al. The effect of irreversible electroporation on the femur: experimental study in a rabbit model. 2015. https://doi.org/10.1038/srep18187
38. Steinbrecher K, Arslan B, Nassin ML, Kent P. Irreversible electroporation in the curative treatment of Ewing's sarcoma. BMJ Case Rep. 2016, 2016:bcr2016216585. https://doi.org/10.1136/bcr-2016-216585.
39. Maughan et al. Safety and efficacy of irreversible electroporation for aggressive fibromatosis: Initial experience. 2018. https://doi.org/10.1200/JCO.2018.36.15_suppl.e23549.

9 Embolization Techniques for Bone Tumors

Jacopo Scaggiante and Gregory Lock

9.1 Introduction

Treatment options for spinal bone tumors include surgery, radiotherapy, and in some cases, chemotherapy. The choice of treatment depends on various factors, including the type and location of the tumor, the patient's overall health, and the presence of neurological symptoms.

Surgery is often the preferred treatment for spinal tumors, especially those causing neurological compromise. However, surgical resection of spinal tumors, particularly those that are highly vascular, can be associated with significant blood loss. Excessive blood loss can obscure the surgical field, increase operative time, and potentially lead to complications such as hematoma formation and infection.

With recent medical advances, to mitigate the risks associated with blood loss during surgery, preoperative embolization has emerged as a valuable adjunctive procedure associated with improved surgical outcomes and easier facilitation of surgical resection [1].

9.2 Embolization for Spinal Bone Tumors

Embolization is a minimally invasive procedure that involves the selective occlusion of feeding vessels of hypervascular spinal lesions using various embolic agents. It is intended to promote devascularization and reduce blood flow to decrease the

J. Scaggiante (✉)
Department of Radiology, Radiation Oncology and Hematology, Fondazione Policlinico Universitario Agostino Gemelli IRCCS, Rome, Italy

G. Lock
Department of Radiology, Princess Alexandra Hospital, Woolloongabba, Australia

C. Pusceddu, S. Marsico (eds.), *Malignant Bone Lesions and Beyond*,
https://doi.org/10.1007/978-3-032-00018-7_9

risks of diffuse bleeding. In 1974, Benati et al. first introduced transarterial embolization of spinal lesions in four cases involving a spinal cord angioma, a hemangioma, a glomus tumor of the petrosal bone, and a dural vascular malformation of the occipital bone [2].

Since then, there have been significant advancements in embolization techniques, including the development of newer embolic agents, microcatheters, and improved imaging modalities. These advancements have led to increased safety and efficacy of the procedure, making it an integral part of the management of spinal tumors.

9.2.1 Benefits of Preoperative Endovascular Embolization

Preoperative embolization offers several benefits, including reduced intraoperative blood loss: By decreasing tumor vascularity, embolization helps minimize bleeding during surgery, leading to a clearer surgical field, shorter operative times, and a reduced need for blood transfusions. In patients who do not undergo preoperative embolization, intraoperative blood loss estimates range from 4350 to 8750 ml for various primary and secondary spinal tumors [3–5]. In contrast, in patients who undergo preoperative embolization, intraoperative blood loss estimates range from 300 to 4300 ml [3, 6, 7]. Patients who underwent preoperative embolization had a more favorable outcome than the patients who did not undergo preoperative embolization [8].

Improved surgical outcomes: Improved surgical outcomes are a key benefit of bone tumor embolization. By reducing blood loss and improving the visualization of the surgical field, embolization can contribute to complete tumor resection and better overall surgical outcomes [9].

Palliation of symptoms: In cases of unresectable tumors, embolization can be used as a palliative measure to reduce tumor size and alleviate symptoms such as pain and neurological deficits. This can start within 24 h of embolization and may last 3–9 months [10].

Facilitates complete tumor resection: Tumors that might have been considered too risky or difficult to remove before embolization could become resectable after the procedure. This is a major benefit for patients, as it opens up the possibility of a more complete treatment and potentially better outcomes [11].

Reduced mass effect and spinal cord compression: While embolization is primarily used to reduce blood loss during surgery, it can also have an effect on tumor size and spinal cord compression by causing tumor necrosis and shrinkage [12].

Slow tumor growth: Embolization of spinal tumors can slow tumor growth [13].

Reduced complications and surgical operating time: Reducing intraoperative bleeding improves visualization of the operative field and decreases complications and surgical operating time [14].

9.2.2 Preoperative Planning and Spinal Angiogram Technical Overview

Spinal digital subtraction angiography (DSA) remains the gold standard for the imaging of the arterial and venous systems supplying the spinal cord, nerve roots, vertebral bodies, and surrounding paraspinal tissues, guiding therapeutic interventions [15].

Real-time fluoroscopic imaging, coupled with digital subtraction techniques that eliminate bony and soft tissue structures, allows for the precise visualization of the arteriovenous system.

The anatomical complexity of the spinal vasculature contributes to the potentially lengthy duration of the procedure, particularly when a comprehensive evaluation is required.

Indeed, the human vertebral column, typically composed of 33 vertebrae (7 cervical, 12 thoracic, 5 lumbar, 5 sacral, and 4 coccygeal), is supplied by a segmental arrangement of arteries. Most vertebral levels receive one or two individual arteries that branch off the aorta or its segmental branches [16], such as the intercostal and lumbar arteries.

Thus, a comprehensive visualization of the entire spinal vasculature, requiring the selective catheterization and imaging of numerous individual arteries from the cervical to the sacral region, may be necessary in certain clinical scenarios, such as extensive vascular malformations or diffuse spinal arteriovenous shunts. However, for a more focused study of spinal tumors, targeting specific regions of the spine suspected to harbor pathology is often sufficient. A useful guiding principle is to visualize normal spinal cord vessels both above and below any identified lesion affecting the cord.

When a complete spinal angiogram is necessary, considering the relatively small caliber of the spinal arteries, general anesthesia may be required, especially if patients are uncomfortable maintaining an uncomfortable position for 1–2 h.

This minimizes patient movement, resulting in higher spatial resolution, but also allows for control of the patient's breathing and peristalsis, further reducing motion artifacts and optimizing image acquisition.

The procedural steps of spinal angiography follow a well-established protocol. The patient is carefully positioned on the angiography table. A thin, flexible catheter is introduced into the arterial system, most commonly via the femoral artery in the groin, using a minimally invasive percutaneous technique. Under fluoroscopic guidance, the catheter is advanced through the aorta to the level of the spinal arteries of interest. Various specialized catheters, with different shapes and sizes (see Table 9.1), are then employed to selectively catheterize individual spinal arteries, one after another.

Once the tip of the catheter is positioned within the target artery, a small amount of iodinated contrast material is carefully injected under fluoroscopy, acquiring

Table 9.1 Most commonly used catheters during spinal angiograms

Catheter	Size (French)	Primary use	Additional details
Angled taper	5F	Supra-aortic vessels	Excellent versatile catheter for vessels that branch from the main aortic artery
Mikaelsson	5F	Intercostal and lumbar arteries	Excellent general-purpose catheter for selecting specific segmental arteries
Simmons 1-2	5F	Intercostal and lumbar arteries	An alternate design to the Mikaelsson, possibly helpful in complex anatomical structures
Cobra 2	4F or 5F	Intercostal and lumbar arteries in younger patients	The smaller 4F size might be preferred for younger patients with narrower blood vessel diameters

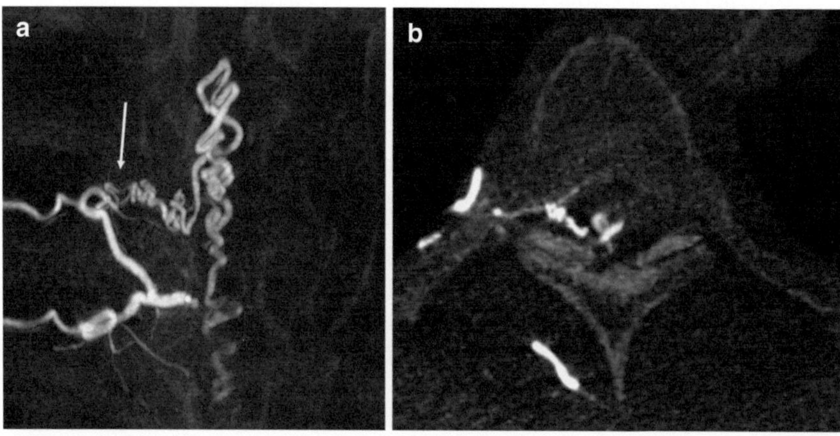

Fig. 9.1 High resolution cone-beam CT (DynaCT) obtained during spinal angiogram, showing a spinal dural arteriovenous fistula (oblique (**a**) and axial (**b**) reconstruction pointing at the foot of the fistula (arrow))

images during the contrast wash-in and wash-out phases to assess the vascular anatomy, flow characteristics, and the presence of any tumor angiographic blush [17]. In case of any doubts, especially for vascular malformations but also for spinal tumors, high-resolution cone-beam CT (HR-CBCT; Fig. 9.1 below) improves the understanding of the disease and helps guide therapeutic decisions [18].

Upon completion of the angiographic runs, the catheter is carefully withdrawn from the arterial system. The access site in the femoral artery is then closed using either manual compression or by the deployment of a vascular closure device.

Ideally, diagnostic spinal angiography can be integrated with therapeutic neurointerventional procedures. Indeed, if a tumor lesion is identified during the diagnostic angiogram, the interventional neuroradiologist may proceed with treatment, such as embolization, reducing the need for separate procedures.

9.2.3 Practical Anatomy and Vascular Supply

Although the fundamental principles of spinal angiography apply broadly, a detailed understanding of regional spinal vascular anatomy is essential for optimizing the procedure, ensuring accurate interpretation, and minimizing complications [19].

Evaluation of spinal cord vascularization frequently requires selective angiography [20], targeting specific arteries based on the vertebral level being examined. The arteries selected for catheterization vary by region:

Cervical region: Typically involves the vertebral arteries, along with branches originating from the thyrocervical (i.e., ascending cervical artery) and costocervical trunks (i.e., deep cervical artery) of the subclavian arteries, or branches of the external carotid artery (i.e., occipital or ascending pharyngeal artery) for upper cervical lesions.

Thoracic and lumbar regions: The intercostal and lumbar arteries, respectively, are the primary vascular feeders to the spinal cord and vertebrae at these levels. Identification of the artery of Adamkiewicz (AKA) is critical.

Sacral region: Vascular supply involves contributions from the lateral and medial sacral arteries.

Precise identification of the artery of Adamkiewicz (AKA) is critical during procedures involving the thoracolumbar spine (Fig. 9.2). The AKA provides the major blood supply to the anterior spinal cord in this segment, and its iatrogenic injury during surgery or angiography can lead to devastating complications, including

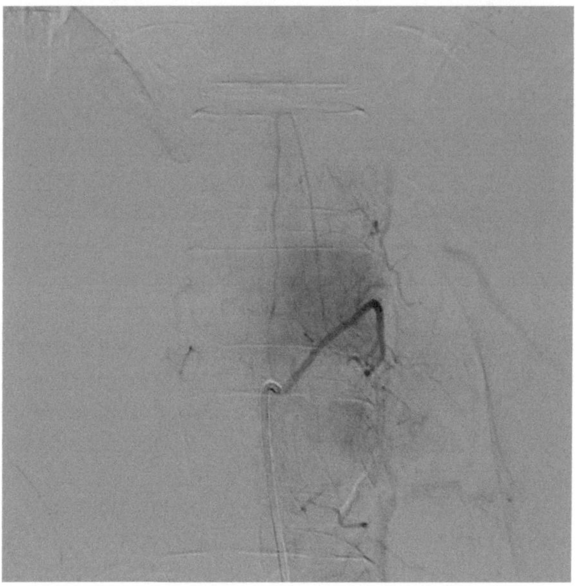

Fig. 9.2 The artery of Adamkiewicz (AKA) with its classic "hairpin" turn

paraplegia due to spinal cord infarction [21]. Therefore, preoperative localization is paramount. The AKA typically arises from a left intercostal or lumbar artery between T8 and L1. Angiographically, it is often identified by its characteristic "hairpin" turn where the feeding anterior radiculomedullary artery ascends before turning sharply downward to join and form the anterior spinal artery. It usually has a larger caliber compared to other radiculomedullary arteries [22].

9.3 Complementary Imaging Techniques

Beyond traditional digital subtraction angiography (DSA), advanced noninvasive imaging modalities such as computed tomography angiography (CTA) and magnetic resonance angiography (MRA) provide powerful tools for assessing the vasculature of the spine. These techniques have proven particularly effective for preoperative diagnosis and planning.

MRA presents several benefits, including potentially better visualization of key arteries (like the artery of Adamkiewicz) and excellent image contrast, while avoiding ionizing radiation. However, MRA scans generally take longer to acquire than CTA scans. CTA, on the other hand, offers the advantage of speed but involves patient exposure to radiation. Although MRA and CTA represent significant advancements for noninvasive evaluation, DSA remains the benchmark ("gold standard") technique due to its superior spatial and temporal resolution. It is considered essential before undertaking any endovascular treatment. Therefore, MRA, CTA, and DSA often play complementary roles in the thorough assessment of spinal vascular anatomy and pathology.

Embolization Techniques:

The choice of embolic agent for transarterial bone tumor embolization depends on several factors, including tumor type, location, size, blood supply, and the operator's experience. The goal is to devascularize the tumor with subsequent tissue necrosis and tumor lysis, while avoiding nontarget embolization.

9.4 Embolic Materials (Table 9.2)

9.4.1 Polyvinyl Alcohol (PVA) Particles

Polyvinyl alcohol (PVA) particles are a type of embolic agent capable of penetrating the tumor blood supply. PVA particles are permanent embolic agents, meaning that they will remain in the blood vessels and continue to block blood flow to the tumor. They work by mechanically occluding the diseased vessels, preventing blood from reaching the tumor.

PVA particles are made of a biocompatible material, easy to deliver through a microcatheter, relatively inexpensive, and available in a variety of sizes, ranging from 40 to 1200 μm. The size of the particles used will depend on the size of the

Table 9.2 Embolic agents

Feature	PVA particles	Embosphere microspheres	Gelfoam (gelatin sponge)	Liquid embolic agents (NBCA, Onyx, Obtura)	Embolization coils
Material/ composition	Polyvinyl alcohol	Tris-acryl copolymer	Gelatin sponge	N-butyl cyanoacrylate (NBCA), ethylene-vinyl alcohol copolymer (EVOH), Onyx (EVOH copolymer with tantalum powder), Obtura (iodinated particles)	Stainless steel, platinum
Size range (μm)	40–1200	40–1200	Variable (blocks, slurry)	Variable (liquid)	Variable (coil size)
Permanence	Permanent	Permanent	Temporary (7–10 days/2–4 weeks)	Permanent	Permanent
Key characteristics	Mechanically occludes vessels, biocompatible, radiopaque	Compressible, uniform size distribution, size stable in liquids, biocompatible, radiopaque	Dissolvable, used for temporary occlusion, adaptable forms (blocks, slurry), radiopaque	Rapid polymerization (NBCA), varied viscosities (Onyx), radiopacity loss (Obtura)	Larger-vessel occlusion, variety of detachable coils, radiopaque coils, embolization can assist other techniques
Primary use	Tumor embolization, vascular malformations, portal vein embolization (PVE)	Uterine fibroid treatment, hepatic artery embolization (HAE)	Stasis before coil embolization, temporary occlusion of vessels	Vascular malformations, tumor embolization	Larger-vessel occlusion, tumor embolization, fistula embolization

(continued)

Table 9.2 (continued)

Feature	PVA particles	Embosphere microspheres	Gelfoam (gelatin sponge)	Liquid embolic agents (NBCA, Onyx, Obtura)	Embolization coils
Advantages	Variety of sizes, relatively inexpensive, biocompatible, newer versions have improved delivery	Compressible, uniform size, stable in liquids, biocompatible, radiopaque, good for small vessels	Temporary occlusion, adaptable forms, safe and effective in various applications, can be used in conjunction with others	Rapid action (NBCA), varied viscosity (Onyx), improved imaging (Obtura)	Effective for larger vessels, various detachable options, can be used in conjunction with others
Disadvantages/ limitations	Irregular shape can lead to aggregation (traditional), may not be as effective for large vessels as others	None significantly mentioned	Temporary occlusion, risk of nontarget embolization, may not be as effective for large vessels as others	Risk of reflux and catheter blockage (NBCA), catheter removal difficulty (Onyx), limited use in bone tumors, may not be as effective for large vessels as others	Primarily for larger vessels, may not be suitable for all tumor embolization scenarios
Packaging and sterility	Sterile, disposable syringes, vials	Sterile, disposable syringes, vials	Sterile, dry, or pre-wetted	Sterile, premixed, or single components	Sterile, single use, detachable coils
Additional considerations	Risk of non-target embolization, requires experience for proper delivery	Less risk of nontarget embolization compared to PVA particles	Lower risk of nontarget embolization compared to liquid embolics	Requires precise placement, may cause inflammation	May migrate or compress surrounding structures

tumor and the vessels that supply it. Different options are available on the market. The traditional contour PVA particles (Boston Scientific, Marlborough, MA) are known for their irregular shape, leading to particle aggregation and occlusion of vessels larger than their diameter [23, 24].

Newer PVA preparations have a smoother outline, reducing catheter occlusion. Contour SE and Bead Block (Biocompatibles, Surrey, UK) are engineered PVA particles with more uniform size and compressibility, aiding delivery through smaller catheters [25].

9.4.2 Embosphere® Microspheres

Embosphere microspheres (Biosphere Medical Inc., Rockland, MA, USA), composed of a clear acrylic copolymer known as tris-acryl, were initially utilized as a microcarrier in cell cultures, establishing their biocompatibility. These microspheres, similar to polyvinyl alcohol (PVA) particles, are available in a size range from 40 to 1200 micrometers, and their application is prevalent in the treatment of uterine fibroids due to several advantageous properties [26]. Notably, these spheres are compressible, facilitating their passage through microcatheters with a luminal diameter smaller than the sphere's actual size. They exhibit a more uniform size distribution compared to PVA particles, and their size remains stable in liquid environments.

9.4.3 Gelfoam (Gelatin Sponge)

Gelfoam, or gelatin sponge, is a dissolvable, sponge-like material used in surgery for many years. It is available in flat rectangular blocks, adaptable for various applications. It can be cut into elongated rectangles or rolled into pledgets for catheter injection, or processed into a slurry for syringe delivery [27]. Gelfoam acts as a temporary occluding agent, with recanalization typically occurring within 7–10 days, though some sources suggest 2–4 weeks [28]. It is often used to achieve stasis before final vessel occlusion with coil embolization. Embolization targets as many branches as safely feasible, avoiding vital structures. Complications primarily arise from nontarget embolization [29, 30]. Studies demonstrate its safety and efficacy in various applications, including splenic hemorrhage and pelvic trauma [31, 32].

9.4.4 Liquid Embolic Agents (LEA)

Liquid embolic agents are crucial tools in endovascular embolization, used to treat various vascular abnormalities and tumors. These agents work by occluding blood vessels, either as a primary treatment or to reduce hemorrhagic risks before surgery. Common liquid embolic agents include N-butyl cyanoacrylate (NBCA) glues, absolute alcohol, Ethibloc, sodium tetradecyl sulfate, and Onyx, with emerging options and applications continuously being explored.

NBCA, approved by the FDA in 2000 for cerebral arteriovenous malformations (AVMs), polymerizes rapidly upon contact with ionic substances in the blood, forming a solid cast. This rapid action is vital in acute hemorrhage treatment. However, its use requires skill to prevent reflux and microcatheter blockage. To address limitations like controlling polymerization and potential toxicity, clinicians often mix lipiodol with NBCA to increase viscosity and slow polymerization [33, 34].

Onyx (Medtronic, Irvine, CA, USA), a commercially available agent since 2005, is composed of ethylene-vinyl alcohol copolymer (EVOH) and dimethyl sulfoxide (DMSO) solvent, solidifying in a "lava-like" flow. Available in various viscosities, Onyx offers versatility for different embolization purposes and forms a sponge-like gel that entraps tantalum powder for radiopacity. Unlike NBCA, Onyx is nonadhesive, reducing the risk of catheter blockage, but it may be difficult to remove the microcatheter in tortuous arteries.

Newer agents like Squid (Balt, Montmorency, France) and PHIL (Precipitating Hydrophobic Injectable Liquid; MicroVention, Aliso Viejo, USA) aim to improve upon existing options. Squid uses micronized tantalum powder for a more homogenous mixture and reduced artifacts in postinterventional imaging compared to Onyx. PHIL, approved for clinical use in Europe, employs a copolymer dissolved in DMSO, with iodine chemically bonded for radiopacity and fewer glare artifacts in CT.

Obtura (Iberhospitex, Lliçà de Vall, Spain) is a novel liquid embolic agent (LEA) used for neurovascular embolization, designed to improve penetration and visualization during the procedure. A key feature of Obtura is its postprocedure radiopacity loss, which significantly enhances anatomical understanding, especially in multi-staged procedures, and reduces postprocedural imaging artifacts. This radiopacity loss is a result of the gradual elimination of iodine from the embolic material after the procedure. The process involves the deconjugation of iodine and its diffusion out of the vascular lesion, leaving behind the radiolucent EVOH. The rate of radiopacity loss with Obtura is notable. In the CLARIDAD trial [35], complete loss of radiopacity was observed from 74.3% of the sessions at 30 days to 100% at 1 year. This progressive radiopacity loss with Obtura facilitates improved visualization in follow-up imaging and staged procedures, without the artifacts associated with other embolic agents.

While the use of liquid embolic agents in bone tumors is limited, they are being explored for this purpose. In non-end organs like bone with multiple arterial feeders, liquid agents may increase the risk of nontarget embolization. However, agents like ethylic, cyanoacrylates, and Onyx have been successfully used for tumor embolization and may be considered for potential curative treatments. In general, for devascularizing tumors as a palliative or presurgical procedure, there is little advantage over particulate embolization.

9.4.5 Coils

Stainless steel fibered coils and platinum coils have been used for many years for vascular occlusion. Coils can be delivered through standard catheters or microcatheters, and the adoption of neurointerventional techniques has led to the development of a variety of detachable coils specifically designed for use outside the central nervous system. Coils are usually reserved for larger-vessel occlusion, but do have a role in tumor embolization after particulate emboli have been used and in the emergency situation where either the expertise or time is lacking for other forms of embolization.

9.4.6 Timing Between Preoperative Endovascular Embolization and Surgery

Preoperative embolization is frequently employed as an adjunctive treatment before surgical resection of spinal tumors, particularly hypervascular ones, with the primary goals of minimizing intraoperative blood loss and facilitating surgery [36]. However, determining the optimal time interval between endovascular embolization and the subsequent surgery is controversial.

9.4.7 Evidence Favoring Early Intervention (< 24 H)

Multiple studies, including systematic reviews and meta-analyses, suggest that performing surgery soon after embolization yields the best results.

Indeed, especially in hypervascular spinal metastases, many authors conclude that complete embolization followed by spinal surgery, keeping the interval as short as possible, ideally less than 24 h, may effectively reduce intraoperative bleeding [37, 38]. The primary rationale behind this is to operate during the period of maximal tumor devascularization before potential revascularization or collateral blood supply develops [12]. Additionally, this helps to mitigate risks related to potential complications like post-embolization swelling.

9.4.8 Alternative Timeframes (24–72 H)

While some evidence points to operating within 24 h, some studies suggest slightly longer intervals may still be acceptable or practical.

One retrospective comparative study specifically evaluating same-day versus next-day surgery suggested operating on the next day or at maximum within 72 h allows benefiting from optimal devascularization [39]. Others usually perform decompressive surgery within 48 h post embolization [12].

Thus, while less than 24 h is often considered ideal, particularly to maximize blood loss reduction in hypervascular tumors, operating within a 2–3 day window might still confer benefits compared to delaying surgery further.

The slightly longer timeframes mentioned (up to 72 h) likely reflect logistical challenges of coordinating embolization and surgery or findings that significant revascularization might not occur immediately within the first few days, though the principle remains to operate promptly.

9.4.9 Possible Complications of Endovascular Embolization

Preoperative endovascular embolization for spinal tumors aims to reduce intraoperative blood loss and facilitate surgery, but it carries risks and potential complications [40].

Neurological complications are a primary concern:

Spinal cord ischemia/infarction: Reported as the most frequent adverse event leading to neurological abnormalities [41]. This can occur through several mechanisms related to the procedure itself, including nontarget embolization, reflux or unintended vessel cannulation, and flowdynamics.

Avoiding spinal cord ischemia during embolization procedures is crucial and requires meticulous technique and careful planning. Precautions aiming to minimize the risk of accidentally compromising the spinal cord's vital blood supply come from deep vascular anatomical knowledge and operator experience with different devices and include:

Thorough angiographic assessment: Before proceeding with endovascular embolization, detailed spinal angiography is crucial to identify critical arteries supplying the spinal cord, such as the artery of Adamkiewicz or cervical enlargement arteries, and understand potential anastomoses [42]. Recognizing complex flow dynamics that might mask spinal arteries is also important.

Superselective catheter placement: Ensure the microcatheter tip is positioned safely within the target vessel, distal to the origin of any identified critical spinal arteries, before injecting embolic material.

Choice of embolic agent: Consider the type and size of embolic material. Small particles and liquid agents might carry a higher risk of penetrating deeply or refluxing into spinal arteries; avoiding them may be prudent if the goal is purely preoperative devascularization rather than tumor necrosis [43]. Larger agents like coils, which stay contained within the target vessel, may have less risk of reflux.

Controlled injection: Inject embolic material slowly under careful fluoroscopic monitoring to prevent reflux into non-target vessels, including spinal arteries.

Swelling from tumor necrosis: Although the procedure is generally considered safe, post-embolization tumor swelling is a recognized potential complication, caused by tumor necrosis [44].

In the limited space of the spinal canal, even moderate swelling can lead to significant consequences. This can manifest as neurological symptoms, such as transient lower extremity weakness, due to compression of the spinal cord or nerve roots.

As reported, symptoms may be transient and can resolve completely; however, prompt surgical intervention following embolization is often recommended, potentially to allow for decompression if significant swelling occurs.

Guidelines and findings related to embolization in other anatomical areas or for general postembolization syndrome shed some light on the potential role of steroids (e.g., dexamethasone following TransArterial ChemoEmbolization for liver tumors [45]). However, results lack direct evidence or explicit recommendations regarding their routine use to prevent swelling after spinal tumor embolization.

Common sense suggests considering the tumor's size, location near critical structures, and the anticipated delay before surgery.

Cerebral stroke: Serious, albeit uncommon, neurologic complications include not only spinal cord ischemia but also cerebral stroke. This risk is primarily associated with the existence of complex vascular connections known as "dangerous anastomoses," which represent natural pathways linking the extracranial arterial system (supplying structures outside the skull, such as the face, scalp, neck muscles, and upper spine) with the intracranial vascular system (supplying the brain).

During the embolization of spinal tumors, particularly those located in the cervical region, the arteries targeted for occlusion (e.g., branches from the vertebral arteries, thyrocervical trunk, or costocervical trunk) may participate in these anastomotic networks [46]. In particular, the vertebral artery is a key vessel supplying both the spinal cord (via spinal branches) and the posterior intracranial circulation. Dangerous anastomoses relevant during spinal tumor embolization often involve connections between branches of the external carotid artery (e.g., the occipital artery and ascending pharyngeal artery) and the vertebral artery.

Embolizing cervical branches of the vertebral artery that supply spinal structures could allow embolic material to inadvertently travel through these connections or directly up the vertebral artery into the intracranial circulation, potentially causing stroke or cranial nerve injury [47].

Other reported more common complications include issues related to the arterial access site (e.g., groin hematoma or femoral artery thrombosis), as well as bleeding, and, rarely, cardiac events potentially related to anesthesia.

9.5 Case Report

A 67-year-old male presented with a several-month history of progressively worsening mid-thoracic back pain. The pain was described as severe, constant, and notably worse at night. Over a few weeks, he developed numbness radiating in a band-like fashion around his upper chest and reported increasing difficulty with balance while walking.

Preoperative magnetic resonance imaging (MRI) of the thoracic spine was performed. Sagittal Short tau inversion recovery (STIR) and T1-weighted sequences demonstrated an aggressive lesion centered within the right T2 vertebral peduncle (Fig. 9.3). The lesion showed extensive involvement of the vertebral body and posterior elements, associated with cortical destruction. Marrow-replacing characteristics were evident, with low signal intensity on T1-weighted images and high signal intensity on STIR sequences. A significant soft tissue component extended posteriorly into the paraspinal muscles. The overall MRI appearance was highly suspicious for a vertebral metastasis, although an aggressive primary bone tumor was considered in the differential diagnosis.

Subsequent computed tomography (CT) of the thoracic spine provided further details (Fig. 9.4). Bone window (right) confirmed extensive lytic bone destruction involving the right T2 vertebral body and posterior elements. Soft tissue window (right) clearly showed the extent of the soft tissue mass, which extended posteriorly into the paraspinal region, medially into the spinal canal, and laterally to the pleura.

For vascular characterization and potential treatment planning, preoperative sagittal and coronal 3D time-resolved MR angiography (MRA) using a time-resolved angiography with interleaved stochastic trajectories (TWIST) sequence was performed (Fig. 9.5). This demonstrated early and intense enhancement of the right T2 lesion during the arterial phase of contrast injection, confirming the hypervascular nature of the lesion (arrow).

The combined imaging findings from MRI, CT, and MRA strongly suggested a hypervascular metastatic lesion to the right T2 vertebral bone. The hypervascularity identified on MRA is particularly relevant for surgical planning, often prompting consideration of preoperative embolization to reduce intraoperative blood loss.

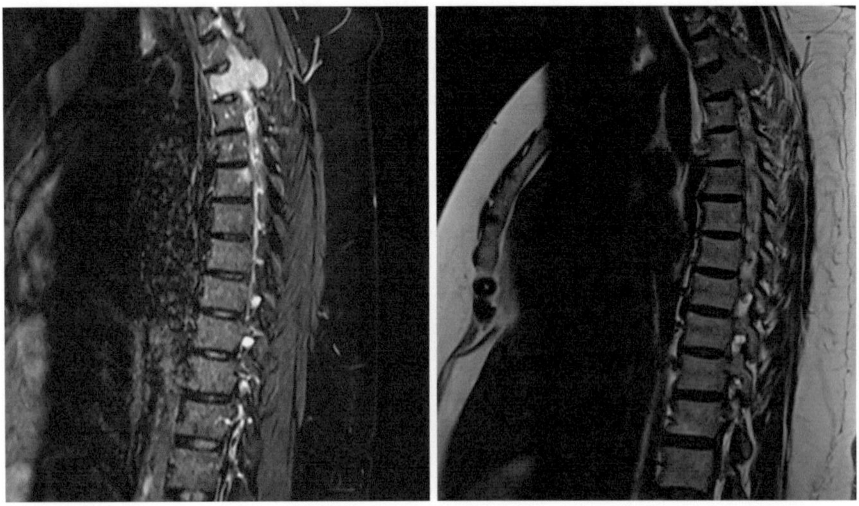

Fig. 9.3 Preoperative MRI-sagittal STIR and T1-weighted sequences of the thoracic spine

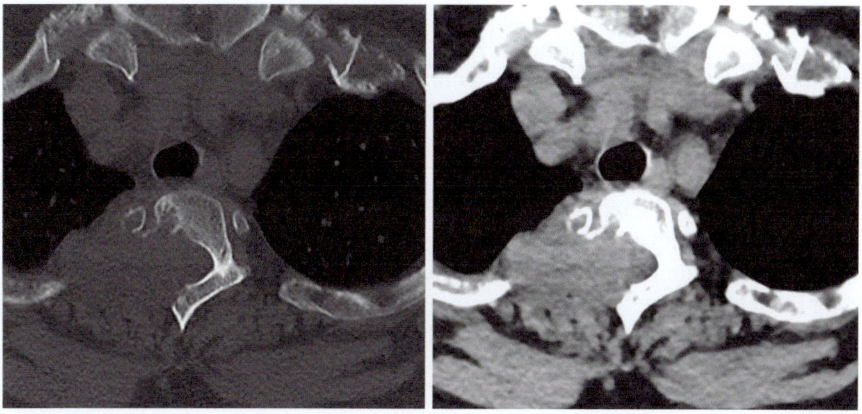

Fig. 9.4 CT of the thoracic spine

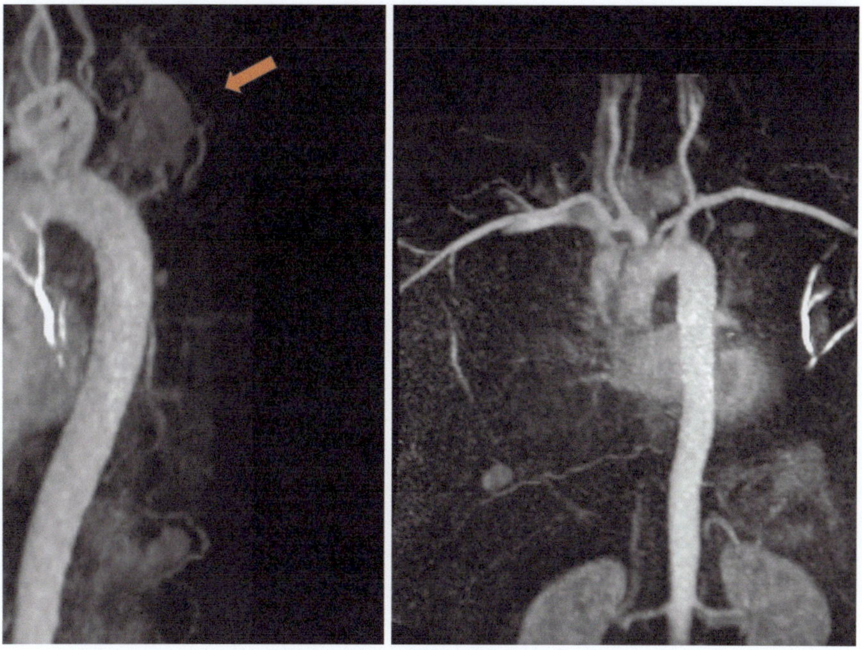

Fig. 9.5 Sagittal and coronal 3D time-resolved MR angiography (MRA) using a TWIST sequence

Thus, a spinal angiogram was performed.

Following the explanation of the benefits, risks, and alternatives for the procedure, consent was obtained from the patient. The risks, including but not limited to stroke, spinal cord ischemia, post-embolization tumor swelling, vascular injury to the cervical or femoral vessels, and groin hematoma, were discussed with the patient.

The patient was brought to the angiographic suite and placed under general anesthesia. A time-out was performed. Both groins were prepped in the usual sterile fashion using Chloraprep and sterilely draped. A single-wall puncture of the right femoral artery was performed, and a 6-Fr short sheath was inserted into the right common femoral artery, maintained on heparinized flush.

A 5-Fr Cobra-2 was advanced over a Guidewire 0.035″ into the aortic arch, and with the aid of roadmapping and digital fluoroscopy, the right T2 intercostal artery was selectively catheterized. The angiogram (Fig. 9.6a) showed a robust tumor blush corresponding to the right T2 vertebral lesion and a proximal origin of the right bronchial artery.

Using the coaxial technique, through the Cobra-2, an Excelsior 1018 microcatheter (Stryker, Fremont, California, USA) was advanced distal to the right bronchial artery. The following superselective angiogram confirmed the tumor blush and also showed reflux into the right T1 intercostal artery via a longitudinal anastomosis (Fig. 9.6b). Based on the angiographic findings, the decision was made to proceed with particle embolization.

Once the proper position was confirmed, a mixture of contrast, non-heparinized saline, and 355–500 μm contour particles (Boston Scientific, Marlborough, MA) was slowly injected into the distal T2 intercostal artery. Injection was carried out in small volumes, and contrast was allowed to wash out before the next small bolus was administered. Contrast reflux was avoided.

In total, 3 cc of a mixture of contrast and particles was injected before significant contrast stagnation was noted in the artery. The microcatheter was flushed with

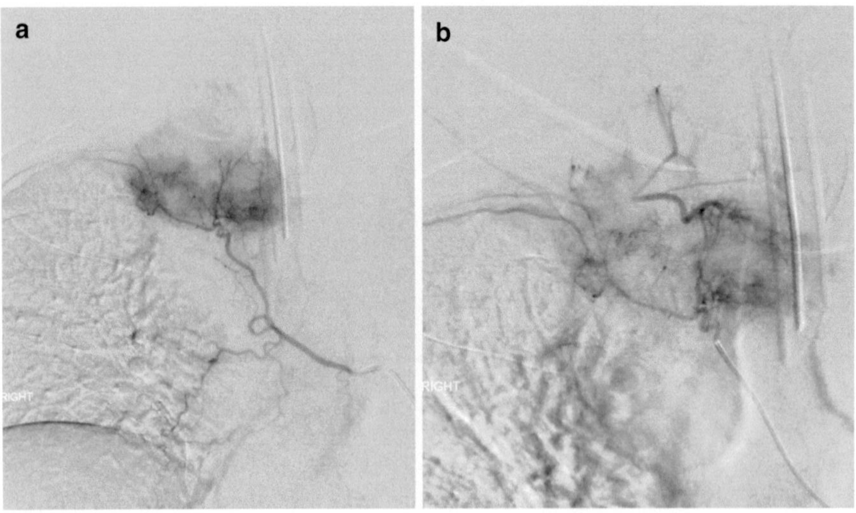

Fig. 9.6 (**a**) Robust tumor blush corresponding to the right T2 vertebral lesion and a proximal origin of the right bronchial artery; (**b**) contrast reflux into the right T1 intercostal artery via a longitudinal anastomosis; (**c**) pre-embolization angiogram; (**d**) post-embolization angiogram; (**e**) coiling pack at the origin of the deep cervical artery; (**f**) final angiogram

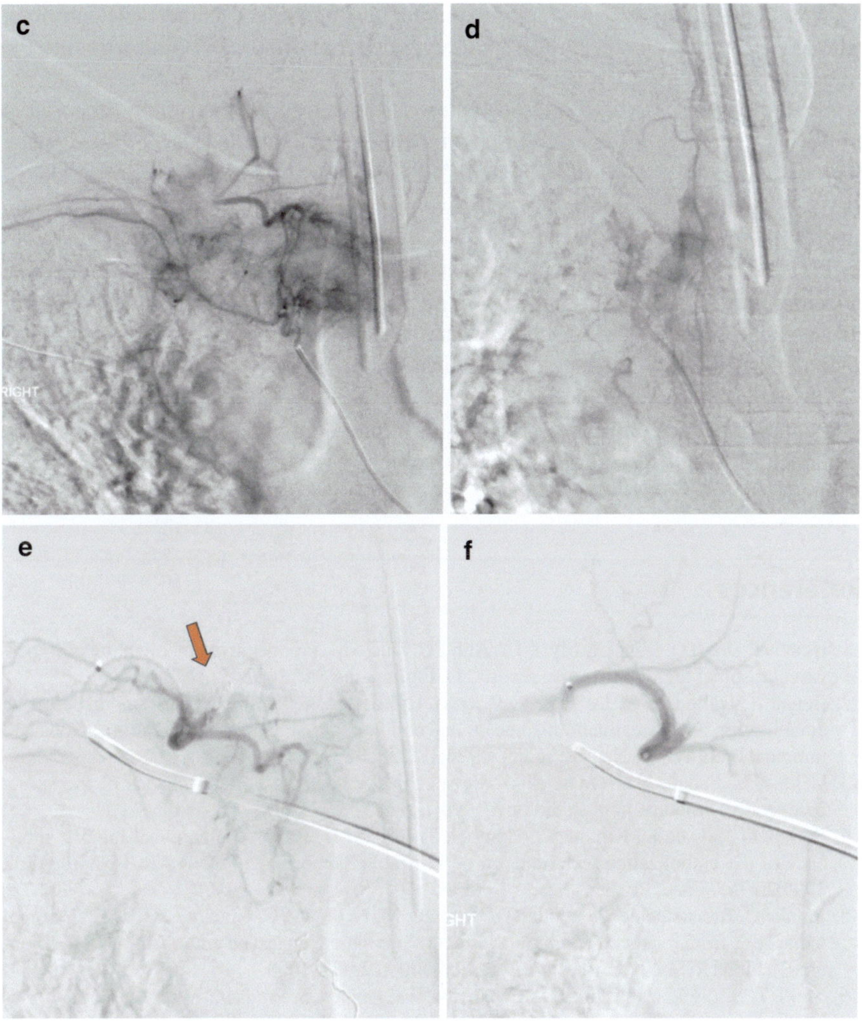

Fig. 9.6 (continued)

saline in the same careful manner, and then loose coiling of the segment, distal to the bronchial artery, completed the embolization.

Compared with the preoperative angiogram (Fig. 9.6c), the follow-up run (Fig. 9.6d) of the right T2 intercostal artery demonstrated significantly diminished capillary blush in the metastatic lesion. However, a subtle blush into the superior lesion compartment, likely coming from the right T1 intercostal artery/supreme intercostal artery, was seen.

Using the coaxial technique, the right T1 intercostal artery was seen branching off the right supreme intercostal artery via the right costocervical trunk.

Therefore, using the coaxial technique, a Benchmark catheter (Penumbra, Alameda, CA) was advanced over a Select catheter over a 0.035″ Glidewire into the right costocervical trunk.

First, the Excelsior 1018 microcatheter was advanced via the right costocervical trunk to the origin of the deep cervical artery and used to obtain a dense coiling pack (Fig. 9.6e, arrow) (Target Detachable Coils, Stryker, Fremont, California, USA). The rationale was promoting the selective push of particles in the tumor, avoiding steal from non-target vessels.

Finally, 1.5 cc of a mixture of contrast, non-heparinized saline, and particles was injected before significant contrast stagnation was noted in the artery. The last follow-up angiogram (Fig. 9.6f) showed an absence of anterograde flow to the metastatic lesion, without evidence of complications.

Following the successful preoperative embolization, the patient underwent subsequent surgical resection of the T2 lesion. Intraoperative estimated blood loss was limited to 800 ml. Spinal stability was achieved with a C5–T5 posterior instrumented fusion.

References

1. Binh NT, Hoa TQ, Linh LT, My T-TT, Anh PQ, Duc NM. Preoperative embolization of hypervascular spinal tumors: two case reports. J Clin Imaging Sci. 2022;12:21.
2. Benati A, Dalle Ore G, Da Pian R, Bricolo A, Maschio A, Perini S. Transfemoral selective embolisation in the treatment of some cranial and vertebro-spinal vascular malformations and tumours. Prelim Res J Neurosurg Sci. 1974;18:233–8.
3. Gellad FE, Sadato N, Numaguchi Y, Levine AM. Vascular metastatic lesions of the spine: preoperative embolization. Radiology. 1990;176:683–6.
4. Berkefeld J, Scale D, Kirchner J, Heinrich T, Kollath J. Hypervascular spinal tumors: influence of the embolization technique on perioperative hemorrhage. AJNR Am J Neuroradiol. 1999;20:757–63.
5. Manke C, Bretschneider T, Lenhart M, Strotzer M, Neumann C, Gmeinwieser J, et al. Spinal metastases from renal cell carcinoma: effect of preoperative particle embolization on intraoperative blood loss. AJNR Am J Neuroradiol. 2001;22:997–1003.
6. Smith TP, Gray L, Weinstein JN, Richardson WJ, Payne CS. Preoperative transarterial embolization of spinal column neoplasms. J Vasc Interv Radiol. 1995;6:863–9.
7. Prabhu VC, Bilsky MH, Jambhekar K, Panageas KS, Boland PJ, Lis E, et al. Results of preoperative embolization for metastatic spinal neoplasms. J Neurosurg. 2003;98:156–64.
8. Ozkan E, Gupta S. Embolization of spinal tumors: vascular anatomy, indications, and technique. Tech Vasc Interv Radiol. 2011;14:129–40.
9. Sare A, Jain N, Chandra V, Beidas A-K, Kumar A, Shukla PA. Perioperative blood loss after embolization of hypervascular musculoskeletal tumors outside of the spine: a single-center ten year experience and systematic review of the literature. Clin Imaging. 2021;79:24–9.
10. Owen RJT. Embolization of musculoskeletal bone tumors. Semin Intervent Radiol. 2010;27:111–23.
11. Westbroek EM, Pennington Z, Ahmed AK, Xia Y, Boone C, Gailloud P, et al. Comparison of complete and near-complete endovascular embolization of hypervascular spine tumors with partial embolization. J Neurosurg Spine. 2020;33:245–51.
12. Zhang B, Yu H, Zhao X, Cao X, Cao Y, Shi X, et al. Preoperative embolization in the treatment of patients with metastatic epidural spinal cord compression: a retrospective analysis. Front Oncol. 2022;12:1098182.

13. Kickuth R, Waldherr C, Hoppe H, Bonel HM, Ludwig K, Beck M, et al. Interventional management of hypervascular osseous metastasis: role of embolotherapy before orthopedic tumor resection and bone stabilization. AJR Am J Roentgenol. 2008;191:W240–7.
14. Al-Mistarehi A-H, Slika H, El Baba B, Sattari SA, Weber-Levine C, Jiang K, et al. Optimizing surgical strategies: a systematic review of the effectiveness of preoperative arterial embolization for hyper vascular metastatic spinal tumors. Spine J. 2025; https://doi.org/10.1016/j.spinee.2024.12.032.
15. Gailloud P. Introduction to diagnostic and therapeutic spinal angiography. Neuroimaging Clin N Am. 2019;29:595–614.
16. Shimizu S, Tanaka R, Kan S, Suzuki S, Kurata A, Fujii K. Origins of the segmental arteries in the aorta: an anatomic study for selective catheterization with spinal arteriography. AJNR Am J Neuroradiol. 2005;26:922–8.
17. Herdt JR, Shimkin PM, Ommaya AK, Chiro G. Angiography of vascular intraspinal tumors. Am J Roentgenol Radium Therapy, Nucl Med. 1972;115:165–70.
18. Raz E, Nossek E, Sahlein DH, Sharashidze V, Narayan V, Ali A, et al. Principles, techniques and applications of high resolution cone beam CT angiography in the neuroangio suite. J Neurointerv Surg. 2023;15:600–7.
19. Gailloud P. Spinal vascular anatomy. Neuroimaging Clin N Am. 2019;29:615–33.
20. Leather RP, Williams GM, Perler BA, Burdick JF, Osterman FA, Mitchell SA, et al. Angiographic localization of spinal cord blood supply and its relationship to postoperative paraplegia. J Vasc Surg. 1991;13:23–35.
21. Taterra D, Skinningsrud B, Pękala PA, Hsieh WC, Cirocchi R, Walocha JA, et al. Artery of Adamkiewicz: a meta-analysis of anatomical characteristics. Neuroradiology. 2019;61:869–80.
22. Hoshiai S, Shiigai M, Konishi T, Nakai Y, Masumoto T. Detection of the artery of Adamkiewicz using multidetector row computed tomography in patients with spinal arteriovenous shunt disease. Pol J Radiol. 2020;85:e163–8.
23. [cited 15 Mar 2025]. Available: https://www.bostonscientific.com/content/dam/bostonscientific/pi/portfolio-group/embolization/contour/Resources/Contour.
24. Lewis AL. Embolisation devices from biomedical polymers for intra-arterial occlusion and drug delivery in the treatment of cancer. In: Park K, editor. Biomaterials for cancer therapeutics. Elsevier; 2013. p. 207–239e.
25. Wáng Y-XJ, De Baere T, Idée J-M, Ballet S. Transcatheter embolization therapy in liver cancer: an update of clinical evidences. Chin. J Cancer Res. 2015;27:96–121.
26. Sofy AA, Tsui S. Comparison of polyvinyl alcohol particles and tris-acryl gelatin microspheres embolic agents used in uterine artery embolization: a systematic review and meta-analysis. J Turk Soc Obstet Gynecol. 2023;20:74–84.
27. Nota T, Kageyama K, Yamamoto A, Jogo A, Sohgawa E, Yonezawa H, et al. Feasibility of gel-like radiopaque embolic material using gelatin sponge and contrast agent for tract embolization after percutaneous treatment. PLoS One. 2023;18:e0281384.
28. Gottfried ON, Schloesser PE, Schmidt MH, Stevens EA. Embolization of metastatic spinal tumors. Neurosurg Clin N Am. 2004;15:391–9.
29. Miyayama S, Yamakado K, Anai H, Abo D, Minami T, Takaki H, et al. Guidelines on the use of gelatin sponge particles in embolotherapy. Jpn J Radiol. 2014;32:242–50.
30. Jander HP, Russinovich NA. Transcatheter gelfoam embolization in abdominal, retroperitoneal, and pelvic hemorrhage. Radiology. 1980;136:337–44.
31. Loya MF, Mangat S, Santoro GC, Martynov A, Shah SS. Prophylactic absorbable gelatin sponge embolization for angiographically occult splenic hemorrhage. Radiol Case Rep. 2018;13:753–8.
32. Alali M, Cao C, Shin JH, Jeon G, Zeng CH, Park J-H, et al. Preliminary report on embolization with quick-soluble gelatin sponge particles for angiographically negative acute gastrointestinal bleeding. Sci Rep. 2024;14:6438.
33. Jiang Y, Zhang Y, Lu Z, Wang X, Bai S, Chen Y, et al. Liquid embolic agents for interventional embolization. Chem Phys Mater. 2022;1:39–50.

34. Vollherbst DF, Chapot R, Bendszus M, Möhlenbruch MA. Glue, Onyx, squid or PHIL? Liquid embolic agents for the embolization of cerebral arteriovenous malformations and Dural arteriovenous fistulas. Clin Neuroradiol. 2022;32:25–38.
35. Llibre-Guerra JC, Guimaraens L, Kadziolka KB, Siddiqui AH, Chapot R, Gil A. Obtura: a novel liquid embolic agent with post-embolization radiopacity loss, in endovascular treatment of brain arteriovenous malformations, dural arteriovenous fistulas, and tumors: CLARIDAD trial. J Neurointerv Surg. 2025; https://doi.org/10.1136/jnis-2023-021442.
36. Griessenauer CJ, Salem M, Hendrix P, Foreman PM, Ogilvy CS, Thomas AJ. Preoperative embolization of spinal tumors: a systematic review and meta-analysis. World Neurosurg. 2016;87:362–71.
37. Yuh WT, Han J, Lee C-H, Kim CH, Kang H-S, Chung CK. The optimal time between embolization and surgery for hypervascular spinal metastatic tumors : a systematic review and meta-analysis. J Korean Neurosurg Soc. 2023;66:438–45.
38. Motov S, Stengel F, Ringel F, Bozinov O, Stienen MN. Current state of preoperative embolization for spinal metastasis - a survey by the EANS spine section. Brain Spine. 2023;3:102712.
39. Tang B, Ji T, Guo W, Tang X, Jin L, Dong S, et al. Which is the better timing between embolization and surgery for hypervascular spinal tumors, the same day or the next day?: a retrospective comparative study. Medicine (Baltimore). 2018;97:e10912.
40. Onishi E, Hashimura T, Ota S, Fujita S, Tsukamoto Y, Matsunaga K, et al. The efficacy and complications of preoperative embolization of metastatic spinal tumors: risk of paralysis after embolization. Spine Surg Relat Res. 2022;6:288–93.
41. Faiella E, Santucci D, Vertulli D, Russo F, Vadalà G, Papalia R, et al. Preoperative embolization of vertebral metastasis: comprehensive review of the literature. Diseases. 2023:11. https://doi.org/10.3390/diseases11030109.
42. Patsalides A, Leng LZ, Kimball D, Marcus J, Knopman J, Laufer I, et al. Preoperative catheter spinal angiography and embolization of cervical spinal tumors: outcomes from a single center. Interv Neuroradiol. 2016;22:457–65.
43. Cloft HJ, Jensen ME, Do HM, Kallmes DF. Spinal cord infarction complicating embolisation of vertebral metastasis: a result of masking of a spinal artery by a high-flow lesion: a result of masking of a spinal artery by a high-flow lesion. Interv Neuroradiol. 1999;5:61–5.
44. Houten JK, Swiggett SJ, Hadid B, Choueka DM, Kinon MD, Buciuc R, et al. Neurologic complications of preoperative embolization of spinal metastasis: a systemic review of the literature identifying distinct mechanisms of injury. World Neurosurg. 2020;143:374–88.
45. Ishikawa T. Prevention of post-embolization syndrome after transarterial chemoembolization for hepatocellular carcinoma-is prophylactic dexamethasone useful, or not? Hepatobiliary Surg Nutr. 2018;7:214–6.
46. Ehlers LD, McMordie J, Lookian P, Surdell D, Puccioni M. Cervical spine aneurysmal bone cyst in a pediatric patient: embolization considerations and potential pitfalls. World Neurosurg. 2020;139:163–8.
47. Geibprasert S, Pongpech S, Armstrong D, Krings T. Dangerous extracranial-intracranial anastomoses and supply to the cranial nerves: vessels the neurointerventionalist needs to know. AJNR Am J Neuroradiol. 2009;30:1459–68.

Integrating Interventional Oncology with Other Cancer Treatment Options for Bone Tumors: Pain Management

10

Luis Moltó García, Olga Comps Vicente, David Bande Julián, Uxía Rodríguez Rivas, Paolo Cossu, and Antonio Montes Pérez

Abbreviations

IO	Interventional Oncology
RT	Radiotherapy
SBRT	Stereotactic Body Radiotherapy
RFA	Radiofrequency Ablation
MWA	Microwave Ablation
IRE	Irreversible Electroporation
CPN	Celiac Plexus Neurolysis
PSN	Peripheral Somatic Neurolysis
DRG	Dorsal Root Ganglion
PNS	Peripheral Nerve Stimulation
SCS	Spinal Cord Stimulation
WHO	World Health Organization
VAS	Visual Analog Scale
QoL	Quality of Life
CR	Complete Response
PR	Partial Response
SD	Stable Disease
PD	Progressive Disease

L. M. García (✉) · O. C. Vicente · D. B. Julián · U. R. Rivas · A. M. Pérez
Anesthesiology Service, Pain Unit, Hospital del Mar, Barcelona, Spain
e-mail: lmolto@hmar.cat; Ocomps@hmar.cat; Dbande@hmar.cat; Urodriguez@hmar.cat; Amontes@hmar.cat

P. Cossu
Anesthesiology Service, Pain Unit, Mater Olbia Hospital, Olbia, Italy
e-mail: Paolo.cossu@materolbia.com

C. Pusceddu, S. Marsico (eds.), *Malignant Bone Lesions and Beyond*, https://doi.org/10.1007/978-3-032-00018-7_10

CT	Computed Tomography
MRI	Magnetic Resonance Imaging
PET	Positron Emission Tomography
NSAIDs	Non-steroidal Anti-inflammatory Drugs
TENS	Transcutaneous Electrical Nerve Stimulation
IV	Intravenous
EMR	Electronic Medical Record

10.1 Introduction

Oncologic pain is a highly prevalent symptom in patients with cancer and hematologic malignancies, with most individuals experiencing pain at some point during the disease course. Pain is present in 70–90% of patients in advanced or terminal stages. Among those undergoing active treatment, prevalence is around 30%, reaching up to 60% in some studies [1]. According to several reports, 38% of patients experience moderate to severe pain, with higher prevalence in specific tumor locations such as the pancreas, head, and neck, as well as in hematologic malignancies like multiple myeloma and lymphomas [2, 3].

Oncologic pain can be classified in various ways:

- Based on its pathophysiological mechanism:
  - Nociceptive pain (most common), caused by activation of peripheral nociceptors in somatic or visceral tissues.
  - Neuropathic pain, resulting from damage to the peripheral or central nervous system.
  - Psychogenic or psychological pain.
- Based on its origin:
  - Tumor-related pain (80%), directly caused by tumor growth and invasion.
  - Treatment-induced pain (20%), secondary to surgical, radiotherapeutic, or chemotherapeutic interventions.
- Based on temporal progression:
  - Acute pain, presenting as an alarm symptom, is typically triggered by a single causative factor.
  - Chronic pain, persisting for more than 3 months, is often multifactorial in nature.

Approximately 48% of oncologic pain cases exhibit characteristics of breakthrough pain, defined as a transient exacerbation occurring over a stable baseline pain [4]. Additionally, one-third of patients present with neuropathic pain, which may reach 45% in terminal stages [5]. Up to 40% of patients report mixed pain with both nociceptive and neuropathic components [6].

Multidisciplinary Approach to Oncologic Pain Management
The management of oncologic pain requires a multidisciplinary approach, involving pain specialists, oncologists, palliative care physicians, interventional radiologists, radiation oncologists, surgeons, and orthopedic specialists. This collaborative strategy ensures optimal pharmacological and nonpharmacological interventions, particularly in cases of complex oncologic pain. Pain management must address both chronic and acute pain, aiming to control pain intensity, enhance functionality, and improve patient quality of life [7].

Clinical examination and imaging techniques aid in identifying the underlying cause of pain, allowing for tailored therapeutic strategies. Due to the complex nature of oncologic pain, treatment must be individualized to minimize side effects while maximizing patient autonomy and quality of life. It is crucial to address both cancer-related pain and pain resulting from treatment sequelae (e.g., surgery, radiotherapy, and chemotherapy).

Pharmacological Management and Interventional Alternatives
All patients should initiate pharmacological pain management, following the WHO Analgesic Ladder. However, pain specialists increasingly advocate for the "Analgesic Elevator" approach, which prioritizes rapid and effective pain relief without necessarily progressing through non-steroidal anti-inflammatory drugs (NSAIDs) and/or weak opioids. Although this chapter does not focus on pharmacological therapy, it is important to highlight that strong opioids are the mainstay of oncologic pain management, particularly for moderate to severe nociceptive pain (e.g., bone pain and soft tissue pain).

The most potent opioids include morphine, fentanyl, oxycodone, hydromorphone, methadone, buprenorphine, and tapentadol. These agents can be administered via multiple routes, including oral, buccal, sublingual, transdermal, subcutaneous, intramuscular, intravenous, nasal, topical, and peripheral. This chapter, however, will specifically address spinal administration. In addition to opioids, patients often receive adjuvant analgesics such as antiepileptics, antidepressants, corticosteroids, NSAIDs, and COX-2 inhibitors [6, 7].

When pain is insufficiently controlled with medication alone or when the side effects compromise the patient's quality of life, interventional alternatives should be considered. The following sections will explore various interventional procedures that may benefit patients with oncologic pain.

10.2 Sympathetic Block

10.2.1 Celiac Plexus Block

10.2.1.1 Introduction
The celiac plexus, along with the splanchnic nerves, is the sympathetic nerve plexus responsible for transmitting sensory information from the upper hemiabdomen. It is located in the retroperitoneum, anterior to the aortic wall, and near the celiac trunk.

Its neurolysis or blockade can relieve pain secondary to oncological processes occurring in the upper abdomen, such as gastric, esophageal, biliary, duodenal, or pancreatic cancer [8]. Due to its high prevalence and the difficulty of surgical resection in many cases, pain secondary to pancreatic cancer is currently one of the main indications for this technique.

In this chapter, we will analyze the role of celiac plexus neurolysis techniques, their efficacy, complications, and limitations in the treatment of severe and refractory pain in patients with oncological disease.

Indications

Celiac plexus neurolysis (CPN) is indicated in the following cases: [9, 10]

1. Uncontrolled pain despite the use of indicated analgesic drugs, including major opioids.
2. The occurrence of adverse effects that significantly impair the patient's quality of life, such as nausea, persistent constipation, drowsiness, cognitive impairment, dependence, or addiction development.
3. Pain with predominantly visceral characteristics localized in the upper hemiabdomen.
4. Pain that does not respond to chemotherapy and/or radiotherapy.
5. Unresectable oncological lesion with a shortened life expectancy.

The following contraindications have been described: [8]

Absolute

1. Coagulopathy or thrombocytopathy that cannot be corrected.

Relative

1. Presence of an intra-abdominal aortic aneurysm.
2. Aortic mural thrombosis.
3. Intra-abdominal infection/sepsis.
4. Intestinal obstruction.

CPN is useful in the following oncological conditions: esophageal cancer, gastric cancer, biliary cancer, hepatocellular carcinoma, proximal small intestine cancer (duodenum, jejunum), pancreatic cancer, and nodal invasion in the upper hemiabdomen. Among these, pancreatic cancer has the strongest evidence supporting effective pain relief following CPN [9].

Pancreatic cancer is the fourth leading cause of cancer-related death in Europe and the United States and the seventh worldwide. [1, 12] There is a clear association between increased pain intensity and persistence and a poorer prognosis in pancreatic ductal adenocarcinoma [13].

The efficacy of CPN is well established during the first month after the procedure in patients with pancreatic cancer, whereas in other upper hemiabdominal cancers, further research is required [9, 14]. Pain relief in pancreatic cancer patients is estimated at 70–80% during the first month [9, 10]. Currently, there is no clear evidence to determine whether one approach technique is superior to others [3].

10.2.1.2 Anatomical Overview

The celiac plexus is a sympathetic plexus typically located at the level of the T12 and L1 vertebral bodies [14, 15]. Posteriorly, it is separated from the vertebral column by the diaphragmatic crura. This is an important anatomical feature, as the diaphragmatic crura serve as a barrier between the celiac plexus (anterior to the crura) and the splanchnic nerves (posterior to the crura) [8, 14, 15]. The network of ganglia within the celiac plexus is located anterior or lateral to the aorta, generally below the origin of the celiac trunk.

The sympathetic nervous system is part of the peripheral nervous system and is responsible for regulating certain involuntary physiological functions. It consists of both afferent and efferent neurons. In general, it is structured as a network of two neurons: a preganglionic neuron located in the central nervous system and a postganglionic neuron situated in a peripheral nervous system structure. Preganglionic neurons originate from the dorsal horn of the spinal cord at thoracic and lumbar levels, from T2 to L2. Most of these neurons synapse with neurons in the paravertebral ganglia of these anatomical regions. Others pass through the paravertebral ganglia without synapsing and reach the postganglionic neuron in nerve plexuses located much closer to the target tissue, as is the case with the celiac plexus [17, 18].

At the thoracic level, nerve fibers originating from preganglionic neurons in the dorsal horn from T5 to T12 form the splanchnic nerves. These nerves are divided into the greater, lesser, and least splanchnic nerves. They contain both efferent motor fibers and afferent sensory fibers. All three nerves cross the thoracic sympathetic ganglionic chain without synapsing, traverse the diaphragm, and reach their target organs. The greater splanchnic nerve (neurons from T5 to T9) and the lesser splanchnic nerve (neurons from T10 to T11) synapse in the celiac plexus. Additionally, some fibers of the lesser splanchnic nerve synapse in the superior mesenteric and aorticorenal plexuses. The least splanchnic nerve (neurons from T11 to T12), which is not always present in all individuals, typically synapses in the aorticorenal ganglion [15, 19, 20].

Postganglionic fibers emerging from the celiac plexus innervate the esophagus, stomach, gallbladder, pancreas, and duodenum. They also influence liver function, regulating glycogenolysis, gluconeogenesis, and hepatic glucose release. At the splenic capsule level, the celiac plexus transmits nociceptive afferent fibers [19].

Classically, the celiac plexus is described as one of the largest autonomic plexuses, composed of two celiac ganglia located at the T12-L1 level, anterior to the celiac trunk and the superior mesenteric artery. Each ganglion is situated medial to the ipsilateral adrenal gland and anterior to the diaphragmatic crura [15]. The left ganglion is positioned posterior to the origin of the splenic artery, while the right ganglion is posterior to the inferior vena cava.

Recent anatomical studies have demonstrated significant variation in the anatomical arrangement of the celiac plexus among individuals. The presence of more than two celiac ganglia is a common finding. Studies conducted since the early 2000s indicate that the celiac ganglia are more frequently located lateral to the aorta rather than anterior, as previously described in classical anatomical texts. Most left celiac ganglia are found between the left adrenal gland and the left diaphragmatic crus. Right celiac ganglia are commonly located at the superior angle formed by the entry of the left renal vein into the inferior vena cava and, in many cases, are covered by the inferior vena cava itself [16, 21].

10.2.1.3 Celiac Plexus Block/Neurolysis Techniques

Various approaches and imaging techniques can be used to access the celiac plexus. The plexus can be reached via an anterior approach, accessing the retroperitoneal space through the peritoneal cavity, or a posterior approach. Imaging modalities include fluoroscopy, computed tomography (CT), magnetic resonance imaging (MRI), ultrasound, or endoscopic ultrasound (EUS). Additionally, direct intraoperative neurolysis can be performed during laparotomy.

10.2.1.4 Approaches

For the posterior approach, the following four techniques can be used [3]: (Fig. 10.2)

1. Antecrural approach. This is the most commonly used approach. The needle entry point is approximately 7.5 cm from the midline (spinous processes). The needles are advanced beyond the diaphragmatic crura at an angle of approximately 60° toward the midline.
2. Retrocrural approach. The needle tip is placed posterior to the diaphragmatic crura. This approach primarily blocks the splanchnic nerves, rather than the celiac plexus itself.
3. Transaortic approach. Performed only from the left side, at the level of the L1 vertebral body. The needle is advanced through both the posterior and anterior aortic walls, with confirmation of arterial blood return followed by its cessation. The drug is then administered at this antecrural location.
4. Transdiscal approach. The needle traverses the T12-L1 intervertebral disc, with its tip positioned anterior to the diaphragmatic crura. This approach is generally used when transverse processes or ribs obstruct a paravertebral approach. It may reduce the risk of visceral puncture (liver, kidney, or pancreas). The incidence of adverse events is low. All events were mild, and no serious adverse events were observed. The efficacy and safety of Neurolytic Splanchnic Nerve Block (NSNB) via trans intervertebral disc approach for patients with intractable cancer pain were demonstrated.

The anterior approach has regained popularity in recent years, particularly with the introduction of CT guidance for its execution. However, it carries risks such as hollow viscus perforation, secondary peritonitis, hemorrhage, and viscerovascular fistula formation [15]. Therefore, it is only indicated in patients for whom a posterior approach is not feasible.

Regardless of the approach, the final needle tip position should be the same:

- Anterior to the aorta and diaphragmatic crura.
- Between the origin of the celiac plexus and the superior mesenteric artery [8].

10.2.1.5 Neurolytic Agents

Currently, two neurolytic agents are available: 50–70% ethyl alcohol and 6–10% phenol. In Spain, phenol is generally unavailable [10]. Below is a comparison of both agents [8, 11, 23] (Table 10.1).

Ethyl alcohol is preferred for longer-lasting neurolytic effects, despite its painful administration. Phenol, while less commonly used, has a smoother onset and can be combined with contrast, but requires larger gauge needles due to its high viscosity.

10.2.1.6 Classic Technique Using Fluoroscopy or CT

Once the possible approaches have been described, we will now detail the classic posterior antecrural approach using fluoroscopy or computed tomography (CT). This technique allows for a quick and straightforward neurolysis or blockade by visualizing bony structures and assessing the distribution of iodinated contrast.

At our center, the patient is admitted on the morning of the procedure. Before entering the operating room, we ensure proper preparation, including fasting for 6 hours for solid foods and 2 hours for liquids. We also confirm hemodynamic stability, an adequate platelet count of over 50,000 cells/μL, correct coagulation parameters with a prothrombin time above 50% and an International Normalized Ratio (INR) below 1.2, and the suspension of any antiplatelet or anticoagulant medication if the patient is undergoing such treatment.

Once in the operating room, the patient is monitored for pulse oximetry, blood pressure, and electrocardiographic activity. Supplemental oxygen is administered

Table 10.1 Comparison of ethyl alcohol and phenol use

Characteristic	50–70% ethyl alcohol	6–10% phenol
Mechanism of action	Causes Wallerian degeneration: Disrupts lipids and precipitates neural proteins	Causes coagulation and necrosis of all neural elements
Baricity (relative to CSF)	Hypobaric	Hyperbaric
Pain on administration	Painful	Painless
Dilution and radiopaque contrast	Does not require a diluent; cannot be mixed with radiopaque contrast	Diluted in glycerin; can be mixed with radiopaque contrast but is highly viscous, requiring ≥20G needles
Onset of action	Immediate to 3–5 days	15 min to 1 day
Duration of effect	12–24 weeks	8–12 weeks
Specific risks	Vasospasm	Arrhythmias, seizures, destruction of Dacron prostheses, and potential vascular wall damage (protein alteration)

through nasal cannulas. The procedure is typically performed under local anesthesia at the needle insertion sites, using 1–2% lidocaine, which may be alkalinized with 1 M bicarbonate. Additionally, mild intravenous sedation is provided. Baseline fluid therapy is administered based on the patient's hemodynamic needs.

Following the procedure, the patient remains hospitalized for at least 48 hours to monitor and rule out any potential complications.

The patient is positioned in a prone decubitus position. Placing a pillow under the iliac crests may be helpful to reduce lumbar lordosis and facilitate the approach. Percutaneous needles with a caliber between 20 and 22G and 10–15 cm in length are used. Using fluoroscopy, in both anteroposterior and lateral projections, the T12 and L1 vertebral bodies are located. The needle is inserted bilaterally, 7.5 cm from the midline of the spine, at a 60° angle toward the midline. The tip of the needle should be positioned laterally to the aorta and anterior to the diaphragm pillars. To confirm the needle's position, we first perform a gentle aspiration to ensure there is no blood, cerebrospinal fluid, or urine. Then, a small amount of radiopaque contrast is administered, and using a posteroanterior view from a C-arm fluoroscopy, we verify that it distributes correctly: anterolateral to the aorta. Afterward, the neurolytic agent is administered: ethyl alcohol (50–60–70%) or phenol (6–10%). Typically, about 15–20 ml is injected on each side [8, 10].

This technique can be performed using either CT or fluoroscopy. Fluoroscopy is simpler and is generally readily available in operating rooms. However, it does not allow for visualization of soft tissues. On the other hand, CT enables the visualization of all anatomical references needed to locate the celiac plexus. It can even allow visualization of the plexus itself [8] and the correct distribution of the radiopaque contrast. The disadvantages of CT include higher radiation risk and less availability, as it is typically not available in the operating room and is generally confined to the interventional radiology suite.

10.2.1.7 Other Imaging Methods

The use of ultrasound as an imaging technique for celiac plexus neurolysis is very recent, first described in 1996. Its effectiveness and the evaluation of the best approach for its use are still under discussion. The most commonly used technique is transgastric ultrasound, using endoscopic ultrasound to explore the celiac trunk and the aorta. Doppler ultrasound helps identify major retroperitoneal vessels [24].

MRI can also be used. MRI allows for proper visualization of all retroperitoneal anatomical structures, with a higher resolution than CT, including the celiac plexus itself. The needle trajectory can be guided in real time with open MRI systems, and there is no need for radiopaque contrast [25, 26]. Its main limitation is the scarcity of availability of such radiological facilities [8].

10.2.1.8 Complications

Celiac plexus neurolysis is a relatively safe procedure with a low complication rate, around 2% [1]. The most common complication is dorsal-lumbar pain and shoulder pain, present in about 96% of patients [8, 27]. Dorsal and lumbar pain usually results from celiac nerve denervation and is often accompanied by shoulder pain due to phrenic nerve irritation. These pains typically persist for about 72 hours after the procedure [8].

Diarrhea and constipation occur with an incidence close to 44% [8]. However, patients typically experience less constipation compared to those who have not undergone celiac plexus neurolysis and continue to take high doses of opioid medication [2].

Other frequent complications include dorsal-lumbar pain and shoulder pain, as mentioned above.

Since the celiac plexus is a sympathetic plexus, its denervation can lead to orthostatic hypotension. It is generally recommended to ensure proper hydration of patients both before and after the procedure to minimize this risk.

In about 1% of patients, serious complications may occur, either from hemorrhage or neurological damage [22, 24, 28]. Vertebral artery spasm due to the neurolytic agent or mechanical damage can lead to spinal cord ischemia, causing lower limb weakness, even paralysis, loss of sensation, or atony of the detrusor muscle [8, 27].

Celiac plexus neurolysis is considered an intermediate-risk bleeding procedure [29]. The transfusion rate associated with celiac plexus neurolysis is around 1%. For patients on antiplatelet drugs, aspirin at a dose of 100 mg should generally not be discontinued, but doses of 300 mg or higher should be suspended. P2Y12 inhibitors should be suspended 5–7 days before the procedure. The most commonly used drug, clopidogrel, should ideally be suspended 7 days prior. As for anticoagulants, an INR of at least 1.2 should be guaranteed before performing the procedure. In cases of low molecular weight heparin or new anticoagulants (dabigatran, rivaroxaban, etc.), it is essential to ensure that at least two half-lives of the drug have passed before the procedure [22].

Currently, there is no international consensus on the exact platelet count, and most oncological patients have hematologic alterations that make it difficult to establish these thresholds. In the future, viscoelastic tests may help determine them [21].

It is important to note that injury to major retroperitoneal vessels may go unnoticed in the immediate aftermath of the procedure. A retroperitoneal hematoma can cause neurological deficits due to nerve compression, even before abdominal pain or a drop in blood pressure occur [21]. Therefore, continuous hemodynamic and neurological monitoring is recommended in the first few hours following the procedure [8, 27, 28].

Other reported complications include hematuria, pneumothorax, pericarditis, pleuritis, intervertebral disc damage, and retroperitoneal abscess [8, 27].

10.2.1.9 Conclusions

Celiac plexus neurolysis is a palliative analgesic technique for patients with oncological pain due to upper abdominal lesions that do not respond to conventional pharmacological treatments and whose tumors are not resectable. It has shown effectiveness of around 70–80% during the first month after the procedure. It is a safe technique, with a low incidence of serious complications (about 1%). Depending on the technique employed, it is relatively simple and widely available in different hospital centers.

10.2.2 Impar Ganglion Block

10.2.2.1 Introduction

The impar ganglion, also known as Walther's ganglion, is a structure of the sympathetic nervous system located in the midline anterior to the sacrococcygeal ligament. This ganglion plays a key role in transmitting pain signals from the distal rectum, anus, distal urethra, distal third of the vagina, vulva, and penis to the central nervous system. Its blockade is an effective therapeutic tool in managing chronic pelvic and perineal pain, both of oncological and non-oncological origin, especially in cases that are refractory to conservative therapies. Since its initial description by Plancarte et al. [30], it has gained importance in managing intractable pain associated with cancer and other non-oncological conditions.

10.2.2.2 Anatomy of the Impar Ganglion and Its Role in Visceral Pain

The impar ganglion, also known as Walther's ganglion, is a key structure in the sympathetic nervous system situated in the midline, anterior to the sacrococcygeal junction. It serves as the convergence point of the bilateral sympathetic chains and participates in transmitting nociceptive signals from the distal rectum, anal canal, distal urethra, vulva, vagina, and penis to the central nervous system. Its postganglionic sympathetic fibers innervate these areas, modulating both sensory and autonomic functions.

Its involvement in pain transmission makes it an important therapeutic target, particularly in cases of pelvic and perineal pain, both oncological and non-oncological in origin. Moreover, the impar ganglion interacts with other pelvic nerve plexuses, such as the superior hypogastric plexus, enabling joint modulation of pain. For this reason, it is often used in combination with other blocks to effectively manage refractory pain affecting extensive areas of the pelvis.

10.2.2.3 Indications and Effectiveness of the Impar Ganglion Block

The impar ganglion block (IGB) is an interventional technique indicated for treating pelvic and perineal pain of various etiologies, especially in cases where conservative therapies have been insufficient. Its use is particularly relevant in managing pain related to cancer, such as perineal pain caused by colorectal, gynecological, or urological tumors, as well as complications derived from treatments such as radiation therapy, including radiation proctitis and vulvodynia [30–33]. It is also effective in relieving postoperative pain related to oncological interventions and neuropathic pain associated with cancer [34]. According to the American Society of Pain and Neuroscience, the IGB should be considered a key tool in patients with intractable oncological pain.

Additionally, the IGB is indicated in treating chronic nonmalignant pelvic pain, such as coccygodynia, vulvodynia, chronic prostatitis, and chronic pelvic pain syndrome. It is also used in cases of postherpetic neuralgia affecting the perineal area [35–37]. These conditions are often refractory to conventional treatments, making the IGB an effective therapeutic option for providing lasting pain relief.

In the context of cancer-related pain, the IGB not only significantly alleviates pain intensity in many patients but also helps reduce opioid dependency, improving quality of life [34, 35]. Although scientific evidence mainly comes from clinical cases and case series, the results support its use as an effective and safe therapeutic tool for managing refractory pain.

10.2.2.4 Approaches for Impar Ganglion Block (IGB)

The impar ganglion can be approached using various techniques, each with its own characteristics and benefits:

Anococcygeal Approach

The anococcygeal approach for the impar ganglion block, initially described by Plancarte et al. in 1990, involves inserting a needle through the anococcygeal ligament and directing it toward the sacrococcygeal junction under fluoroscopic guidance. This procedure aims to position the needle tip in front of the sacrococcygeal joint, allowing precise access to the impar ganglion for the administration of the therapeutic agent. To prevent complications, the operator uses the nondominant hand at the rectal level, which helps avoid accidental perforations.

Despite its effectiveness, this approach has significant limitations due to associated risks. These include rectal perforation, which can lead to serious complications, trauma to the operator during manipulation, fragmentation of the angled needle during the procedure, and the possibility of intraosseous injection, in addition to patient discomfort. These factors contribute to a procedure failure rate of up to 30% in some cases, limiting its clinical application. To mitigate some of these problems, the use of curved needles has been proposed, which has been shown to reduce tissue trauma and minimize the risk of needle fragmentation. Although this technical modification offers certain advantages, the anococcygeal approach remains less commonly used in clinical practice due to the potential complications and inherent difficulties of the procedure.

Transsacrococcygeal Approach (Midline Approach)

The transsacrococcygeal approach, described by Wemm and Saberski in 1995, is a widely used technique for the impar ganglion block due to its simplicity, safety, and efficacy [2]. This method involves inserting a needle through the sacrococcygeal ligament and carefully advancing it toward the precoccygeal region, where the impar ganglion is located. By following a direct midline trajectory, the procedure avoids manipulating sensitive structures such as the rectum or highly vascular tissues, making it less invasive than other approaches.

The procedure is performed with the patient in the prone position, identifying the sacrococcygeal junction using anatomical landmarks and confirming it with fluoroscopy. A needle is inserted along the midline, crossing the sacrococcygeal ligament at an appropriate angle until it reaches the precoccygeal region. Once properly positioned, a radiological contrast is injected, and the lateral projection reveals the "comma sign," an inverted apostrophe on the anterior face of the joint. This contrast should remain dorsal to the rectal gas pattern but anterior to the coccyx. In an Anterior-Posterior (AP) projection, a rounded image is observed at the joint level. After verifying the location, the neurolytic agent is administered.

Intercoccygeal Approach

The intercoccygeal approach is a technique that provides direct access to the impar ganglion through the joint spaces between the coccygeal vertebrae (Fig. 10.1). It is especially useful in older patients with ossification of the sacrococcygeal ligament, as it avoids complications associated with this rigid tissue [30, 31].

The procedure is performed under fluoroscopic or computed tomography (CT) guidance, where a needle is inserted through the selected intercoccygeal space, advancing it toward the precoccygeal region until it is positioned in front of the impar ganglion. Once positioned, a radiological contrast is injected, and after verification (similar distribution to the transsacrococcygeal approach), the neurolitic agent is administered.

Lateral Approach Guided by CT

Proposed by Agarwal-Kozlowski et al., this method involves introducing a needle laterally, without crossing the sacrum or coccyx. The lateral approach reduces the risk of infection by moving the insertion point away from contaminated areas, such as the anal opening [3]. Although technically more demanding, its effectiveness has been reported in patients with complex anatomies [32].

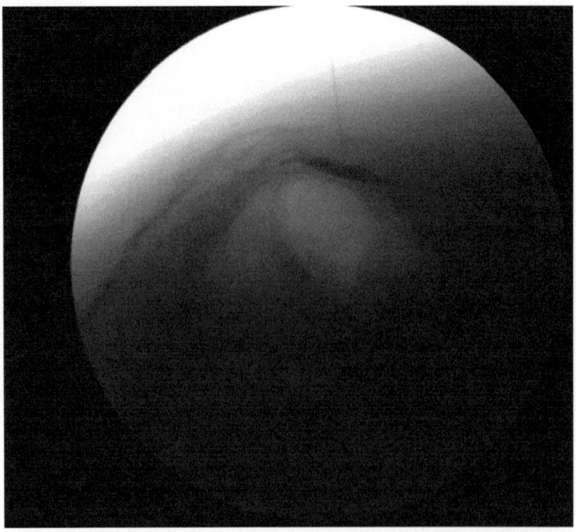

Fig. 10.1 Intercoccygeal approach. The contrast agent is visualized below the coccygeal vertebrae. Dr. Moltó's own work

10.2.2.5 Imaging Techniques

Most of the procedures described in the literature for ganglion impar block (GIB) are performed under fluoroscopic guidance, with more than 95 documented procedures supporting its use. Fluoroscopy is the most commonly used technique due to its wide availability and its ability to confirm the needle's position in real time during the procedure, ensuring greater safety and efficacy [30, 31].

In addition to fluoroscopy, other imaging modalities such as computed tomography (CT) and ultrasound (US) have been explored. CT stands out for offering greater precision in locating the ganglion impar, being particularly useful in patients with fibrosis or anatomical alterations that make access difficult with other techniques [3]. Due to its ability to generate detailed images, CT is a valuable tool in complex cases.

Ultrasound, although less studied, presents itself as an interesting alternative. It allows for the identification of the ganglion impar without exposing the patient to radiation, making it an ideal option for diagnostic and non-neurolytic therapeutic blocks [37]. Its use is particularly advantageous in situations where minimizing radiation risks and optimizing procedural logistics is desired.

10.2.2.6 Comparisons Between Techniques

There are no randomized controlled trials directly comparing the approaches for GIB. However, the transsacrococcygeal approach seems to offer the best balance between simplicity and safety, being the most commonly used [31]. On the other hand, the CT-guided and ultrasound-guided approaches have shown specific advantages in terms of precision and risk reduction in selected cases [32, 37].

10.2.2.7 Conclusion

GIB can be performed using different approaches and imaging techniques. The choice of method depends on patient characteristics, the operator's experience, and available resources. Despite the differences between techniques, all are effective in relieving pelvic and perineal pain. Further studies are needed to establish direct comparisons between approaches and optimize selection according to clinical needs.

10.2.3 Superior Hypogastric Plexus Block (SHPB)

10.2.3.1 Introduction

Superior hypogastric plexus block (SHPB) is an interventional technique used to treat visceral pain in the pelvic region, particularly in patients with oncological pain or refractory chronic pain [38, 40]. This procedure allows the interruption of visceral pain transmission to the central nervous system, providing significant relief in patients with difficult-to-control pelvic pain [41, 42]. It is especially relevant in the management of oncological pain, where conventional treatments such as opioid analgesics may be insufficient or cause unwanted side effects [43–45].

10.2.3.2 Anatomy of the Superior Hypogastric Plexus (SHP) and Its Role in Visceral Innervation

The superior hypogastric plexus is located in the retroperitoneum, anterior to the vertebral body of the fifth lumbar vertebra (L5) and the first sacral vertebra (S1) [40, 43]. It is composed of sympathetic fibers originating from the lumbar splanchnic nerves, which connect to the inferior hypogastric plexuses through the hypogastric nerves [44]. This nervous system is responsible for the sympathetic innervation of organs such as the uterus, ovaries, bladder, distal rectum, prostate, and external genital structures [43]. The nociceptive fibers of the plexus transmit deep visceral pain, making it a key therapeutic target in the management of pelvic pain associated with cancer and other pathologies [41, 45].

10.2.3.3 Indications and Efficacy of SHP Block

The superior hypogastric plexus block is primarily indicated in the treatment of pelvic visceral pain, a condition that can have various etiologies, both malignant and nonmalignant. Major indications include:

Cancer-Related Pain

It is the most common indication, especially in patients with advanced gynecological, colorectal, or urological cancer. In these conditions, the pain is often visceral and mediated by sympathetic fibers that converge in the superior hypogastric plexus [1].

Refractory Chronic Pain

Nonmalignant pathologies such as endometriosis, interstitial cystitis, chronic post-surgical pain, or chronic pelvic pain syndrome, in which previous treatments have failed and the patient experiences significant impairment of quality of life [40].

10.2.3.4 Efficacy of Superior Hypogastric Plexus Block (SHPB)

Studies have shown that SHPB provides significant pain relief in a large proportion of patients. In the context of malignant pain, data suggest that up to 70% of patients experience significant pain reduction after a neurolysis procedure with alcohol or phenol [42, 43]. For nonmalignant pain, although results may be less consistent, relief has been reported in approximately 50% of patients who undergo a diagnostic block followed by therapeutic neurolysis [44]. In addition to reducing pain intensity, the procedure also helps reduce opioid consumption, improving quality of life and reducing associated side effects [45].

10.2.3.5 Techniques for SHP Block

The SHP block is performed using various techniques, each with its own indications, advantages, and limitations. The most commonly used techniques are described below:

Paravertebral Approach

The superior hypogastric plexus block (SHPB), first described in 1990 by Plancarte et al. [43], is a percutaneous technique widely used for managing refractory pelvic pain, especially that of neoplastic origin.

The procedure is performed with the patient in the prone position, placing a support under the lower abdomen to optimize lumbar curvature. The L4-L5 intervertebral space is located and verified using fluoroscopy. The needle entry point is identified 5–7 cm laterally from the midline, at the level of the L4-L5 intervertebral space. A 22G, 15 cm Chiba needle is used, which is inserted through the skin at a 30-degree caudal and 45-degree medial angle. The needle tip is directed toward the anterolateral region of the L5-S1 junction (Fig. 10.2). During needle advancement, contact with structures such as the L5 transverse process and sacral wing should be avoided to prevent obstruction of the needle's trajectory. If the L5 transverse process is encountered during advancement, the needle should be withdrawn into the subcutaneous tissue and redirected to avoid contact. It is then advanced again until it reaches the vertebral body of L5.

Once in contact with the vertebral body, the needle trajectory is adjusted so that it smoothly slides along the bone surface toward the anterolateral portion, a position confirmed by fluoroscopy in a lateral projection. The needle is advanced approximately 1 cm beyond the vertebral body's edge, at which point a loss of resistance can be felt. This indicates that the needle tip has passed through the anterior fascia of the ipsilateral psoas muscle and is in the retroperitoneal space.

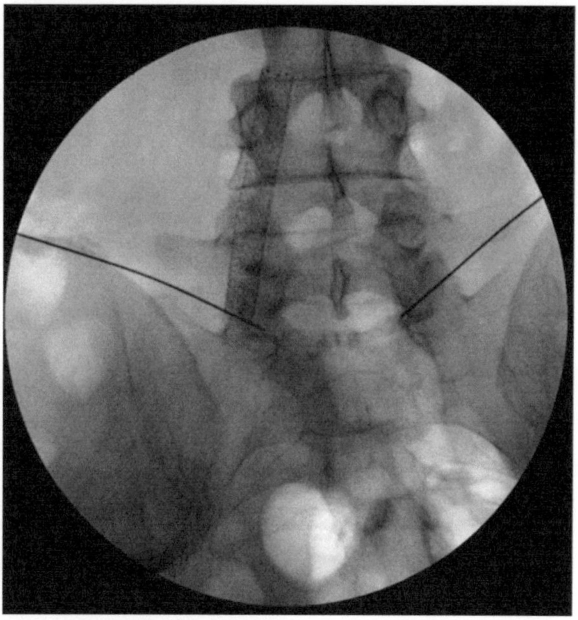

Fig. 10.2 Paravertebral approach for hypogastric plexus block. Anteroposterior fluoroscopic image. Needles guided by fluoroscopy positioned in the anterolateral region of the L5 vertebral body. Dr. Moltó's own work

With the correct position confirmed via fluoroscopy, the contrast medium is injected, followed by the neurolytic agent (Figs. 10.3 and 10.4). This bilateral approach ensures adequate coverage of the superior hypogastric plexus.

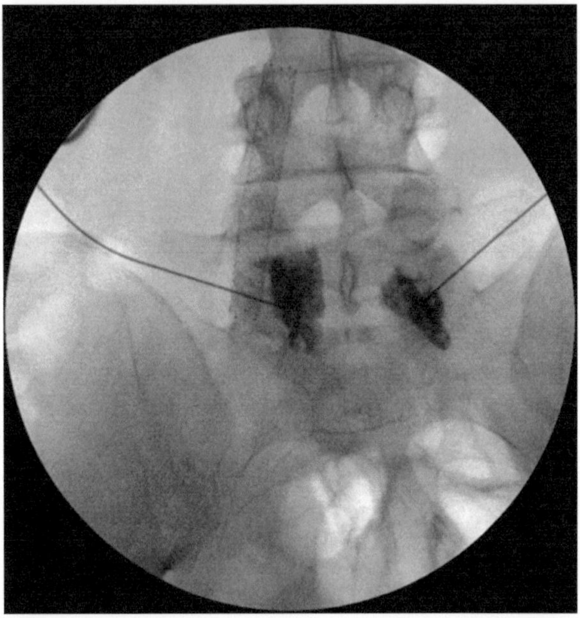

Fig. 10.3 Paravertebral approach. Anteroposterior fluoroscopic image showing appropriate spread of iodinated contrast. Dr. Moltó's own work

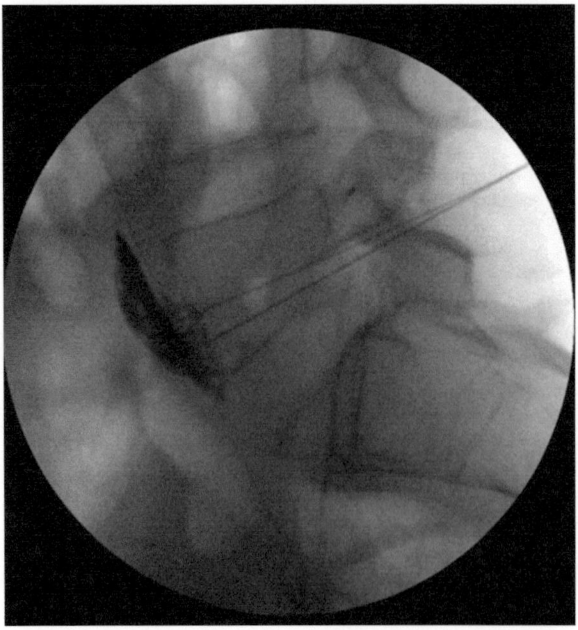

Fig. 10.4 Paravertebral approach. Lateral fluoroscopic image showing appropriate spread of iodinated contrast. Dr. Moltó's own work

Transdiscal Approach

The transdiscal technique, described by Ina et al. in 1992 [43], uses a more direct approach to reach the superior hypogastric plexus by traversing the intervertebral disc between L5 and S1. This technique allows precise anatomical access but requires specific prophylactic measures, such as the prior administration of 1 g of ceftriaxone, to reduce the risk of discitis (4%).

The patient is positioned in the prone position with support under the iliac crest, optimizing the alignment of the lumbar spine. Fluoroscopy is used to adjust the viewing angle, first in the cephalic direction to align the vertebral endplates, and then in an oblique tilt of 15–25 degrees, which allows optimal visualization of the L5-S1 intervertebral disc.

The Chiba needle, typically 15–20 cm in length and 20-22G in gauge, is introduced through an entry point marked laterally from the midline, 5–7 cm away. The insertion follows a controlled trajectory using a "tunnel vision" technique (Fig. 10.5), guiding the needle laterally to the inferior aspect of the facet joint.

Once the needle reaches the disc, a small amount of contrast is injected to confirm its precise location inside the disc. From there, the needle is carefully advanced to penetrate the disc, which is identified by a loss of resistance indicating that the tip has reached the retroperitoneal space.

Once the needle position is confirmed in the retroperitoneal space, it is verified by administering contrast (Figs. 10.6 and 10.7), followed by the injection of the neurolytic agent.

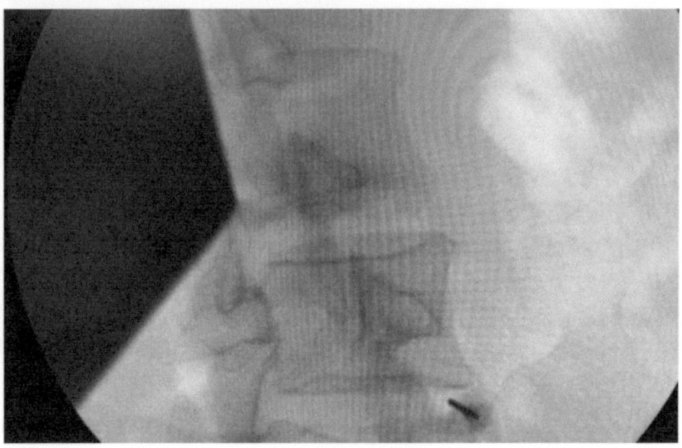

Fig. 10.5 Transdiscal approach. "Tunnel vision" technique, guiding the needle laterally to the inferior aspect of the facet joint. Dr. Moltó's own work

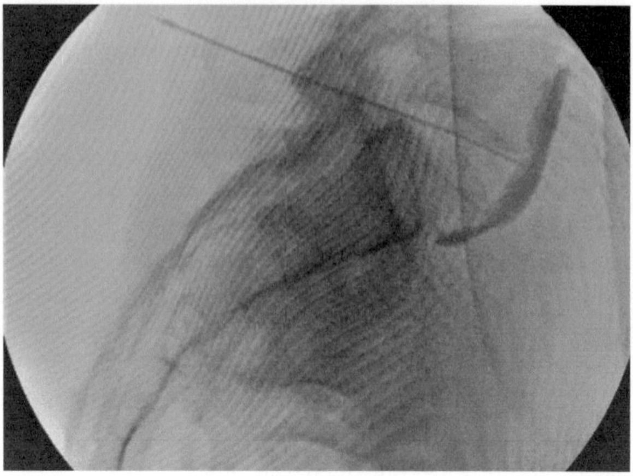

Fig. 10.6 Transdiscal approach. Anteroposterior (6) and lateral (7) fluoroscopic images showing appropriate spread of iodinated contrast. Dr. Moltó's own work

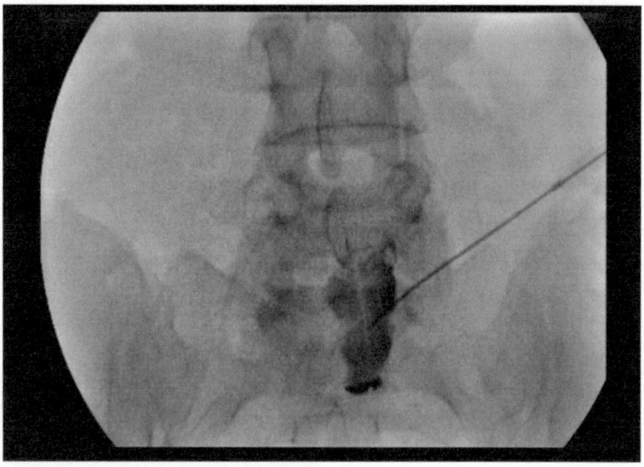

Fig. 10.7 Transdiscal approach. Anteroposterior (6) and lateral (7) fluoroscopic images showing appropriate spread of iodinated contrast. Dr. Moltó's own work

Transdiscal Approach

The transdiscal approach is considered equally effective as the paravertebral approach in terms of pain relief, according to studies such as those by Erdine et al. [44], although its implementation requires rigorous technical management and additional safety measures. The transdiscal technique represents a valuable option in the management of pelvic pain related to cancer, especially useful in patients with significant vertebral deformities or large transverse processes, conditions that may hinder the use of classical techniques such as the Plancarte approach [42].

Ultrasound-Guided Anterior Approach

The neurolysis technique for the superior hypogastric plexus (SHPN) guided by ultrasound is performed with the patient in the supine position, under aseptic conditions, and after an 8-hour fast, complemented with intestinal preparation using bisacodyl and activated charcoal. Before the procedure, patients are asked to empty their bladder to reduce complications during the intervention [45, 46]. Using a

5–2 MHz curved transducer, the bifurcation of the abdominal aorta into the common iliac arteries is identified, followed by the body of the fifth lumbar vertebra (L5). Color Doppler is used to confirm the location of the iliac vessels, ensuring precise visualization of the vascular structures [46].

Once the anatomical landmarks are identified, 2% lidocaine (3–4 ml) is administered for subcutaneous local anesthesia, typically about 3–4 cm below the umbilicus [44]. A Chiba needle is then inserted using an out-of-plane technique under ultrasound guidance, carefully advancing it toward the most anterior point of the L5 vertebral body. The needle is slightly withdrawn after contacting the bone to avoid injecting the medication into the periosteum, and aspiration is performed to confirm the absence of blood, minimizing the risk of intravascular injection [45, 46].

The procedure includes a diagnostic phase in which bupivacaine is administered as an anesthetic agent to assess the initial effectiveness of the block. If no complications or significant changes in vital signs occur, neurolysis is performed by injecting a neurolytic agent. Depending on the protocol, 50% ethanol or 10% phenol can be used, always in combination with a local anesthetic, to ensure uniform distribution of the medication along the anterior curvature of the L5 vertebral body. The injection is performed slowly and in a controlled manner, confirming its distribution in real time using ultrasonography.

During and after the procedure, the patient's vital signs are monitored, with the patient remaining fully conscious. Any complications or adverse effects related to the procedure or the neurolytic agent are recorded and treated accordingly. The technique described stands out for its precision and efficacy in managing cancer-related pelvic pain, as noted by Mishra et al. [45] and Abdelghaffar et al. [47], who have documented its effectiveness and safety under these controlled conditions.

Anterior Approach Guided by X-Ray

The technique begins with the patient in the supine position under sterile conditions. The L5-S1 intervertebral space is identified using fluoroscopy (Fig. 10.8). The entry point is marked on the skin with a radiopaque object, and 2% lidocaine (3–4 ml) is administered for subcutaneous local anesthesia, below the umbilicus.

A 22G, 20 cm Chiba needle is inserted under fluoroscopic guidance toward the anterior portion of the L5 vertebral body. Upon reaching bone resistance, aspiration is performed to confirm that there is no blood in the needle. Then, 2–5 ml of contrast is injected to visualize its distribution, confirming that no vascular structure is involved. A lateral view (Fig. 10.8) then confirms the correct diffusion of the contrast in the anterior region of the vertebral body.

Once the needle position is secured, a preliminary test is performed by injecting 3 ml of 0.5% bupivacaine. If no changes in neurological status or vital signs are observed, the neurolytic agent is injected, with intermittent aspirations to avoid intravascular injection. During the injection, slight forward pressure is applied to the needle to maintain its position. The procedure concludes with real-time monitoring of the distribution of the neurolytic agent using fluoroscopy, ensuring proper coverage of the target region.

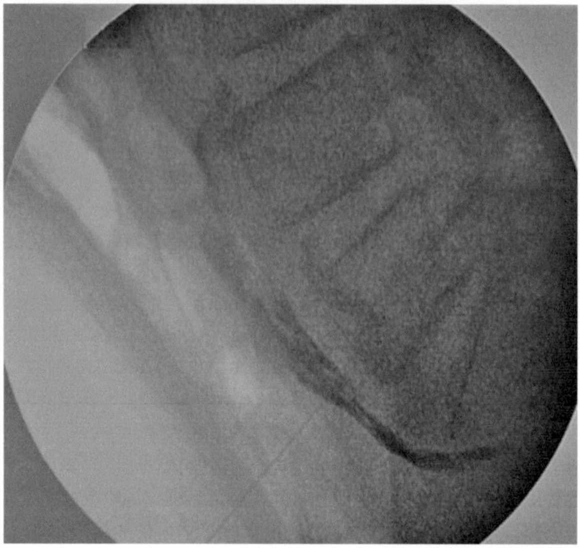

Fig. 10.8 Anterior approach guided by X-ray. A lateral view then confirms the correct diffusion of the contrast in the anterior region of the vertebral body. Dr. Moltó's own work

CT-Guided Approach

Computed tomography (CT) has revolutionized interventional techniques by providing precise and detailed visualization of anatomical structures, allowing for safer and more effective procedures. In the case of superior hypogastric plexus blockade, CT facilitates the identification of the plexus and ensures accurate needle placement, minimizing the risk of complications [48].

Among the CT-guided approaches for this procedure are the unilateral anterior approach, which allows for needle insertion from an anterior position [48]; the bilateral transdiscal approach, described by Dooley et al. [49], which uses the L5-S1 intervertebral disc as the access route; the posterior paramedial approach, which introduces needles from a posterior and lateral position relative to the spine; and the single-needle approach, a modified technique that simplifies the procedure by using only one needle [50]. These methods stand out for their precision and effectiveness, with CT being key to their success.

10.2.3.6 Comparison of Techniques

Different techniques for superior hypogastric plexus blockade offer varying levels of efficacy, safety, and accessibility. The paravertebral approach remains the most commonly used due to its proven efficacy and lower complication rate. However, techniques such as the transdiscal approach and CT guidance offer specific advantages in complex cases.

The paravertebral approach, guided by fluoroscopy, is particularly effective in patients with normal pelvic anatomy, as it provides real-time guidance to ensure precise needle placement. In comparison, the transdiscal approach offers more direct access to the superior hypogastric plexus, but at the cost of a higher risk of intervertebral disc infections.

The ultrasound-guided anterior approach, although technically more challenging, is highlighted for its safety in patients with significant anatomical distortion. Ultrasound allows for clear visualization of surrounding structures, minimizing the risk of vascular perforation or visceral damage.

On the other hand, CT, although costly and with greater radiation exposure, is particularly useful in cases where anatomical precision is critical. Unlike fluoroscopy, CT provides detailed three-dimensional images, which are essential in patients with large pelvic tumors or complex anatomy.

10.2.3.7 Conclusion

Superior hypogastric plexus blockade (SHPB) is an effective intervention for managing pelvic pain associated with cancer. Each technique presents advantages and disadvantages that should be evaluated based on the individual characteristics of the patient, the experience of the healthcare staff, and the available resources. The paravertebral approach is the most commonly used due to its efficacy and low complication risk, while ultrasound and CT-guided methods are useful options in patients who cannot tolerate the prone position or have anatomical abnormalities that contraindicate the posterior approach. Currently, there are no conclusive studies determining which technique is most effective for superior hypogastric plexus blockade.

10.2.4 Stellate Ganglion Block

10.2.4.1 Anatomy

The stellate ganglion is one of the three ganglia that form the sympathetic trunk at the cervical level. In 80% of cases, the inferior cervical ganglion fuses with the first thoracic ganglion, forming the cervicothoracic or stellate ganglion. This ganglion provides sympathetic fibers to the upper limb through the C7, C8, and T1 branches. It is laterally related to the anterior and middle scalene muscles, medially to the longus colli muscle, anteriorly to the carotid artery, and posteriorly to the transverse process of C6 or C7 and the prevertebral fascia. The vertebral artery is found at the C7 level [51].

10.2.4.2 Indications

The block is indicated in the presence of oncologic pain in the head, neck, and upper limb, as well as in postoperative pain following breast cancer surgery. In non-oncologic patients, it is indicated for sympathetically mediated pain syndromes in the head, neck, and upper limb; complex regional pain syndrome in the upper limb and face; atypical facial pain; facial herpes zoster and postherpetic neuralgia; and precordial pain due to angina [52].

10.2.4.3 Approach

The approach has been described using fluoroscopic or ultrasound guidance. This procedure is performed under sterile conditions, with sedation and local anesthesia at the injection site. Ultrasound guidance has the advantage of visualizing adjacent structures such as the esophagus, carotid artery, thyroid vessels, as well as the real-time dispersion of the administered medication.

In the fluoroscopic approach, the patient is placed in a supine position, either in a neutral position or with slight rotation to the opposite side of the procedure. The vertebral bodies and transverse processes of C6 and C7 are identified, with a slight craniocaudal tilt to eliminate double contour. The needle should be advanced toward the junction of the transverse process and the vertebral body, below the uncinate process. The procedure can be performed at either C6 or C7 using a BD Yale™ Quicke (Franklin Lakes, NJ, USA) 22-gauge needle. Once the needle reaches the bone surface, iodinated contrast is administered.

It will show a paraspinal (fusiform) pattern, neither radicular nor intravascular. At this level, infiltration is performed with a local anesthetic and corticosteroid [51].

For the use of ultrasound, the patient is placed in a supine or lateral decubitus position. A BD Yale™ Quicke (Franklin Lakes, NJ, USA) 22-gauge needle is used. The approach is performed "in-plane" using a linear probe, allowing continuous visualization of the needle tip. The needle is advanced to the deep cervical fascia above the longus colli muscle, where a local anesthetic and corticosteroid are administered [53].

The administered dose for this procedure ranges from 7 to 10 mL of 0.25% bupivacaine (2 mL) without epinephrine, combined with 8 mg of dexamethasone or 12 mg of betamethasone. If effective, a pulsed radiofrequency ablation of the stellate ganglion may be considered, performed at 42 °C for 4 min, which provides a longer-lasting effect compared to corticosteroids.

There are indirect signs of a successful stellate ganglion block, including an increase in temperature of at least 1 °C in the affected limb due to cervical sympatholysis, and the presence of unilateral Horner's syndrome: ptosis, miosis, enophthalmos, anhidrosis, nasal and conjunctival congestion, and venodilation.

Although it is a safe technique, as with any interventional procedure, complications may occur, including Horner's syndrome, brachial plexus block, recurrent laryngeal nerve block, hematoma, vascular or thyroid injury, and esophageal puncture.

There is insufficient evidence to favor performing the procedure under ultrasound guidance versus fluoroscopy. However, the availability of ultrasound equipment in our units has led to an increased preference for ultrasound guidance.

10.2.5 Glossopharyngeal Nerve Block

10.2.5.1 Anatomy

The glossopharyngeal nerve is a nerve that originates from the brainstem at the level of the medulla oblongata, exiting the skull through the jugular foramen. It is a mixed nerve with motor, sensory, and parasympathetic functions. It provides innervation to the external ear, the posterior pharynx, the soft palate, and the epiglottis, as well as the posterior third of the tongue, the carotid body, and the carotid sinus. Its motor innervation includes muscles of the pharynx and stylopharyngeus for swallowing, as well as secretory fibers to the parotid gland. Tumors of the tongue, pharynx, and base of the skull may lead to glossopharyngeal neuralgia.

10.2.5.2 Clinical Presentation

Glossopharyngeal neuralgia has been associated with carcinomas of the parapharyngeal space, pharyngeal, nasopharyngeal, or tongue cancers.

The involvement of the glossopharyngeal nerve is characterized by severe paroxysmal pain located in the throat, external auditory canal, posterior part of the tongue, and the angle of the mandible. The pain is typically sharp, stabbing, and can be triggered by swallowing, coughing, speaking, or chewing.

10.2.5.3 Approach

Glossopharyngeal neuralgia can cause intense pain that may not be controlled with pharmacological treatment, possibly requiring advanced neurosurgical interventions. Microvascular decompression has a high success rate (80–90%), although its use is limited in cancer patients due to the risks of permanent damage to lower cranial nerves. An alternative to neurosurgical approaches is radiofrequency ablation, which selectively targets the branches of the glossopharyngeal nerve [54].

The development of radiofrequency has enabled its application through tomography-guided, fluoroscopy-guided, and ultrasound-guided approaches. According to the reviewed work, pain relief has been found in over 50% of patients with oropharyngeal cancer treated [55]. The most frequent complications are the onset of dysphagia and hypoesthesia.

The use of ultrasound in glossopharyngeal nerve blockade has minimized the risk of complications and improved efficacy [55]. Ultrasound-guided extracranial approaches have proven effective in reducing pain and opioid consumption in patients with oropharyngeal cancer, with success rates greater than 90% in the short term. The use of anatomical references such as the internal carotid artery and the curved transducer has enabled safer identification and treatment of the nerve. Recent techniques such as the posterior approach to the mandibular branch minimize complications by avoiding critical structures such as the parotid gland, the vagus nerve, or the hypoglossal nerve [55]. In cases of fibrosis or the presence of tumor masses, parapharyngeal approaches using ultrasound and nerve stimulation have been developed, allowing safe access to the glossopharyngeal nerve [56].

The treatment of glossopharyngeal neuralgia continues to evolve toward less invasive and safer techniques, integrating advances in imaging and ablation technology. While these interventions offer significant pain relief, complications remain a major challenge, highlighting the need for careful patient selection and multidisciplinary management.

10.3 Radiofrequency for Osteoarticular Pain in Oncology Patients

10.3.1 Introduction

Osteoarticular pain in oncology patients is very common, especially in those with advanced disease and/or undergoing certain oncological treatments, such as chemotherapy, hormone therapy, or radiotherapy [57–59]. In fact, the skeleton is the third most common site for metastasis, after the lungs and liver [57].

Despite its high incidence and the availability of multiple treatments, controlling osteoarticular pain remains a significant clinical challenge. In this chapter, we will review the origin of oncological osteoarticular pain, provide a brief overview of conventional treatments, and discuss therapeutic options for patients who do not respond to conventional therapies, specifically radiofrequency techniques.

10.3.2 Incidence, Pathophysiology, and Clinical Features of Oncological Osteoarticular Pain

The estimated incidence of osteoarticular pain in oncology patients is 75% [58]. The majority of this pain is secondary to metastases and multiple myeloma, as the incidence of primary bone tumors is very low, approximately 1 per 100,000 people per year [59]. The tumors that most commonly metastasize to bone include: breast cancer (70%), prostate cancer (85%), lung cancer (40%), and kidney cancer (40%). Multiple myeloma affects the bone in 95% of cases [60]. Estrogen receptor-positive breast cancer can present with bone metastasis late, even up to 10 years after completing successful oncological treatment [61].

Bones rich in bone marrow and trabecular structure are most affected, with a clear preference for the vertebrae, ribs, pelvis, epiphyses of long bones, and the skull [60, 61]. Elderly patients are at higher risk due to the dynamics of their bone metabolism: reduced osteoblast activity, increased osteoclast activity, and osteocyte apoptosis [61].

Oncological bone pain occurs through four main mechanisms: [62]

1. The destruction of bone tissue caused by tumor invasion and growth. This phenomenon stimulates the nerve fibers of the endosteum and leads to the release of various inflammatory mediators.
2. Stretching of the periosteum secondary to tumor growth, which stimulates the numerous nerve fibers of this tissue, causing pain.
3. Tumor growth itself can invade or compress adjacent sensory fibers at the site of metastasis.
4. The alteration of bone architecture can lead to pathological fractures.

Therefore, it has a mixed origin, both inflammatory and neuropathic. All the mechanisms described lead to central hyperexcitability, initially at the dorsal root ganglion and the dorsal horn of the spinal cord. The presence of this phenomenon makes it challenging to control symptoms such as allodynia, hyperalgesia, and breakthrough pain [58].

Patients typically present with moderate to severe pain [58]. Initially, pain is often nocturnal and worsens with load or movement of the affected area. In more advanced stages, episodes of breakthrough pain are common, along with difficulty or even inability to move, neurological deficits related to nerve compression, and pathological fractures [57].

10.3.3 Conventional Treatment of Oncological Bone Pain

The main treatment objectives are to prevent disease progression and to adequately control symptoms. For pain management, a multidisciplinary approach is essential.

Pharmacological treatment should be tailored to the intensity and characteristics of the pain. The use of anti-inflammatory drugs cannot be employed chronically due to potential cardiovascular and renal damage [63]. Therefore, opioid medications will be one of the most important pillars of treatment. As always, their use is limited by adverse effects, especially in patients with chronic oncological pain and a long life expectancy. The use of anticonvulsants and antidepressants effective against neuropathic pain should also be employed. Bisphosphonates and denosumab are used as bone resorption inhibitors to prevent pathological fractures and treat hypercalcemia [64, 65].

The most effective invasive technique is radiotherapy, both for pain control and for disease control. One-third of treated patients experience complete pain relief. The use of radionuclides has also proven useful in the treatment of bone metastases secondary to follicular thyroid cancer, prostate cancer, and breast cancer. Orthopedic surgery is useful for correcting unstable spinal lesions or pathological fractures in long bones, for example [60–62].

10.3.4 Role of Radiofrequency Techniques in Oncological Osteoarticular Pain

Despite the various therapeutic options described, a significant percentage of patients, around 50%, do not achieve adequate pain relief [58]. In this context, minimally invasive approaches for effective pain control are being developed. Currently, the radiofrequency technique with the highest level of scientific evidence, albeit limited, is ablative radiofrequency for vertebral metastases [66–68]. Other radiofrequency techniques with published case series applied to oncological osteoarticular pain include: radiofrequency of the dorsal root ganglion in vertebral metastases with nerve compression, radiofrequency of the dorsal root middle branch (RMRD), radiofrequency of the sacroiliac joints, radiofrequency of the intercostal nerves, and radiofrequency of the femoral and obturator nerves. The following outlines their possible clinical applications.

10.3.5 Vertebral Metastases

Thermal Ablation

Thermal ablation is a minimally invasive technique useful in the treatment of vertebral metastases and the pain they cause. It may or may not be associated with a vertebral augmentation technique such as vertebroplasty or kyphoplasty.

It is recommended in the following cases: [68–70]

1. Vertebral fracture causing spinal deformity or compromising respiratory function.
2. Vertebral fracture significantly increasing the patient's pain.
3. Asymptomatic pathological vertebral fracture.
4. Inability to apply an optimized radiotherapy protocol with curative and/or palliative intent.
5. Poor response to conventional analgesic treatments.

Generally, it is recommended for cases of single tumors less than 3 cm that are inoperable or in cases of oligometastatic disease (fewer than three to five metastatic lesions, each less than 3 cm in size). In some highly selected cases, it can also be used as a curative technique. In cases of significant spinal instability, a Spinal Instability Neoplastic Score (SINS) greater than 7, or spinal cord compression due to epidural metastases, its use is not recommended [70–72].

10.3.5.1 Procedure

Before the procedure, proper hemostasis will be ensured (platelet count >50,000/μL, INR > –1.2). The procedure is performed under general anesthesia or sedation and analgesia with regional technique. All ablation modalities cause intense pain during the procedure and for the following 24 hours [69]. At our center, it is currently performed under light sedation with bilateral erector spinae muscle block at the site to be treated (20 ml of 0.25% levobupivacaine and 4 mg of dexamethasone per side, under ultrasound control).

Under CT and fluoroscopy guidance, a bone biopsy needle (between 10 and 14 G) is placed at the lesion site, with prior infiltration of the periosteum with 1% lidocaine. Radiofrequency cannulas are then introduced (Fig. 10.9). The following modalities can be performed [69, 70]:

- *Ablative Radiofrequency*: Administration of alternating current (between 400 and 500 KHz) to achieve a temperature at the lesion site between 60 °C and 100 °C.
- *Microwave Ablation*: Administration of electrical current generating a non-ionizing electromagnetic field, causing molecular damage through particle friction.
- *Laser Photocoagulation*: Tissue destruction is caused by thermal injury.

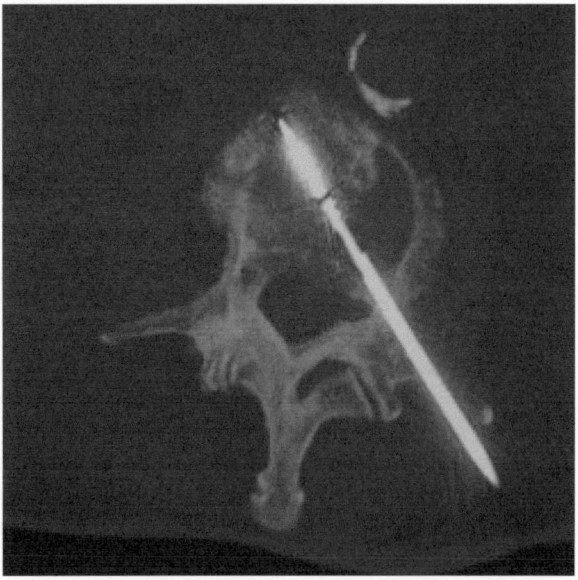

Fig. 10.9 Left transpedicular access cannula positioned at the vertebral level. Coaxially, a microwave ablation needle is identified, located centrally within the vertebral body, corresponding to the previously identified lesional area. Dr. Moltó's own work

- *High-Intensity Focused Ultrasound*: High-energy ultrasound causing thermal tissue damage.
- *Cryoablation*: Tissue temperatures around −180 °C causing rupture of cellular membranes and organelles.

10.3.5.2 Efficacy

Different thermal ablation techniques have been shown to reduce pain intensity in patients with vertebral fractures in over 80% of cases. Various clinical trials report a 50% reduction in pain intensity on the Visual Analog Scale (VAS) or NRS (Numerical Rating Scale), with a significant improvement in quality-of-life scores as well [73–76].

10.3.5.3 Radiofrequency of the Dorsal Root Ganglion

Pulsed radiofrequency techniques applied to the dorsal root ganglion (DRG) are used in patients with chronic lumbar or dorsal radicular pain, leading to significant improvements both in pain intensity and quality of life. The use of pulsed radiofrequency (an electric current that generates tissue temperatures not exceeding 42 °C) ensures that the procedure is not neuroablative, maintaining an adequate safety profile [77, 78].

In the context of oncological pain secondary to vertebral metastases, DRG radiofrequency is also being applied in patients with axial pain. Case series are available, such as the one published by Arai et al. in 2015 [79] and the randomized prospective study published by Fanous et al. in 2021 [80]. In the Arai et al. publication, 15 patients with dorsal pain secondary to intractable vertebral metastases underwent bilateral pulsed radiofrequency on the DRG at the levels to be treated. A significant improvement in pain levels was observed 3 weeks after the procedure.

In Fanous et al.'s study [80], a group of patients with axial dorsal pain from vertebral metastases lasting over 6 months, unresponsive to conventional analgesic treatment, and without neurological deficits, were divided into three groups of 23 subjects. The efficacy of betamethasone injection at the DRG level, conventional radiofrequency (80 °C tissue temperature for 90 s), and pulsed radiofrequency (42 °C tissue temperature for 460 s) was compared. In all groups, significant reductions in pain intensity and opioid consumption were achieved. The conventional radiofrequency group showed the greatest efficacy, although four patients experienced symptoms of neuritis.

In both studies, the technique was performed under fluoroscopic control, with 20G cannulas placed bilaterally at the DRG of the targeted level [79, 80].

10.3.5.4 Radiofrequency of the Dorsal Root Median Branch (RMRD)

RMRD radiofrequency is a widely used technique for treating lumbar facet syndrome, showing effectiveness in chronic non-oncological pain contexts [81]. Its use in oncological pain is not well-studied, even though lumbar pain is often one of the first clinical signs reported by cancer patients. A case series published by Kim et al. in 2022 [82]describes three cases of patients with primary tumors located in the upper hemiabdomen (gastric, pancreatic head, and biliary duct) at an advanced stage with peritoneal dissemination and implants near the celiac and superior mesenteric plexuses. All patients experienced severe lower lumbar pain, required high doses of opioids, and presented characteristics of facet syndrome. Prior to lumbar facet radiofrequency, test blocks were performed with positive results. Two cases underwent pulsed radiofrequency, and one received conventional radiofrequency. After 1 month, all patients reported a pain improvement of 70% or more. Quality of life and ambulation capacity were not assessed.

Given the prevalence of lower lumbar pain in the general population, researching its incidence in oncological patients and evaluating potential minimally invasive treatments would be valuable.

10.3.5.5 Sacral and Pelvic Metastases

As explained in the section on the incidence, pathophysiology, and clinical aspects of oncological osteoarticular pain, the pelvis is a frequent site for metastases. These lesions can, among other causes, lead to sacroiliac joint dysfunction, resulting in intense low back pain radiating to the buttocks. The incidence of sacroiliac joint dysfunction in patients with non-oncological chronic pain is estimated between 15% and 30%, but no data exists on the incidence in oncological patients [83].

Sacroiliac pain in cancer patients can arise from the same etiologies as in non-cancer patients. However, it generally presents as multifactorial, involving [83, 84]:

- Tumor or metastatic invasion of the joint.
- Chemotherapy and radiotherapy treatments.

- Pathological fractures.
- Joint instability.
- Inflammation of the surrounding periosteum.
- Bone marrow extraction causing damage to joint tissues.

When conventional treatment (rehabilitation, analgesic drugs, including opioids) is ineffective, radiofrequency techniques play an important role. Literature describes case series using various radiofrequency techniques: conventional, pulsed, and cooled. These address the posterior rami of L4, L5, S1, S2, and S3 bilaterally [84–86].

Hutson et al. [84] present a series of six cancer patients with metastases localized to the sacrum and other bones in the pelvic ring, as well as lumbar vertebrae. Initially, all patients underwent ultrasound-guided injections of corticoids (40 mg of triamcinolone and 4 mL of 0.25% bupivacaine) into both sacroiliac joints with confirmed efficacy. In some cases, a test block of the posterior rami of L4, L5, S1, S2, and S3 was performed bilaterally, while in others, conventional radiofrequency was directly applied to the targeted rami. After these initial cases, data from 25 patients with the same oncological pathology were collected, and six patients required other invasive analgesic techniques, such as implantation of an intrathecal morphine, bupivacaine, and clonidine pump, implantation of a spinal cord stimulator, or sacroplasty.

In the cases published by Ramabusa et al. [86] and Yi et al. [87], the use of cooled radiofrequency and pulsed radiofrequency, respectively, following a positive test block, showed improvements of over 50% in pain intensity and significant improvements in ambulation. Both patients also had metastases in the spine and other bones in the pelvic ring.

At present, no randomized clinical trials are providing stronger scientific evidence for this technique. Based on the studies presented, any form of radiofrequency applied to the posterior rami of L4, L5, S1, S2, and S3 can be very effective in controlling sacroiliac joint pain in oncological patients, with a minimal complication rate.

10.3.5.6 Extraaxial Metastases

As discussed in the previous section, radiofrequency techniques are available for controlling sacroiliac joint dysfunction pain, but the iliac bone is also a common site for metastases. Long bones, particularly the femur, also frequently present metastatic lesions.

In the literature, we find case series and retrospective clinical studies on radiofrequency techniques for controlling pain from these metastases. Ablative radiofrequency techniques stand out, although with lower clinical evidence compared to vertebral metastases. We also find cases of radiofrequency applied to peripheral nerves such as the obturator nerve or the suprascapular nerve. Below, we present the clinical application of each.

10.3.5.7 Ablative Radiofrequency for the Control of Extraaxial Metastases

Ablative radiofrequency for the treatment of pain secondary to oligometastases (one or two well-localized lesions) has recently been recognized as a highly useful technique [87]. Initially developed as a treatment for osteoid osteomas in both children and adults, it is now the treatment of choice. Over the past 14 years, its use has expanded to treat metastases in various locations [88, 89].

Similar to the treatment of vertebral metastases, the procedure is guided by CT. Various radiofrequency modalities can be chosen, with microwave radiofrequency being the most commonly used. If the periosteum is intact, the radiofrequency cannula is inserted through a bone biopsy needle; if the periosteum is compromised, the cannula is inserted directly into the lesion. Depending on the size of the lesion, a single active tip cannula (for lesions 3–4 cm) or needles with multiple cannulas may be used. It is recommended that the lesion size exceeds the metastasis size by 2 mm [89, 90]. After performing the ablative technique, the procedure is often accompanied by percutaneous osteoplasty to prevent pathological fractures. That is, a cement volume is injected to fill the space left in the bone after the ablation. The cement volume will vary depending on the lesion size [90, 91].

These techniques reduce patient pain levels by 50% within 24 hours post-procedure, lasting up to 3 months. They also improve the Oswestry Disability Index in 60–80% of patients. The complication rate is low, with the most common being skin burns, infection at the puncture site, or nerve injuries [91]. Intense local pain often occurs during the intervention, so sedation and proper intravenous analgesia are recommended [90].

10.3.5.8 Radiofrequency of the Obturator and Femoral Nerves

In the field of non-oncological chronic pain, radiofrequency of the obturator and femoral nerves, typically conventional and fluoroscopically guided, has been shown to be effective in treating refractory hip joint pain, even after hip prosthesis implantation. Pain intensity improvements range from 30% to 90%, depending on the study, though a few report some functional improvement data [92].

Few studies have been conducted on patients with oncological pain, but case series such as the one published by Kawaguchi et al. in 2001 [93]and the clinical case by Stone et al. in 2014 [94] are notable. In both, a conventional block was performed before applying conventional radiofrequency guided by fluoroscopy, with Stone's case also using ultrasound assistance. In Kawaguchi's study, one femoral metastasis case was treated with radiofrequency solely on the obturator nerve, without achieving pain relief. However, pain relief was achieved in the patient treated on both the femoral and obturator nerves. Stone et al. performed both the prognostic block and conventional radiofrequency on both nerves, resulting in a 50% reduction in pain intensity and improved joint mobility.

10.3.5.9 Radiofrequency of the Suprascapular Nerve

The suprascapular nerve is the main target for controlling chronic shoulder pain, even being used before starting rehabilitation treatments to improve tolerance.

Recently, ultrasound has surpassed fluoroscopy as the most commonly used imaging technique to guide these procedures. Both pulsed and conventional radiofrequency techniques are used at the suprascapular level.

Recent reviews on radiofrequency techniques for shoulder joint pain do not show a strong consensus on the need for prognostic blocks, the use of conventional or pulsed radiofrequency, or the duration of pulsed treatments. In the 3-month follow-ups, there is a trend toward significant pain reduction compared to conventional conservative treatment, though not statistically significant. Moreover, it remains to be studied whether radiofrequency applied solely to the suprascapular nerve is effective or if it benefits from targeting additional nerves, such as the axillary nerve [95, 96].

In the field of oncological pain, evidence is much scarcer. Chang et al. published a case series in which a test block of the suprascapular nerve was followed by conventional radiofrequency. A total of six patients were included, five with metastases in the humeral head and one with brachial plexus infiltration. All patients experienced a pain improvement of 50% or more on the EVA, and there was a significant improvement in shoulder joint mobility [97].

10.3.5.10 Conclusion

Osteoarticular pain in cancer patients is frequent and often refractory to conventional treatments. The severity of the pain and short life expectancy require rapid escalation in analgesic treatment intensity. Radiofrequency techniques are highly useful as minimally invasive procedures with low complication rates and good results both in pain control and quality of life. Therefore, we should be familiar with and apply them promptly when indicated.

10.4 Neuroaxial Techniques

10.4.1 Intrathecal Therapy in Cancer Pain

10.4.1.1 Introduction

Cancer is one of the leading causes of death worldwide, with 19.96 million new cases diagnosed in 2022 and 9.7 million deaths [98].

Traditionally, cancer pain management has relied on high-dose opioids. In recent years, this approach has evolved due to advances in oncological treatment, allowing patients to live longer with a relatively preserved quality of life.

It is estimated that cancer pain treatment is inadequate in up to 51% of patients [99]. In this context, therapeutic alternatives such as intrathecal (IT) therapy have emerged for pain management.

The administration of drugs via the intrathecal route has been considered a safe and effective treatment for refractory chronic pain for over 40 years.

Intrathecal drug administration for pain management is based on the pharmacodynamic interactions of these agents with central nervous system receptors. The pharmacological targets of these analgesic drugs are located in the dorsal horn of the spinal cord. This system consists of a catheter placed in the intrathecal space, connected to a delivery pump. IT therapy has demonstrated its effectiveness in treating pain refractory to oral analgesics, bypassing first-pass hepatic metabolism and the blood-brain barrier. IT therapy also allows for the use of smaller drug doses compared to systemic administration, resulting in fewer adverse effects and better pain control.

The FDA has approved only two drugs for intrathecal use: an opioid (morphine) and a nonopioid (ziconotide), both as monotherapy for chronic pain treatment.

There is evidence that IT therapy in cancer pain patients is effective, reduces adverse effects, and improves survival [100–106].

10.4.1.2 Indications and Contraindications

The Polyanalgesia Consensus Conference (PACC) expert panel, established in 2000, aims to improve the efficacy and safety of IT therapy. This group periodically publishes guidelines, with the latest update on cancer pain published in 2024 [100].

PACC considers IT therapy an appropriate treatment for cancer pain in carefully selected patients and recommends psychological evaluation and treatment, as long as it does not delay its implementation (Consensus Points 1 and 2 of PACC) [100].

If life expectancy is less than 3 months, IT therapy with a subcutaneous port (port-a-cath) may be considered instead of an infusion pump.

As with any invasive spinal procedure, special attention must be given to coagulation status (e.g., altered hepatorenal function and anticoagulant use). It is essential to follow evidence-based guidelines for managing drugs that affect coagulation [103].

The presence of an active chronic infection is a contraindication for implantable device placement [107–109].

10.4.1.3 Test Dose

Performing a test dose before IT implantation has been standard practice. Following the latest PACC review, experts continue to recommend the test dose. In cancer pain cases, it is optional and at the discretion of the physician and patient (Consensus Point 14 of PACC) [100].

Regarding the administration of the test dose, it can be performed as a single injection, bolus test, or continuous infusion; there is no evidence proving the superiority of one method over another.

10.4.1.4 Recommendations for Medication Selection and Dosing

The FDA has authorized the intrathecal infusion of ziconotide and morphine for pain treatment. Other drugs in monotherapy or combination therapy may be considered off-label after FDA-approved drugs have failed or are contraindicated.

Commonly used drugs for cancer pain include opioids (morphine, hydromorphone, fentanyl, sufentanil), ziconotide, bupivacaine, clonidine, and baclofen. Drug selection should be based on pain characteristics, catheter tip location, and the pharmacokinetic and pharmacodynamic properties of each drug.

The different algorithms for cancer pain treatment, according to the latest PACC review, are based on life expectancy: a more limited prognosis (less than 6 months) (Table 10.2) or a more favorable prognosis (more than 6 months) (Table 10.3) [100].

The recommended starting doses for IT drugs in opioid-naïve patients (Table 10.4).

Table 10.2 Commonly used drugs for cancer pain with a more limited prognosis (less than 6 months)

Line	Treatment options
1st line	Morphine or hydromorphone ± bupivacaine/fentanyl ± bupivacaine
2nd line	Morphine or hydromorphone or fentanyl + low doses of ziconotide ± bupivacaine
3rd line	Hydromorphone or morphine or fentanyl + clonidine ± bupivacaine/ziconotide + bupivacaine/ziconotide + clonidine/clonidine as a secondary or tertiary adjuvant/ sufentanil as primary or secondary
4th line	Opioid + ziconotide/sufentanil + bupivacaine/baclofen as a secondary or tertiary adjuvant/sufentanil + clonidine/bupivacaine + clonidine + ziconotide
5th line	Refractory pain, consider multiple drug combinations

Table 10.3 Commonly used drugs for cancer pain with a more favorable prognosis (more than 6 months)

Line	Treatment options
1st line	Morphine or hydromorphone or fentanyl ± bupivacaine/ziconotide
2nd line	Hydromorphone or morphine or fentanyl + bupivacaine + ziconotide/ hydromorphone or morphine or fentanyl + clonidine
3rd line	Hydromorphone or morphine or fentanyl + bupivacaine + clonidine/ziconotide + bupivacaine/ziconotide + clonidine/sufentanil
4th line	Refractory pain, consider multiple drug combinations

Table 10.4 Recommended starting doses for IT drugs in opioid-naïve patients

Drug	Recommended initial dose/24 h
Morphine	0.1–0.5 mg
Hydromorphone	0.02–0.1 mg
Fentanyl	25–75 mcg
Sufentanil	10–20 mcg
Ziconotide	0.5–1 mcg
Bupivacaine	1–4 mg
Clonidine	40–100 mcg
Baclofen	25 mcg (50 mcg for spasticity)

10.4.1.5 Adverse Effects

Adverse effects depend on the administered drug. The most commonly used drugs present the following risks:

- Opioids: The most severe adverse effect is respiratory depression, with a potentially higher risk when using hydrophilic opioids and when combined with other central nervous system depressants such as benzodiazepines. Sudden discontinuation of opioid infusion may cause withdrawal syndrome. Other adverse effects include pruritus, constipation, urinary retention, lower limb edema, and endocrine dysfunction.
- Ziconotide: The most common side effects include nausea, mental status changes (confusion and memory loss), hallucinations, nightmares, and psychotic thoughts. Cases of muscle degradation and elevated creatine kinase (CK) levels have also been reported [110].
- Bupivacaine: Urinary incontinence, numbness, weakness, respiratory depression, and hypotension induced by sympathectomy. Rarely, toxic myelitis and arachnoiditis [100].

10.4.1.6 Complications

The main complications reported include:

1. Infection: Meningitis and encephalitis.
2. Hemorrhage: Epidural hematoma, spinal hematoma, pocket hematoma.
3. Granuloma formation at the tip of the intrathecal catheter: Reports suggest an incidence of up to 8%, though the actual prevalence is unknown. Granuloma formation has been identified following intrathecal administration of morphine, hydromorphone, bupivacaine, sufentanil, baclofen, and tramadol.
4. Intrathecal catheter rupture.
5. Hygroma or seroma formation.

10.4.1.7 Surgical Technique

The intrathecal infusion system is implanted in the operating room following standard aseptic measures. Prophylactic antibiotics are administered 30 min before implantation.

The patient is placed in the lateral decubitus position, preferably on the right side. Using fluoroscopy, the spinal needle entry point is marked at the pedicle of the vertebra, two segments below the selected spinal puncture site.

A preliminary spinal puncture is performed using a 22G Quincke spinal needle to confirm proper access to the intrathecal space. Once confirmed, a lumbar incision is made, and the fascia is exposed. A spinal cannula is then inserted until cerebrospinal fluid (CSF) is obtained, after which the intrathecal catheter is introduced, positioning its tip in the area of greatest pain under fluoroscopic guidance.

Recently, Chen et al. provided specific guidelines on intrathecal catheter tip placement based on pain location [111] (Table 10.5).

Table 10.5 Guidelines on intrathecal catheter tip placement based on pain location

Pain location	Catheter tip placement
Face	C1-C2
Brachial plexus	C3-C5
Upper limbs	C3-C5
Upper thoracic wall	T3-T4
Visceral abdomen	T5-T6
Lower thoracic wall	T6-T7
Abdominal wall	T6-T7
Back	T8-T11
Pelvis	T9-T12
Lower limbs	T10
Sacrum	Vertebral body level corresponding to conus medullaris

After catheter implantation, the cannula and guide are removed, and the catheter is secured to the fascia. An abdominal pocket is created to house the pump, and the catheter is tunneled subcutaneously to connect it to the pump.

The pumps are prefilled with the corresponding medication before implantation. The reservoir must be emptied before filling.

The pump can be either programmable or fixed-rate. Programmable pumps offer the advantage of faster dose titration without the need to empty the reservoir. Some pumps allow patient-administered bolus doses for breakthrough pain control.

Finally, the incisions are closed.

10.4.1.8 Conclusions

The use of IT therapy for cancer pain management has been widely demonstrated. The path forward involves improving clinical practice, including optimal patient selection, appropriate drug choice and dosing, and management of comorbidities.

10.4.1.9 Spinal Neuromodulation Techniques

Neuromodulation techniques are selective treatments targeting different areas of the nervous system (brain, spinal cord, or peripheral) involved in the transmission of nociceptive stimuli, aiming to reversibly modify neural activity [112]. The most commonly used therapies in pain management units for chronic pain treatment include spinal cord stimulation (SCS), dorsal root ganglion stimulation (DRGS), and intrathecal drug infusion [113].

Spinal Cord Stimulation: Posterior Columns and Dorsal Root Ganglion

Spinal cord stimulation (SCS) involves the implantation of a device that delivers electrical impulses to the spinal cord to block or modulate nociceptive stimuli [114]. SCS and dorsal root ganglion (DRG) stimulation techniques have been developed over the past two decades [115].

In SCS, electrodes are placed in the posterior columns of the spinal cord to attenuate the transmission of nociceptive stimuli at the spinal level [115] (Fig. 10.10). Its

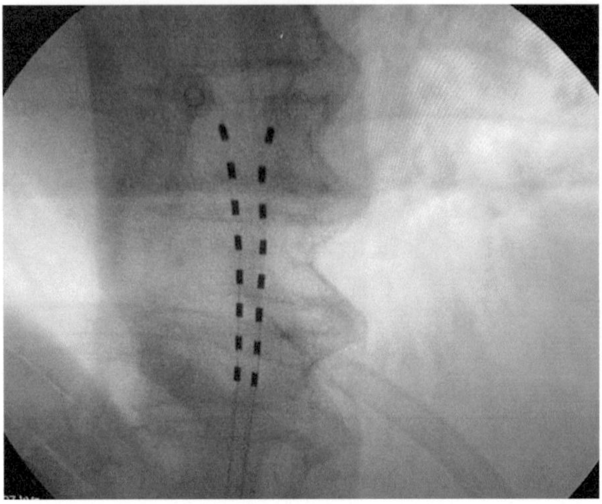

Fig. 10.10 Posterior cord stimulation electrodes. Dr. Moltó's own work

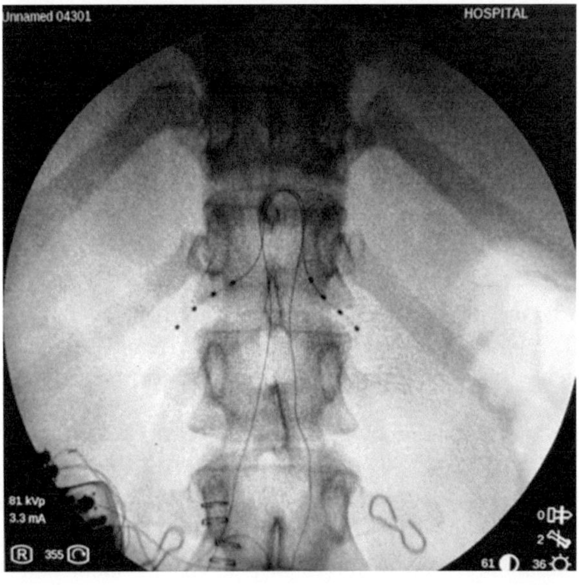

Fig. 10.11 Dorsal root ganglion stimulation electrodes. Dr. Moltó's own work

indications are well-defined, primarily for chronic pain refractory to other treatments [6]. The main indications include: chronic neuropathic pain, persistent spinal pain syndrome, complex regional pain syndrome, and chronic ischemic pain, including refractory angina and Raynaud's syndrome [113].

Dorsal root ganglion stimulation (DRGS) is a therapy that delivers electrical impulses to the dorsal root ganglion (Fig. 10.11), a key structure in transmitting pain signals from the periphery to the central nervous system [118]. The main indications include: complex regional pain syndrome, localized neuropathic pain, post-surgical pain syndrome, refractory peripheral pain, failed back surgery syndrome, localized ischemic pain, and postamputation pain [119].

The advantage of DRGS over SCS is its greater effectiveness for localized pain, particularly neuropathic pain [120]. Although oncologic pain is not a common indication for SCS or DRGS, these techniques may be useful when there is a clear indication, and the cancer is stable or not expected to progress, making them suitable for managing pain in oncological patients, particularly those with refractory chronic pain or difficult-to-treat pain [10]. These therapies are indicated for neuropathic pain and, in some cases, somatic or visceral pain, where conventional treatments are ineffective or cause intolerable side effects. The main indications for oncological patients include:

1. Neuropathic pain associated with cancer: Pain due to tumor invasion of nerve plexuses or spinal roots; chemotherapy-induced neuropathies.
2. Post-surgical oncological pain: Following major surgeries, amputations, thoracotomies, or mastectomies.
3. Failed back surgery syndrome: After surgery for metastases or spinal cord compression.
4. Refractory somatic or visceral chronic pain.

The main advantage of these procedures is the reduction in opioid dosage, improved neuropathic pain control, and enhanced quality of life [118].

Considerations for Implantation in Oncological Patients

When considering implantation in an oncological patient, several factors must be taken into account: [115]

1. Thorough evaluation by a multidisciplinary team to rule out tumor progression as the cause of pain.
2. General condition and prognosis: These therapies should benefit patients with a sufficiently long life expectancy.
3. Trial phase: As with non-oncological patients, a trial phase must be conducted to confirm the effectiveness of the device before permanent implantation.

These procedures are performed on an outpatient basis, with antibiotic prophylaxis, under sedation, and with the patient in a prone position, guided by fluoroscopy [19]. Epidural access is required for electrode placement on the posterior columns in SCS or on the DRG in DRGS [20]. During the procedure, paresthesia is induced in the areas where the electrodes are placed to confirm that they correspond with the patient's pain area. The electrodes are then fixed, and extensions are positioned laterally on the back above the iliac crest to connect to an external generator. This trial phase is used to confirm treatment efficacy, with a positive response defined as pain relief greater than 50%. After 15 days, the final implantation of the generator is performed in the operating room, placed subcutaneously or subfascially. Typically, it is implanted above the gluteal region, as it is well-tolerated during daily activities and minimally mobile, but it can also be positioned in other areas, such as the lower abdominal flank or subclavicular region. Patient preferences regarding lifestyle, activity, nutritional status, access for recharges or programming, and aesthetics must be considered [119, 120].

Complications

The most common complications during implantation include: [117]

- Radicular puncture with secondary neuritis.
- Intravascular or intrathecal puncture.
- Bleeding.
- Infection with the risk of meningitis.
- Electrode migration or breakage.

The implanted generators may be rechargeable, with wireless recharging through a portable device. Depending on usage, they last between 10 and 20 years, while non-rechargeable generators have a lifespan of 3–7 years, depending on programming and use. Non-rechargeable generators require no maintenance from the patient.

These generators offer different stimulation programs to adjust the stimulus and pain control for each case. The International Neuromodulation Society and its consensus group have established recommendations for performing SCS and DRGS techniques, including training requirements, perioperative considerations (such as preparation before the procedure, antibiotic prophylaxis, postoperative complications, and the implantation site of the stimulator) [116, 120].

References

1. Haumann J, Joosten EBA, van den Beuken-van Everdingen MHJ. Pain prevalence in cancer patients: status quo or opportunities for improvement? Curr Opin Support Palliat Care. 2017;11(2):99–104.
2. Beuken-van Everdingen MH, Hochstenbach LM, Joosten EA, Tjan-Heijnen VC, Janssen DJ. Update on prevalence of pain in patients with cancer: systematic review and meta-analysis. J Pain Symptom Manag. 2016;51(6):1070–90.
3. Breivik H, Cherny N, Collett B, de Conno F, Filbet M, Foubert AJ, et al. Cancer-related pain: a pan- European survey of prevalence, treatment, and patient attitudes. Ann Oncol. 2009;20(8):1420–33.
4. Pérez-Hernández C, Blasco A, Gándara Á, Mañas A, Rodríguez-López MJ, Martínez V, et al. Prevalence and characterization of breakthrough pain in patients with cancer in Spain: the CARPE-DIO study. Sci Rep. 2019;9(1):17701.
5. Pignon T, Fernandez L, Ayasso S, Durand MA, Badinand D, Cowen D. Impact of radiation oncology practice on pain: a cross-sectional survey. Int J Radiat Oncol Biol Phys. 2004;60(4):1204–10.
6. Strömgren AS, Groenvold M, Petersen MA, Goldschmidt D, Pedersen L, Spile M, et al. Pain characteristics and treatment outcome for advanced cancer patients during the first week of specialized palliative care. J Pain Symptom Manag. 2004;27(2):104–13.

7. Scarborough BM, Smith CB. Optimal pain management for patients with cancer in the modern era. CA Cancer J Clin. 2018;68(3):182–96.
8. Kambadakone A, Thabet A, Gervais DA, Mueller PR, Arellano RS. CT-guided celiac plexus neurolysis: a review of anatomy, indications, technique, and tips for successful treatment. Radiographics. 2011;31(6):1599–621.
9. Arcidiacono P, Calori G, Carrara S, McNicol E, Testoni P. Celiac plexus block for pancreatic cancer pain in adults. Cochrane Database Syst Rev. 2011;2011(3):CD007519.
10. Herrero Trujillano MM, Mendiola de la Osa A, Insausti Valdivia J, Pérez-Cajaraville J. Revisión de los procedimientos intervencionistas neurolíticos en el dolor asociado al cáncer de páncreas. Propuesta de algoritmo. Rev Soc Esp. Dolor. 2019;26(6):342–58.
11. Gabriel CM. Pancreatic cancer related pain: review of pathophysiology and intrathecal drug delivery Systems for Pain Management. Pain Physician. 2021;24:E583–94.
12. Stoffel EM, Brand RE, Goggins M. Pancreatic cancer: changing epidemiology and new approaches to risk assessment, early detection, and prevention. Gastroenterology. 2023;164(5):752–65.
13. Ceyhan GO, Bergmann F, Kadihasanoglu M, Altintas B, Friess H. Pancreatic neuropathy and neuropathic pain – a comprehensive pathomorphological study of 546 cases. Gastroenterology. 2009;136(1):177–186.e1.
14. Nagar S, Nagar S, Jordan V, Dawson J. Sympathetic nerve blocks for persistent pain in adults with inoperable abdominopelvic cancer. Cochrane Database Syst Rev. 2024;Issue 6:CD015229.
15. Loukas M, Klaassen Z, Merbs W, Tubbs RS, Gielecki J, Zurada A. A review of the thoracic splanchnic nerves and celiac ganglia. Clin Anat. 2010;23(5):512–22.
16. Zhang X, Zhao Q, Zeng N, Cai C, Xie X. The celiac ganglia: anatomic study using MRI in cadavers. AJR Am J Roentgenol. 2006;186(6):1520–3.
17. McCorry LK. Physiology of the autonomic nervous system. Am J Pharm Educ. 2007;71(4):78.
18. Waxenbaum JA, Reddy V, Varacallo MA. Anatomy, Autonomic Nervous System. [Updated 2023 Jul 24]. In: StatPearls [Internet]. Treasure Island (FL): StatPearls Publishing; 2025 Jan-. Available from: https://www.ncbi.nlm.nih.gov/books/NBK539845/
19. Sharabi AF, Carey FJ. Anatomy, Abdomen and Pelvis, Splanchnic Nerves. [Updated 2024 Mar 5]. In: StatPearls [Internet]. Treasure Island (FL): StatPearls Publishing; 2025. Available from: https://www.ncbi.nlm.nih.gov/books/NBK560504/
20. Beveridge TS, Johnson M, Power A, Power NE, Allman BL. Anatomy of the nerves and ganglia of the aortic plexus in males. J Anat. 2015;226(1):93–103.
21. du Plessis M, Loukas M. A comprehensive study of the abdominal ganglia part 1: celiac, phrenic and superior mesenteric ganglia. Clin Anat. 2022;35(7):998–1006.
22. Navarro-Martinez J, Montes A, Comps O, Sitges-Serra A. Retroperitoneal abscess after Neurolytic celiac plexus block from the anterior approach. Reg Anesth Pain Med. 2003;28(6):528–30.
23. Jackson T, Gaeta R. Neurolytic blocks revisited. Curr Pain Headache Rep. 2008;12(1):7–13.
24. Pérez-Aguado G, de la Mata D, Valenciano C, Sainz I. Endoscopic ultrasonography-guided celiac plexus neurolysis in patients with unresectable pancreatic cancer: an update. World J Gastrointest Endosc. 2021;13(10):460–72.
25. Guangxin J, Xiaoxia Q, Min D, Mengjun D, Xuebin Z. Navigated magnetic resonance imaging-guided celiac plexus neurolysis using an open magnetic resonance system for pancreatic cancer patients with upper abdominal pain. J Cancer Res Ther. 2019;15(4):825–30.
26. Hol P, Kvarstein G, Viken O, Smedby O, Tønnessen T. MRI-guided celiac plexus block. J Magn Reson Imaging. 2000;12(4):562–4.
27. Urits I, Jones M, Orhurhu V, Peck J, Corrigan HA. A comprehensive review of the celiac plexus block for the management of chronic abdominal pain. Curr Pain Headache Rep. 2020;24(8):42.
28. Warner N, Moeschler S, Warner M, Hoelzer B, Eldrige J, Bendel. Bleeding complications in patients undergoing celiac plexus block. Reg Anesth Pain Med. 2016;41(4):488–93.

29. Narouze S, Benzon H, Provenzano D, Buvanendran A, De Andres J, Deer T, et al. Interventional spine and pain procedures in patients on antiplatelet and anticoagulant medications (second edition): guidelines from the American Society of Regional Anesthesia and Pain Medicine, the European Society of Regional Anaesthesia and Pain Thera. Reg Anesth Pain Med. 2018;43(3):225–62.
30. Plancarte R, Amescua C, Patt RB, Allende S. Presacral blockade of the ganglion of Walther (ganglion impar). Anesthesiology. 1990;73:NA.
31. Wemm K Jr, Saberski L. Transsacrococcygeal approach to the ganglion impar: a technique to block pelvic pain transmission. Reg Anesth. 1995;20(5):367–72.
32. Agarwal-Kozlowski K, Lierz P, Knitschke M, et al. Blockade of the ganglion impar (ganglion of Walther): a simple and efficient technique for perineal pain. Anesth Analg. 2009;108(2):647–51.
33. Kim YH, Lee CJ, Yoon SH, et al. Ultrasound-guided ganglion impar block: a technical report. Pain Physician. 2015;18(4):E537–45.
34. Ahmed A, Singh D, et al. Combined superior hypogastric plexus and ganglion impar neurolytic block for cancer pain. Pain Pract. 2014;14(1):E57–63.
35. Sir E, Eksert D. Radiofrequency treatment for perineal pain: a comparison of pulsed and conventional techniques. Pain Med. 2017;18(3):533–9.
36. Usmani H, Khan A, et al. Efficacy of radiofrequency ablation for ganglion impar: comparative study between pulsed and continuous techniques. Pain Pract. 2018;18(5):623–30.
37. Bhatnagar S, et al. Bedside ultrasound-guided neurolysis of ganglion impar in patients with advanced pelvic cancer. Indian J Palliat Care. 2014;20(2):153–7.
38. Adas C, et al. Cryoablation of the ganglion impar for cancer-related pelvic pain: a novel approach. J Pain Res. 2021;14:1809–15.
39. Gupta D, et al. Complications and safety of ganglion impar block: a review. Pain Med. 2019;20(4):846–53.
40. Hou S, Novy D, et al. Efficacy of superior hypogastric plexus Neurolysis for the treatment of cancer-related pelvic pain. Pain Med. 2020;21(6):1255–62.
41. Plancarte R, Amescua C, Patt RB, et al. Superior hypogastric plexus block for pelvic pain associated with cancer. Reg Anesth Pain Med. 1990;15(4):200–3.
42. Plancarte R, et al. Neurolytic block of the superior hypogastric plexus in gynecologic cancer pain. Reg Anesth. 1992;17(2):44–7.
43. Ina H, Kobayashi M, Imai S, Fukada Y, Narita M, Otagiri T. A new approach to superior hypogastric plexus block: trans-intervertebral disc (L5-S1 disc) technique. Reg Anesth Pain Med. 1992;17(Suppl 3):123.
44. Erdine S, et al. Transdiscal approach for superior hypogastric plexus neurolysis. Reg Anesth Pain Med. 2000;25(6):610–4.
45. Mishra S, et al. Ultrasound-guided neurolysis of the superior hypogastric plexus for advanced cancer pain. Pain Med. 2013;14(8):1250–6. https://doi.org/10.1111/pme.12198.
46. Abdelghaffar NA, Farahat TE. Fluoroscopic anterior approach versus ultrasound guided superior hypogastric plexus neurolysis in cancer pelvic pain: a randomized controlled study. BMC Anesthesiol. 2022;22(1):403.
47. Kanazi G, Perkins F, Thakur R, Dotson E. New technique for superior hypogastric plexus block. Reg Anesth Pain Med. 1999;24(5):473–6.
48. Cariati M, De Martini G, Pretolesi F, Roy MT. CT-guided superior hypogastric plexus block. J Comput Assist Tomogr. 2002;26:428–31.
49. Dooley J, Beadles C, Ho KY, Sair F, Gray-Leithe L, Huh B. Computed tomography-guided bilateral transdiscal superior hypogastric plexus neurolysis. Pain Med. 2008;9(2):236–2.
50. Waldman SD, Wilson WL, Kreps RD. Superior hypogastric plexus block using a single needle and computed tomography guidance: description of a modified technique. Reg Anesth. 1991;16:286–7.
51. Restrepo-Garces CE, Gómez Bermudez CM, Jaramillo Escobar S, Jazmín Ramirez L, Lopera LM, Vargas JF. Bloqueo ganglio estrellado. Rev Soc Esp Dol. 2012;19(2):101–7.

52. López-Millá JM, Coca-Gamito C, Cámara-Faraig A, Dóaz-Infante E, García Rubira JC. Bloqueo del ganglio estrellado como tratamiento de la tormetna arritmica: estudio observacional. Rev Esp Anestesiol Reanim. 2024;71(1):1.
53. Peng P, Narouze S. Chapter 3: sonoanatomy of the cervical sympathetic chain. In: Ultrasound guidance for interventional pain management of cervical pain syndromes. An anatomical and clinical study. Datawyse I Universitaire Pers Maastricht; 2012. p. 31–44.
54. Bharti N, Chattopadhyay S, Singla N, Bala I, Batra YK, Bakshi J. Pulsed radiofrequency ablation for the treatment of glossopharyngeal neuralgia secondary to oropharyngeal carcinoma. Pain Physician. 2018;21(3):295–302.
55. Kojima Y, Okamoto S, Hirabayashi K. Ultrasound-guided selective glossopharyngeal nerve block: posterior mandibular ramus approach. Pain Med. 2023;25(3):169–72.
56. Punj J, Jain D, Singh LD, Thakur JP, Pandey RK, Darlong V. Combination of peripheral nerve stimulator and ultrasound guidance may improve the efficacy of glossopharyngeal nerve block. J Anaesthesiol Clin Pharmacol. 2023;39(2):318–9.
57. Mercadante S. Malignant bone pain: pathophysiology and treatment. Pain. 1997;69(1–2):1–18.
58. Falk S, Dickenson A. Pain and nociception: mechanisms of cancer-induced bone pain. J Clin Oncol. 2014;32:1647–54.
59. Doncel Cabot A, Majó BJ. Tumores óseos en atención primaria. Med Int. 2003;41(3):145–50.
60. Coleman R, Hadji P, Body J, Santini D, Chow E. Bone health in cancer: ESMO clinical practice guidelines. Ann Oncol. 2020;31(12):1650–63.
61. Fornetti J, Welm A, Stewart S. Understanding the bone in cancer metastasis. J Bone Miner Res. 2018;33(12):2099–113.
62. Milgrom D, Lad N, Koniaris L, Zimmers T. Pain and muscle weakness in cancer patients. Curr Osteoporos Rep. 2017;15(2):76–87.
63. Bindu S, Mazumder S, Bandyopadhyay U. Non-steroidal anti-inflammatory drugs (NSAIDs) and organ damage: a current perspective. Biochem Pharmacol. 2020;180:1141–7.
64. Colvin L, Fallon M. Challenges in cancer pain management – bone pain. Eur J Cancer. 2008;44(8):1083–90.
65. Bennett M, Eisenberg E, Ahmedzai S, BhaskaR A, O'Brien T. Standards for the management of cancer-related pain across Europe-a position paper from the EFIC task force on cancer pain. Eur J Pain. 2019;23(4):660–8.
66. Grosinger A, Alcorn S. An update on the Management of Bone Metastases. Curr Oncol Rep. 2024;26(4):400–8.
67. Aman M, Mahmoud A, Deer T, Sayed D, Hagedorn J. The American Society of Pain and Neuroscience (ASPN) best practices and guidelines for the interventional Management of Cancer-Associated Pain. J Pain Res. 2021;16(14):2139–64.
68. NICE: conditions and diseases – Cancer – Metastases. NICE Guidance: Radiofrequency ablation for palliation of painful spinal metastases. [Online].; April 2023 [cited 2024 Jan 9. Available from: https://www.nice.org.uk/guidance/ipg758
69. Ryan A, Byrne C, Pusceddu C, Buy X, Tsoumakidou G. CIRSE standards of practice on thermal ablation of bone Tumours. Cardiovasc Intervent Radiol. 2022;45(5):591–605.
70. Tomasian A, Levy J, Jennings J. Percutaneous vertebral augmentation and thermal ablation in patients with spinal metastases. Semin Intervent Radiol. 2024;41(2):170–5.
71. Khan M, Jennings J, Baker J, Smolock A, Shah L. ACR appropriateness criteria® Management of Vertebral Compression Fractures: 2022 update. Am Coll Radiol. 2023;20(5S):S102–24.
72. Murtaza H, Sullivan C. Classifications in brief: the spinal instability neoplastic score. Clin Orthop Relat Res. 2019;477(12):2798–803.
73. Buitrago G, Castro E, Garrido JC, Fortea F, Villoria F. Experiencia preliminar en el tratamiento combinado de metástasis vertebrales mediante radiofrecuencia y cifoplastia en sesión única. Rev Soc Esp Dolor Madrid. 2013;20
74. Dupuy D, Liu D, Hartfeil D, Hanna L, Blume J. Percutaneous radiofrequency ablation of painful osseous metastases: a multicenter American College of Radiology Imaging Network trial. Cancer. 2010;116(4):989–97.

75. Tomasian A, Wallace A, Northrup B, Hillen T, Jennings J. Spine Cryoablation: pain palliation and local tumor control for vertebral metastases. AJNR Am J Neuroradiol. 2016;37(1):189–95.
76. Anchala P, Irving W, Hillen T, Friedman M, Georgy B. Treatment of metastatic spinal lesions with a navigational bipolar radiofrequency ablation device: a multicenter retrospective study. Pain Physician. 2014;17(4):317–27.
77. Levy J, Hopkins T, Morris J, Tran N, David E. Radiofrequency ablation for the palliative treatment of bone metastases: outcomes from the multicenter OsteoCool tumor ablation post-market study (OPuS one study) in 100 patients. J Vasc Interv Radiol. 2020;31(11):1745–52.
78. Surbano M, Castroman P. Radiofrecuencia pulsada del ganglio de la raíz dorsal para el dolor radicular lumbosacro: una revisión narrativa. Rev Soc Esp Dolor. 2021;28(4)
79. Arai Y, Nishihara M, Yamamoto Y, Arakawa M, Kondo M. Dorsal root ganglion pulsed radiofrequency for the management of intractable vertebral metastatic pain: a case series. Pain Med. 2015;16(5):1007–12.
80. Fanous S, Saleh E, Abd Elghafar E, Ghobrial H. Randomized controlled trials between dorsal root ganglion thermal radiofrequency, pulsed radiofrequency and steroids for the management of intractable metastatic back pain in thoracic vertebral body. Br J Pain. 2021;15(3):270–81.
81. Cohen S, Bhaskar A, Bhatia A, Buvanendran A, Deer T. Consensus practice guidelines on interventions for lumbar facet joint pain from a multispecialty, international working group. Reg Anesth Pain Med. 2020;45(6):424–67.
82. Kim Y, Kim T, Lee Y, Oh Y, Oh J. Medial branch radiofrequency treatment for low-back pain in cancer patients: a case series. Palliat Med Rep. 2022;3(1):316–21.
83. Roldan C, Javed S, Cata J. Sacroiliitis in cancer patients: a review of current literature. Pain Manag. 2020;10(2):107–15.
84. Hutson N, Hung JC, Puttanniah V, Lis E, Laufer I, Gulati A. Interventional pain management for sacroiliac tumors in the oncologic population: a case series and paradigm approach. Pain Med. 2017;18(5):959–68.
85. YR Y, Lee N, Kwon Y, Jang J, Lim S. Radiofrequency application for the treatment of pain secondary to sacroiliac joint metastases. Korean J Pain. 2016;29(1):53–6.
86. Ramasubba C, Cohen SP. Cooled sacroiliac radiofrequency denervation for the treatment of pain secondary to tumor infiltration: a case-based focused literature review. Pain Physician. 2013;16(1):1–8.
87. Swarm R, Paice J, Anghelescu D, Are M, Gurski L. Adult cancer pain, version 3.2019, NCCN clinical practice guidelines in oncology. J Natl Compr Cancer Netw. 2019;17(8):977–1007.
88. Singh D, Katyan A, Kumar N, Nigam K, Misra R. CT-guided radiofrequency ablation of osteoid osteoma: established concepts and new ideas. Br J Radiol. 2020;93(1114)
89. Posteraro A, Dupuy D, Mayo-Smith W. Radiofrequency ablation of bony metastatic disease. Clin Radiol. 2004;59(9):803–11.
90. Qiu Y, Zhang K, Ye X, Zhang X, Wang J. Combination of microwave ablation and percutaneous osteoplasty for treatment of painful extraspinal bone metastasis. Vasc Interv Radiol. 2019;30(12):1934–40.
91. Cazzato R, de Rubeis G, de Marini P, Dalili D, Gangi A. Percutaneous microwave ablation of bone tumors: a systematic review. Eur Radiol. 2021;31(5):3530–354.
92. Kumar P, Hoydonckx Y, Bhatia A. A review of current denervation techniques for chronic hip pain: anatomical and technical considerations. Curr Pain Headache Rep. 2019;23(6):38.
93. Kawaguchi M, Hashizume K, Iwata T, Furuya H. Percutaneous radiofrequency lesioning of sensory branches of the obturator and femoral nerves for the treatment of hip joint pain. Reg Anesth Pain Med. 2001;26(6):576–81.
94. Stone J, Matchett G. Combined ultrasound and fluoroscopic guidance for radiofrequency ablation of the obturator nerve for intractable cancer-associated hip pain. Pain Physician. 2014;17(1):E83–7.
95. Pushparaj H, Hoydonckx Y, Mittal N, Peng P, Cohen SP, Cao X, Bhatia A. A systematic review and meta-analysis of radiofrequency procedures on innervation to the shoulder joint for relieving chronic pain. Eur J Pain. 2021;25(5):986–1011.

96. MS E, McCormick Z, Beal C, Julia J, Nagpal A. Putting our shoulder to the wheel: current understanding and gaps in nerve ablation for chronic shoulder pain. Pain Med. 2021;22(Suppl 1):S2–8.
97. Chang K, Hung C, Wang T, Yang R, Sun W. Ultrasound-guided proximal suprascapular nerve block with radiofrequency lesioning for patients with malignancy-associated recalcitrant shoulder pain. J Ultrasound Med. 2015;34(11):2099–105.
98. Bray F, Laversanne M, Sung H, et al. Global cancer statistics 2022: GLOBOCAN estimates of incidence and mortality worldwide for 36 cancers in 185 countries. CA Cancer J Clin. 2024;74:229–63.
99. Paice JA, Von Roenn JH. Under- or overtreatment of pain in the patient with cancer: how to achieve proper balance. J Clin Oncol. 2014;32:1721–6.
100. Deer TR, Hayek SM, Grider JS, et al. The polyanalgesic consensus conference (PACC): updates on clinical pharmacology and comorbidity management in intratecal drug delivery for cancer pain. Neuromodulation. 2024;24:00670–6.
101. Smith TJ, Staats PS, Deer TR, et al. Randomized clinical trial of an implantable drug delivery system compared with comprehensive medical management for refractory cancer pain: impact on pain, drug-related toxicity, and survival. J Clin Oncol. 2002;20:4040–9.
102. Rauck RL, Wallace MS, Leong MS, et al. A randomized, double-blind, placebo-controlled study of intratecal ziconotide in adults with severe chronic pain. J Pain Symtom Manage. 2006;31:393–406.
103. Brogan SE, Winter NB, Okifuji A. Prospective observational study of patient-controlled intrathecal analgesia: impact on cancer-associated symptoms, breakthrough pain control, and patient satisfaction. Reg Anesth Pain Med. 2015;40:369–75.
104. Carvajal G, Dupoiron D, Seegers V, et al. Intrathecal drug delivery systems for refractory pancreatic cancer pain: observational follow-up study over an 11-year period in a comprehensive cancer center. Anesth Analg. 2018;126:2038–46.
105. Stearns LJ, Narang S, Albright RE, et al. Assessment of health care utilization and cost of targeted drug delivery and conventional medical management vs conventional medical management alone for patients with cancer-related pain. JAMA Netw Open. 2019;2:e191549.
106. Ma K, Jin Y, Wang L, et al. Intrathecal delivery of hydromorphone vs morphine for refractory cancer pain: a multicenter, randomized, single-blind, controlled no inferiority trial. Pain. 2020;161:2502–10.
107. Deer TR, Smith HS, Cousins M, et al. Consensus guidelines for the selection and implantation of patients with noncancer pain for intrathecal drug delivery. Pain Phys. 2010;13:E175–213.
108. Knight KH, Brand FM, McHaourab AS, Veneziano G. Impantable intrathecal pumps for chronic pain: highlights and updates. Croat Med J. 2007;48:22–34.
109. Deer TR, Provenzano DA, Hanes M, et al. The Neurostimulation appropriateness consensus committee (NACC) recommendations for infection prevention and management. Neuromodulation. 2017;20:31–51.
110. Deer TR, HayeK SM, Grider JS, et al. The polyanalgesic consensus conference (PACC): intrathecal drug delivery guidance on safety and therapy optimization when treating chronic noncancer pain. Neuromodulation. 2024;27(7):1107–39.
111. Chen GH, Spiegel MA, Magram YC, et al. Evaluation of fixed intrathecal bupivacaine infusion doses in the oncologic population. Neuromodulation. 2020;23:984–90.
112. De la Calle Reviriego JL, Villarreal A. Neuromodulación: Estimulador medular e infusión intratecal. Cap 29. Manual de Medicina del dolor. Fundamentos, evaluación y tratamiento. Sociedad Española del dolor. Editorial médica Paramericana; 2016. p 289–99.
113. Rock AK, Truong H, Park YL, Pilitisis J. Spinal cord stimulation. Nerosurg Clin N Am. 2019;30(2):169–94.
114. Molnar G, Barolat G. Principles of cord activation during spinal cord stimulation. Neuromodulation. 2014;17(1):12–21.
115. Deer T, Russo M, Grider J, Pope J, Rigoard P, Hagedorn J, et al. The Neurostimulation appropriateness consensus committee (NACC): recommendations for surgical technique for spinal cord stimulation. Neuromodulation. 2022;1-34:25.

116. Hagedorn JM, Illigens BM-W, Zylka MJ. Targeting the dorsal root ganglion for the treatment of chronic pain: cellular and molecular mechanisms. Pain. 2021;162(5):1103–12.
117. Pope JE, Deer TR, Kramer J. A systematic review: current and future directions of dorsal root ganglion therapeutics to treat chronic pain. Pain Med. 2021;22(5):1039–54.
118. Harrison C, Epton S, Bojanic S, Green AL, FitzGerald JJ. The efficacy and safety of dorsal root ganglion stimulation as a treatment for neuropathic pain: a literature review. Neuromodulation. 2018;21(3):225–33.
119. Davanzo J, Brandmeir N. Surgical technique and patient selection for spinal cord stimulation for chronic pain. Neurol India. 2020;68:S213–7.
120. Chapman KB, et al. Best practices for dorsal root ganglion stimulation for chronic pain: guidelines from the American Society of Pain and Neuroscience. J Pain Res. 2023;16:839–79.

Integrating Interventional Oncology with Other Cancer Treatment Options for Bone Tumors: Radiotherapy

11

Gian Carlo Mattiucci, Francesco Preziosi, Palmira Foro Arnalot, and Martina Iezzi

Abbreviations

SBRT	Stereotactic Body Radiotherapy
EBRT	External Beam Radiotherapy
NSBM	Non-spinal Bone Metastases
SRE	Skeletal-Related Event
OS	Overall Survival
PFS	Progression-Free Survival
ESTRO	European Society for Radiotherapy and Oncology
EORTC	European Organization for Research and Treatment of Cancer
PTV	Planning Target Volume
CTV	Clinical Target Volume
GTV	Gross Tumor Volume
MRI-Linac	Magnetic Resonance Imaging-Linear Accelerator
VMAT	Volumetric Modulated Arc Therapy
IMRT	Intensity Modulated Radiotherapy
ISRS	International Stereotactic Radiosurgery Society

G. C. Mattiucci
Radiation Oncology, Mater Olbia Hospital, Olbia, Italy

Dipartimento di Scienze Radiologiche ed Ematologiche, Università Cattolica del Sacro Cuore, Rome, Italy
e-mail: giancarlo.mattiucci@materolbia.com

F. Preziosi (✉) · M. Iezzi
Radiation Oncology, Mater Olbia Hospital, Olbia, Italy
e-mail: martina.iezzi@materolbia.com

P. Foro Arnalot
Radiation Oncology, Hospital del Mar, Barcelona, Spain
e-mail: pforo@hmar.cat

C. Pusceddu, S. Marsico (eds.), *Malignant Bone Lesions and Beyond*,
https://doi.org/10.1007/978-3-032-00018-7_11

RCT	Randomized Controlled Trial
CI	Confidence Interval
Gy	Gray (unit of radiation dose)
RT	Radiotherapy
CRT	Conventional Radiotherapy
HBI	Hemibody Irradiation
SC24	Canadian Clinical Trials Group Study SC.24
SABR	Stereotactic Ablative Radiotherapy
COMET	Canadian Oligometastases Trial
CT	Computed Tomography
PET-CT	Positron Emission Tomography-Computed Tomography
MRI	Magnetic Resonance Imaging
HT3	5-Hydroxytryptamine-3 (Serotonin) Receptor
3DCRT	Three-Dimensional Conformal Radiotherapy

11.1 Introduction

Bone metastases are a common and debilitating consequence of advanced cancer, significantly affecting patients' quality of life. These lesions can lead to severe pain, pathological fractures, spinal cord compression, and other complications that restrict mobility and diminish overall well-being.

Palliative radiotherapy has long been a mainstay for symptom management. However, with increasing life expectancy in advanced cancer, the treatment paradigm is shifting towards durable control of metastases to optimize both quality of life and survival. Stereotactic body radiotherapy (SBRT) is emerging as a promising modality, especially for patients with oligometastatic disease (limited metastases). SBRT's precise targeting and high-dose delivery in a hypofractionated regimen offer the potential for improved local control and potentially better survival outcomes compared to traditional palliative approaches, while minimizing toxicity.

This chapter will delve into the role of radiotherapy across the spectrum of palliative and oligometastatic disease, analyzing the latest evidence on innovative therapies, including SBRT, and their impact on survival. We will examine the advantages and disadvantages of SBRT, its clinical indications, treatment protocols, and the findings of pivotal clinical trials.

11.2 Role of Radiotherapy in the Treatment of Painful Bone Metastases

Bone metastases are common in advanced cancer and are linked to substantial morbidity, including tumor-induced pain, pathological fractures, and compromise of the neuraxis.

Almost all malignancies have the capacity to spread to the skeleton. Approximately 80% of bony lesions originate from breast, prostate, lung, kidney, and thyroid cancers [1].

The management of bone metastases should focus on alleviating symptoms, preventing the emergence of new ones, as well as potential complications.

Radiotherapy represents an effective treatment option for symptomatic bone metastases, offering prolonged pain relief with minimal toxicity and favorable cost-effectiveness.

Advances in cancer therapies have considerably extended survival in many patients, resulting in a growing emphasis on managing symptomatic lesions to preserve quality of life, and in select cases, potentially improve survival [2]. Furthermore, the likelihood of radiotherapy-induced side effects is reduced with the application of increasingly precise techniques.

Historically, palliative radiotherapy was not administered until the symptoms related to bone metastases manifested. However, as certain patient subsets are surviving long enough for skeletal-related events (SREs) to occur, investigating prophylactic treatment for asymptomatic or minimally symptomatic bone lesions has become essential [3, 4].

In a phase II clinical trial, Gillespie et al. explored the use of prophylactic radiation therapy for asymptomatic high-risk bone metastases (bulky lesions ($\geq$ 2 cm); disease involving the hip (acetabulum, femoral head, and femoral neck), shoulder or sacroiliac joints; disease in long bones occupying one-third to two-thirds of the cortical thickness; disease in the vertebrae of the junctional spine (C7–T1, T12–L1, and L5–S1); and/or disease with posterior element involvement) [4]. The study compared the results with those of systemic therapy or observation alone [5]. Treatments were delivered using conventional radiotherapy or stereotactic techniques. At the one-year follow-up, the radiotherapy group showed a significantly lower incidence of SREs (1.6% versus 29%), and a significant correlation was found between SREs and poor overall survival [5].

An ongoing clinical trial is also investigating the advantages of prioritizing prophylactic radiotherapy in patients with bulky osseous tumors or lesions in the junctional spine [5]. Further research is necessary to identify the optimal dose and treatment strategies for this patient group.

11.3 Indications and Recommended Fractionation Scheme

Focusing on patients with uncomplicated bone metastases (painful, without impending or existing pathological fractures, and absent spinal cord or cauda equina compression, regardless of lesion size [6]), the initial clinical assessment should encompass the following aspects:

- Performance status
- Prognostic evaluation of anticipated survival

- Thorough pain history, encompassing pain intensity and positions that exacerbate discomfort
- Analgesic use and adherence to prescribed therapy
- Medical and surgical history
- Interpretation of radiological imaging in conjunction with the patient's clinical history and physical examination

In contrast, a malignant spinal cord or cauda equina compression secondary to spine lesions warrants an urgent intervention. Radiation oncologists generally defer to open surgery for spinal decompression in surgical candidates, as it provides the best potential for restoring neurological function. However, for patients who are not ideal surgical candidates or who refuse surgery, conventional radiotherapy alone is often utilized for managing symptomatic compression.

Conventional radiotherapy can produce a clinically significant pain response in up to 80% of patients, with a median duration of pain relief ranging from 18 to 21 months [6]. It should be considered for the treatment of uncomplicated painful bone metastases, particularly when pain is insufficiently controlled with analgesics or when a reduction in pain medication is sought.

Numerous randomized studies have compared single-fraction radiotherapy with multiple-fraction radiotherapy for the management of symptomatic bone metastases. **The most common single-fraction regimen is 8 Gy in 1 fraction, while multiple-fraction regimens generally consist of 20 Gy in 5 fractions, 24 Gy in 6 fractions, and 30 Gy in 10 fractions** [7, 8].

An updated systematic review by Rich et al. of 29 trials demonstrated comparable levels of pain relief between single- and multiple-fraction radiotherapy, with overall response rates of 61% versus 62% and complete response rates of 23% versus 24%, respectively. While no significant differences were noted between treatment arms in terms of risk of pathological fractures, spinal cord compression, or acute toxicities, retreatment rates were higher in the single-fraction group (20% versus 8%) [7]. The higher retreatment rate may reflect either differences in the durability of the regimens or greater comfort with retreatment following single-fraction therapy.

Both quality of life and cost-effectiveness have not been comprehensively examined as primary endpoints, and therefore, no definitive conclusions can be drawn in this regard. Nevertheless, the potential advantages of shorter treatment courses should be taken into consideration.

For diffuse pain caused by multiple bone metastases, single-fraction hemibody or wide-field irradiation should be considered due to the significant and rapid pain relief observed in several clinical trials and prospective studies [9–14]. The most frequently used fractionation regimen is 6 Gy in a single fraction for the upper body and 8 Gy in one fraction for the lower body. For the latter, intravenous antiemetic prophylaxis is recommended for at least 12 hours.

Radionuclide therapy (e.g., radium-223, strontium-89, or samarium-153) is a feasible palliative option for patients with painful osteoblastic or mixed-pattern bone metastases, particularly in cases of prostate cancer.

The side effects of radiation therapy depend on the tissues that receive a significant dose. For instance, the treatment of lumbar spine metastases often involves irradiation of the bowel loops, which can lead to nausea and abdominal discomfort.

However, side effects following conventional radiotherapy are generally mild, and most patients do not experience any acute toxicity [15, 16].

In most cases, treatment is associated with fatigue in at least two-thirds of patients [17]. Additionally, up to 44% of patients may experience a pain flare in the first week following treatment, which typically resolves within one to three days [18].

Radiation-induced nausea and vomiting are most effectively managed with 5-hydroxytryptamine-3 (5-HT3) receptor antagonists [67, 68] and possibly with daily dexamethasone [19–21]. Pain flares can be managed with symptomatic treatments, such as paracetamol and dexamethasone, even in the absence of consensus regarding the routine use of the latter [22].

A few studies compare the prophylactic use of glucocorticoids versus placebo [23]. The SC.23 randomized trial demonstrated that prophylactic dexamethasone (8 mg for five days) significantly reduced the incidence of pain flares from 35% (with placebo) to 26% in patients with bone metastases receiving a single dose of 8 Gy [24]. Conversely, the DEXA randomized trial did not find any effect of prophylactic dexamethasone on pain flare incidence after radiation, although an immediate effect on pain was observed [25].

A significant late effect of radiation therapy is the development of radiation-induced vertebral compression fractures. However, reports indicate that with conventional radiation, the risk of these fractures is less than 5% [16, 26].

Clinical evaluation of pain and function remains the most important assessment of response to treatment. Response assessment with imaging is discouraged after the treatment of uncomplicated bone metastases. It could be considered within clinical trials, or for patients treated with the intent of local control or remineralization.

The median time to response is three to four weeks [27, 28].

The response should preferably be measured according to the criteria outlined in the International Consensus Working Party recommendations [29]: patients experiencing a pain reduction of at least two points on an 11-point scale without an increase in analgesic use, or a 25% or greater reduction in opioid requirements without a corresponding increase in pain score, are considered to have had a significant response.

Patients who do not experience pain relief or show progression after initial radiotherapy, or those who relapse after an initial response, should be considered for reirradiation.

In this context, a meta-analysis encompassing seven studies assessed the efficacy of reirradiation for painful bone metastases and reported a pooled overall response rate of 58% (95% CI 0.49–0.67) [30].

A randomized non-inferiority trial involving 850 patients compared the pain-relieving effect of **8 Gy in a single dose** to 20 Gy in multiple fractions of 2.5 or 4 Gy, with treatment administered at least four weeks after initial radiotherapy. In the intention-to-treat population, the response rate two months after single-fraction radiotherapy was found to be non-inferior to that of multiple-fraction radiotherapy (28% vs 32%), with the pain response ranging from 45% to 51%, independent of prior pain response, previous radiotherapy, or the initial fractionation regimen. Moreover, 8 Gy in a single dose was associated with fewer adverse events compared to the fractionated schedule [31].

Various techniques are employed for palliative radiotherapy of bone metastases, ranging from 3-dimensional conformal radiation therapy (3DCRT) to more advanced and conformal approaches such as intensity-modulated radiotherapy (IMRT, see Fig. 11.1) and volumetric modulated arc therapy (VMAT, see Fig. 11.2).

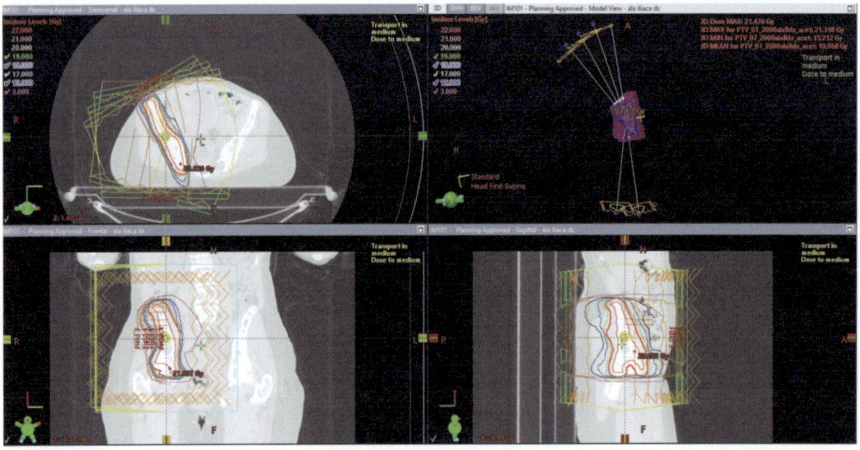

Fig. 11.1 IMRT treatment planning of bony pelvic lesion (Copyright© 2025, Varian Medical Systems, Inc. All rights reserved)

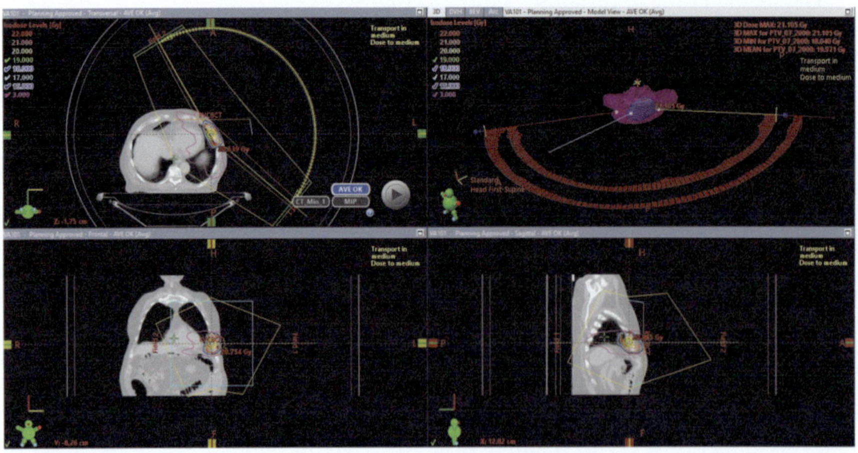

Fig. 11.2 VMAT treatment planning of costal lesion (Copyright© 2025, Varian Medical Systems, Inc. All rights reserved)

Conformal techniques offer the advantage of sparing normal tissues, which theoretically reduces radiation-induced toxicities and allows for dose escalation.

However, these techniques are more expensive and resource-intensive due to their complexity and the need for increased quality control. In contrast, simpler static field treatments reduce the need for contouring and complex dosimetric calculations, making them more time-efficient.

To date, there is no conclusive evidence supporting the superiority of any single technique. Each approach should be considered based on the individual patient's clinical assessment.

Regarding target delineation, the target volumes for bone metastases may vary depending on the type of bone (long, short, flat, sesamoid, or irregular), the presence of extraosseous extension, and, in post-operative cases, the presence of surgical implants and the location of the surgical access.

For conventional radiotherapy, there is no universal consensus or recommendation for defining a specific target. The most commonly used approach is based on portal field simulation. When using 3D-CT or MRI-based target definition, it is strongly recommended to use a contouring approach based on the gross tumor volume (GTV), clinical target volume (CTV), and planning target volume (PTV) [6].

According to ICRU Report 50, the GTV, which represents the macroscopic disease, can be defined using CT, MRI, or PET-CT imaging. The CTV, which accounts for subclinical disease, can be created by isotropic expansion of the GTV or by delineating the affected bone compartment. A retrospective study has shown that compartmental CTVs in pelvic bone metastases are associated with improved pain control and local control [32]. Finally, the PTV is a geometric volume that compensates for setup errors and potential organ motion, and is defined by a CTV expansion that is Center-dependent.

11.4 Role of Radiotherapy in the Treatment of Oligometastatic Bone Disease

Bone metastases are among the most common sites of metastatic spread [33, 34], occurring in a significant number of patients with advanced cancer, and they represent a major cause for referral to radiation oncology services. Historically, the treatment options for bone metastases primarily relied on conventional 2D and 3D external beam radiation therapy (EBRT), which, although effective, often provided limited precision and posed challenges in terms of sparing surrounding healthy tissue. Over the past several decades, however, there has been a dramatic evolution in radiotherapy techniques, leading to more advanced and effective treatment strategies for metastatic disease. One of the most noteworthy developments has been the increasing use of stereotactic body radiation therapy (SBRT), which has emerged as a promising and highly effective treatment modality for bone metastases [35].

SBRT allows for the delivery of highly focused and intense doses of radiation to metastatic tumors with remarkable precision, minimizing radiation exposure to healthy tissues surrounding the target area [36]. This precision is particularly advantageous in the treatment of bone metastases, which are often located near critical structures and organs, making traditional radiation approaches less optimal. In recent years, multiple phase I and II clinical trials have assessed the efficacy of SBRT in the treatment of oligometastatic disease — a stage of cancer where patients have a limited number of metastases, typically fewer than five, in contrast to more widely metastatic disease [37]. These trials have investigated the use of SBRT in various cancers, including non-small cell lung cancer, prostate cancer, and other malignancies, with the results showing improvements not only in progression-free survival (PFS) but also in overall survival (OS), underscoring the potential of SBRT to significantly extend patient lifespans while maintaining a good quality of life.

Recently, a group of experts from the European Society for Radiotherapy and Oncology (ESTRO) and the European Organization for Research and Treatment of Cancer (EORTC) proposed a new classification to better address the heterogeneity observed among patients with oligometastatic disease [38]. This disease can present in several forms, including de novo, which is distinct from recurrent presentations (i.e., consecutive episodes of metastasis) and induced oligometastatic disease, which occurs after a previous polymetastatic disease has been treated. This differentiation is important for tailoring therapeutic strategies and understanding the clinical outcomes for each patient.

To further refine this classification, patients are subdivided into three main categories: oligorecurrence, oligoprogression, and oligopersistence. These categories are based on two key factors: whether the patient is undergoing systemic therapy and the progression status of the lesions. Oligorecurrence refers to cases where metastatic lesions recur after treatment but remain limited in number. Oligoprogression, on the other hand, involves the progression of only a few lesions, while the majority of metastases remain stable. Oligopersistence is used when the lesions persist despite treatment, but they are still limited in extent [39].

The importance of oligometastatic status becomes particularly evident in patients with bone metastases, where the disease is more challenging to manage. In these cases, not only is symptom palliation a primary focus, but improving progression-free survival could also become a critical therapeutic goal. This approach opens up possibilities for more personalized treatment strategies, including local therapies like surgery or radiation, in conjunction with systemic treatments. The idea is that, for some patients, aggressive treatment of oligometastatic disease could delay disease progression, prolong survival, and improve overall quality of life.

This emerging classification system has significant implications for clinical practice, as it allows clinicians to better stratify patients based on the unique characteristics of their disease, ultimately leading to more targeted and effective treatments. Furthermore, it emphasizes the potential of individualized therapeutic regimens that not only aim to control the disease but also to enhance patient outcomes in the long term.

In addition to its success in oligometastatic disease, SBRT has gained increasing support from randomized trials for its use in both spine and non-spine bone metastases [40].

In the phase II SABR-COMET trial [41], patients with well-controlled primary tumors of various histologies and fewer than five oligometastatic foci were treated using SBRT schedules, including 35 Gy in 5 fractions, 60 Gy in 8 fractions, and 54 Gy in 3 fractions. Although bone metastases accounted for 35% of all metastatic sites treated, the protocol specifically excluded femoral bone metastases and any lesions within 3 mm of the spinal cord. After a 5-year follow-up, the results showed a median overall survival benefit of 22 months for patients receiving SBRT compared to those undergoing standard palliative treatment, with an absolute survival benefit of 25% at 5 years [42].

A prominent example is the recent SC24 trial, which focused on patients with painful spinal metastases [43]. The data from this trial have reinforced the clinical utility of SBRT in treating spinal metastases, offering effective pain relief and tumor control with fewer side effects compared to traditional radiation therapies [44]. This has further validated the use of SBRT as a standard treatment option not only in patients with localized spinal disease but also in those with non-spinal bone metastases, contributing to its broader adoption in clinical settings.

The growing body of evidence supporting SBRT has led to its increasing incorporation into clinical practice, especially for patients with oligometastatic disease, where the focus is on achieving long-term control of metastatic lesions and prolonging survival.

Furthermore, by inducing the presentation of cancer antigens to the immune system [13], SBRT is thought to trigger a tumor-targeted immune response (including bystander and abscopal effects), thereby enhancing the therapeutic efficacy of immunotherapies.

For patients with more widely spread metastatic cancer, SBRT is being considered as a complementary strategy in a multidisciplinary approach, often combined with other treatments such as systemic therapies, immunotherapies, or targeted therapies. This integrated approach is part of a shift toward more personalized cancer treatment, where the goal is not only to treat the disease effectively but also to minimize side effects and enhance the patient's quality of life [45].

11.5 Indications, Recommended Fractionation Scheme, and Long-Term Results

In the management of bone metastases, it is crucial to distinguish between spinal and non-spinal bone metastases (NSBM), as each type presents distinct clinical and biological characteristics that influence treatment decisions. The localization of metastases plays a pivotal role in determining the optimal therapeutic approach, particularly when utilizing SBRT, which offers unique advantages in treating bone lesions.

Spinal metastases are particularly complex due to their involvement with critical structures such as the spinal cord and nerve roots. The presence of metastases in this region can lead to severe complications, including intense pain, neurological deficits, and even spinal cord compression, with the risk of paralysis. In these cases, SBRT proves to be essential, as it enables the delivery of high radiation doses with millimeter precision, minimizing the risk of damaging the spinal cord and surrounding nervous structures. Prompt management of spinal metastases can significantly improve patient quality of life by preventing irreversible neurological damage and effectively controlling pain.

On the other hand, non-spinal metastases, which affect peripheral bones (such as the femur, pelvis, and ribs), while not directly involving the spinal cord, can still cause significant pain and bone weakening, increasing the risk of pathological fractures. Here too, SBRT represents a highly effective therapeutic option, as it allows the delivery of high doses of radiation in a precise manner, reducing the risk of collateral damage to surrounding healthy tissues. For non-spinal metastases, SBRT is particularly beneficial for treating lesions located in challenging anatomical areas that are difficult to reach through other techniques, such as surgery, or in patients who are not candidates for invasive interventions.

Moreover, the ability of SBRT to focus on single or multiple lesions while maintaining a high level of precision makes it particularly suitable for the treatment of bone metastases in oligometastatic patients, where the number of metastases is limited. The distinction between spinal and non-spinal metastases thus becomes crucial in selecting the most appropriate treatment strategy, maximizing therapeutic benefits, and minimizing potential side effects.

Regarding NSBM, a recent literature review and meta-analysis conducted by Nguyen et al. [46] includes recommendations from the International Stereotactic Radiosurgery Society (ISRS).

A total of 25 studies were included in the analysis, with 18 suitable for quantitative assessment. The most commonly treated anatomical sites for metastases were the pelvis, ribs, lower extremities and hips, and upper extremities and shoulders.

An example of a metastases to the sternum is shown in Fig. 11.3.

The pooled local control (LC) rate at 1 year was 95% (CI: 89%–98%), ranging from 80% to 100%, with low heterogeneity. At 2 years, the pooled LC rate remained high at 94% (95% CI: 86%–98%), with a similar range of 80% to 100% and low heterogeneity. Local failure was more likely in patients with certain histologies, such as lung cancer, renal cell carcinoma, and melanoma, as well as those who received spine SBRT.

For overall survival (OS), the pooled rate at 1 year was 84% (95% CI: 73%–91%), with a range from 67% to 98%, showing high heterogeneity. At 2 years, the OS rate dropped slightly to 81% (95% CI: 45%–95%), with a range of 45% to 98% and high heterogeneity. In a univariable analysis, prostate cancer patients had better OS at 1 year, while patients with lung cancer, pelvic bone metastases, and rib metastases had worse OS outcomes.

There was notable variability in the dose fractionation protocols across and within studies. While some patients received 40–50 Gy in 10 fractions, other regimens varied from single fractions to multi-fraction schedules, with none exceeding 5 fractions. Common treatment schedules included 18–24 Gy in a single fraction, 27–30 Gy in 3 fractions (see Fig. 11.1), and 30–35 Gy in 5 fractions.

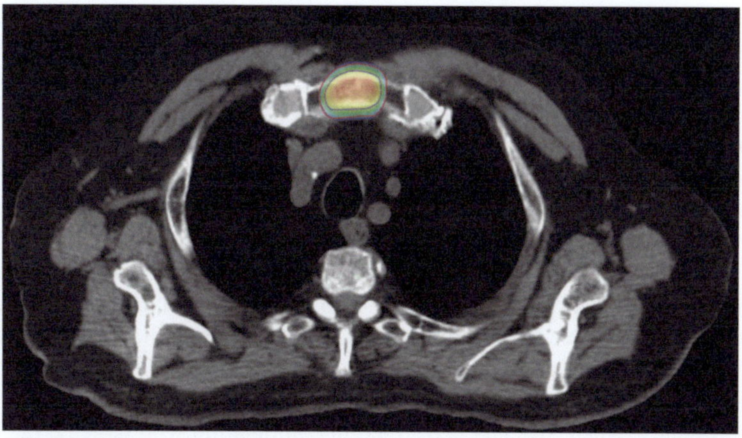

Fig. 11.3 A painful metastasis to the sternum treated with 30 Gy in 3 fractions (Copyright© 2025, Varian Medical Systems, Inc. All rights reserved)

Table 11.1 Dose fractionation for NSBM SBRT

Dose fractionation	Number of fractions
18–24 Gy	1
27–30 Gy	3
30–35 Gy	5

NSBM SBRT was generally well-tolerated, with a low rate of adverse events reported in 12 studies. The most frequent grade 1–2 acute toxicities were fatigue, pain flare, and nausea/vomiting. Fractures were the most common late toxicity, with incidence rates ranging from 0% to 17%.

The ISRS-endorsed consensus recommends the following dose fractionation schedules: 18–24 Gy in 1 fraction, 27–30 Gy in 3 fractions, and 30–35 Gy in 5 fractions (Table 11.1).

Due to the variability in the location and anatomy of NSBM, dose selection should be individualized based on the target site and clinical indication.

Dose de-escalation, defined as the use of multiple fractions with lower doses per fraction, should be considered if the lesion has previously undergone treatment with SBRT or EBRT (provided more than three months have passed between treatments), if the lesion involves weight-bearing bones, or in patients with moderate-to-severe cortical erosion ($\geq$ 30%). Conversely, dose escalation should be considered for metastases with radiation-resistant histologies (e.g., colon, kidney, melanoma, and sarcoma), or in cases with a large mass or extraosseous involvement [47].

Instead, regarding spinal lesions, recent ESTRO guidelines [48] offer important recommendations for managing these lesions, especially in the context of SBRT for vertebral metastases.

For patients with vertebral metastases from solid tumors, SBRT should be administered with a prescribed dose greater than the equivalent of 1 × 18 Gy to ensure optimal therapeutic efficacy. For de novo vertebral metastases, high-dose spine SBRT protocols typically include fractionations such as 1 × 20 Gy, 1 × 24 Gy, 2 × 12 Gy, 3 × 10 Gy, and 5 × 7 Gy (Table 11.2, Fig. 11.2). Based on these dosing schemes, the expected local control rate ranges from 80% to 90% over a 1 to 2-year follow-up period, showing promising results in terms of both efficacy and safety.

An example of a metastasis to D4 is shown in Fig. 11.4.

For patients with painful vertebral metastases from solid tumors who meet the eligibility criteria for spine SBRT, a fractionated approach of 2 × 12 Gy is conditionally recommended as the preferred palliative treatment, offering effective pain relief while minimizing risks. In contrast, for patients with vertebral metastases from solid tumors, single-fraction SBRT with doses of 16 or 18 Gy is not recommended as an alternative to conventional low-dose palliative radiotherapy (1 × 8 Gy), particularly when pain relief and/or improvement in quality of life are the primary treatment objectives.

Additionally, when SBRT is performed in combination with targeted radiotherapy or immunotherapy, it is essential for spine SBRT practitioners to discuss the potential risks of unexpected or increased toxicity with the oncology team. A multidisciplinary approach is key to ensuring that patients receive the most appropriate treatment, carefully considering any potential interactions or complications that may arise from the combination of therapies.

Table 11.2 Dose fractionation for spine bone metastasis SBRT

Dose fractionation	Number of fractions
20–24 Gy	1
24 Gy	2
30 Gy	3
35 Gy	5

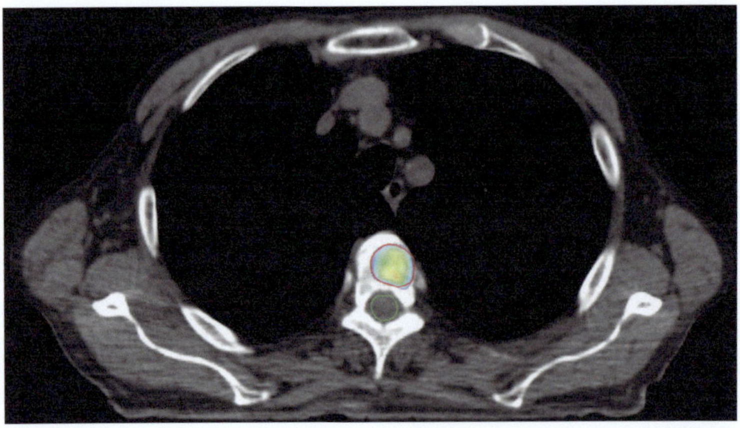

Fig. 11.4 Metastasis from prostate carcinoma to the D4 dorsal vertebra, treated with 35 Gy in 5 fractions. The PTV is contoured in red, and the spinal cord is highlighted in green (Copyright© 2025, Varian Medical Systems, Inc. All rights reserved)

Numerous prospective studies [49] have demonstrated improved pain control with the use of SBRT compared to conventional external beam radiotherapy, along with excellent long-term local control. As a result, the application of SBRT for spinal metastases has been steadily increasing worldwide. This growing interest is supported by promising clinical outcomes, which highlight the potential of SBRT to offer better symptom relief and more effective tumor control.

Furthermore, there is renewed research into the application of new technologies that could further refine and enhance spinal SBRT practices [50]. Among the most promising innovations is MRI-Linac technology, which has been evaluated in various clinical settings. More recently, MRI-Linac has been explored for use in spine SBRT, offering new possibilities for improving treatment precision [51]. This combination of MRI and linear accelerator technology provides real-time imaging during radiation delivery, allowing for more accurate targeting of tumors while minimizing radiation exposure to surrounding healthy tissues.

MRI-Linac technology could significantly improve the efficacy of spine SBRT, particularly in cases where target coverage is often compromised due to the need to avoid critical organs at risk, such as the spinal cord or cauda equina. By providing enhanced imaging capabilities during treatment, MRI-Linac enables clinicians to deliver higher doses of radiation to the tumor while maintaining stringent safety margins. This advancement holds the potential to further optimize outcomes in patients with spinal metastases, reducing treatment-related toxicity and improving overall patient prognosis.

In conclusion, SBRT treatment for both spinal and non-spinal lesions has proven to be a highly effective and safe therapeutic option, demonstrating minimal side effects. It achieves an impressive rate of local control while also contributing to encouraging overall survival outcomes. This is supported by a growing body of evidence, which consistently shows that SBRT provides excellent local control with both rapid and long-lasting effects. As the evidence continues to accumulate, SBRT stands out as a promising approach for managing a wide range of tumors, offering not only effective tumor control but also an improved quality of life for patients. The ongoing advancements in techniques and patient selection further enhance its potential, making SBRT a key component of modern cancer treatment strategies.

References

1. Mundy GR. Metastasis to bone: causes, consequences and therapeutic opportunities. Nat Rev Cancer. 2002;2:584–93. https://doi.org/10.1038/nrc867.
2. Nguyen Q-N, Chun SG, Chow E, et al. Single-fraction stereotactic vs conventional multiple-fraction radiotherapy for pain relief in patients with predominantly nonspine bone metastases: a randomized phase 2 trial. JAMA Oncol. 2019;5(6):872–8. https://doi.org/10.1001/jamaoncol.2019.0192. This is a phase II study that provides the strongest evidence for the use of stereotactic radiotherapy for symptomatic non-spine bone metastases
3. Rosen DB, Benjamin CD, Yang JC, et al. Early palliative radiadion versus observation for high-risk asymptomatic or minimally symptomatic bone metastases: study protocol for a randomized controlled trial. BMC Cancer. 2020;20(1):1115–212. https://doi.org/10.1186/s12885-020-07591-w.

4. Shulman RM, Meyer JE, Li T, Howell KJ. External beam radiation therapy (EBRT) for asymptomatic bone metastases in patients with solid tumors reduces the risk of skeletal-related events (SREs). Ann Palliat Med. 2019;8(2):159–67. https://doi.org/10.21037/apm.2018.10.04.
5. Gillespie EF, Yang JC, Mathis NJ, et al. Prophylactic radiation therapy versus standard of care for patients with high-risk asymptomatic bone metastases: a multicenter, randomized phase II clinical trial. J Clin Oncol. 2023:JCO2300753–JCO2300753. https://doi.org/10.1200/JCO.23.00753. The authors demonstrate a significant reduction in skeletal related events in patients whose asymptomatic bone metastases were treated with prophylactic palliative radiotherapy.
6. van der Velden J, et al. ESTRO ACROP guidelines for external beam radiotherapy of patients with uncomplicated bone metastases. Radiother Oncol. 2022;173:197–206. https://doi.org/10.1016/j.radonc.2022.05.024.
7. Rich SE, Chow R, Raman S, et al. Update of the systematic review of palliative radiation therapy fractionation for bone metastases. Radiother Oncol. 2018;126(3):547–57. https://doi.org/10.1016/j.radonc.2018.01.003.
8. Chow R, Hoskin P, Schild SE, et al. Single vs multiple fraction palliative radiation therapy for bone metastases: cumulative meta-analysis. Radiother Oncol. 2019;141:56–61. https://doi.org/10.1016/j.radonc.2019.06.037.
9. Berg RS, Yilmaz MK, Høyer M, Keldsen N, Nielsen OS, Ewertz M. Half body irradiation of patients with multiple bone metastases: a phase II trial. Acta Oncol. 2009;48:556–61. https://doi.org/10.1080/02841860802488128.
10. Mill WB, Glasgow GP, Ratkin G. Hemi-body irradiation in the palliation of disseminated malignancies. Mo Med. 1980;77:72.
11. Nag S, Shah V. Once-a-week lower hemibody irradiation (HBI) for metastatic cancers. Int J Radiat Oncol Biol Phys. 1986;12:1003–5. https://doi.org/10.1016/0360-3016(86)90398-6.
12. Poulter CA, Cosmatos D, Rubin P, Urtasun R, Cooper JS, Kuske RR, et al. A report of RTOG 8206: a phase III study of whether the addition of single dose hemibody irradiation to standard fractionated local field irradiation is more effective than local field irradiation alone in the treatment of symptomatic osseous metastases. Int J Radiat Oncol Biol Phys. 1992;23:207–14. https://doi.org/10.1016/0360-3016(92)90563-w.
13. Quilty PM, Kirk D, Bolger JJ, Dearnaley DP, Lewington VJ, Masone MD, et al. A comparison of the palliative effects of strontium-89 and external beamradiotherapy in metastatic prostate cancer. Radiother Oncol. 1994;31:33–40. https://doi.org/10.1016/0167-8140(94)90411-1.
14. Tong D, Gillick L, Hendrickson FR. The palliation of symptomatic osseous metastases: final results of the study by the radiation therapy oncology group. Cancer. 1982;50:893–9. https://doi.org/10.1002/1097-0142(19820901)50:5<893::aid-cncr2820500515>3.0.co;2-y.
15. Chow E, Zeng L, Salvo N, Dennis K, Tsao M, Lutz S. Update on the systematic review of palliative radiotherapy trials for bone metastases. Clin Oncol (R Coll Radiol). 2012;24:112–24. https://doi.org/10.1016/j.clon.2011.11.004.
16. Rich SE, Chow R, Raman S, Liang Zeng K, Lutz S, Lam H, et al. Update of the systematic review of palliative radiation therapy fractionation for bone metastases. Radiother Oncol. 2018;126:547–57. https://doi.org/10.1016/j.radonc.2018.01.003.
17. Spencer K, Parrish R, Barton R, Henry A. Palliative radiotherapy. BMJ. 2018;360:k821. https://doi.org/10.1136/bmj.k821.
18. McDonald R, Chow E, Rowbottom L, DeAngelis C, Soliman H. Incidence of pain flare in radiation treatment of bone metastases: a literature review. J Bone Oncol. 2014;3:84–9. https://doi.org/10.1016/j.jbo.2014.10.001.
19. Feyer PC, Maranzano E, Molassiotis A, Roila F, Clark-Snow RA, Jordan K, et al. Radiotherapy-induced nausea and vomiting (RINV): MASCC/ESMO guideline for antiemetics in radiotherapy: update 2009. Support Care Cancer. 2011;19:S5–S. https://doi.org/10.1007/s00520-010-0950-6.
20. Kirkbride P, Bezjak A, Pater J, Zee B, Palmer MJ, Wong R, et al. Dexamethasone for the prophylaxis of radiation-induced emesis: a National Cancer Institute of Canada clinical trials group phase III study. J Clin Oncol. 2000;18:1960–6. https://doi.org/10.1200/JCO.2000.18.9.1960.

21. Wong RKS, Paul N, Ding K, Whitehead M, Brundage M, Fyles A, et al. 5Hydroxytryptamine-3 receptor antagonist with or without short-course dexamethasone in the prophylaxis of radiation induced emesis: a placebo- controlled randomized trial of the National Cancer Institute of Canada ClinicalTrials group (SC19). J Clin Oncol. 2006;24:3458–64.
22. Niglas M, Raman S, Rodin D, Detsky J, DeAngelis C, Soliman H, et al. Should dexamethasone be standard in the prophylaxis of pain flare after palliative radiotherapy for bone metastases? A debate. Ann Palliat Med. 2018;7:279–83. https://doi.org/10.21037/apm.2017.04.08.
23. Fabregat C, Almendros S, Navarro-Martin A, Gonzalez J. Pain flare-effect prophylaxis with corticosteroids on bone radiotherapy treatment: a systematic review. Pain Pract. 2020;20:101–9. https://doi.org/10.1111/papr.12823.
24. Chow E, Meyer RM, Ding K, Nabid A, Chabot P, Wong P, et al. Dexamethasone in the prophylaxis of radiation-induced pain flare after palliative radiotherapy for bone metastases: a double-blind, randomised placebo-controlled, phase 3 trial. Lancet Oncol. 2015;16:1463–72. https://doi.org/10.1016/S1470-2045(15)00199-0.
25. van der Linden YM, Westhoff PG, Stellato RK, van Baardwijk A, de Vries K, Ong F, et al. Dexamethasone for the prevention of a pain flare after palliative radiation therapy for painful bone metastases: the multicenter double-blind placebo-controlled 3-armed randomized Dutch DEXA study. Int J Radiat Oncol Biol Phys. 2020;108:546–53. https://doi.org/10.1016/j.ijrobp.2020.05.007.
26. Sahgal A, Whyne CM, Ma L, Larson DA, Fehlings MG. Vertebral compression fracture after stereotactic body radiotherapy for spinal metastases. Lancet Oncol. 2013;14:e310–20. https://doi.org/10.1016/S1470-2045(13)70101-3.
27. van der Velden JM, van der Linden YM, Versteeg AL, Verlaan J-J, Sophie Gerlich A, Pielkenrood BJ, et al. Evaluation of effectiveness of palliative radiotherapy for bone metastases: a prospective cohort study. J Radiat Oncol. 2018;7:325–33.
28. van der Linden YM, SPDS D, EJA V, CAM M, JWH L, Dutch Bone Metastasis Study Group. Prediction of survival in patients with metastases in the spinal column: results based on a randomized trial of radiotherapy. Cancer. 2005;103:320–8. https://doi.org/10.1002/cncr.20756.
29. Chow E, Hoskin P, Mitera G, Zeng L, Lutz S, Roos D, et al. Update of the international consensus on palliative radiotherapy endpoints for future clinical trials in bone metastases. Int J Radiat Oncol Biol Phys. 2012;82:1730–7. https://doi.org/10.1016/j.ijrobp.2011.02.008.
30. Huisman M, van den Bosch MAAJ, Wijlemans JW, van Vulpen M, van der Linden YM, Verkooijen HM. Effectiveness of reirradiation for painful bone metastases: a systematic review and meta-analysis. Int J Radiat Oncol Biol Phys. 2012;84:8–14. https://doi.org/10.1016/j.ijrobp.2011.10.080.
31. Chow E, van der Linden YM, Roos D, Hartsell WF, Hoskin P, Wu JSY, et al. Single versus multiple fractions of repeat radiation for painful bone metastases: a randomised, controlled, non-inferiority trial. Lancet Oncol. 2014;15:164–71. https://doi.org/10.1016/S1470-2045(13)70556-4.
32. Kim T, Cha HJ, Kim JW, Seong J, Lee IJ. High dose and compartmental target volume may improve patient outcome after radiotherapy for pelvic bone metastases from hepatocellular carcinoma. Oncotarget. 2016;7:53921–9. https://doi.org/10.18632/oncotarget.9767.
33. Chow E, Harris K, Fan G, Tsao M, Sze WM. Palliative radiotherapy trials for bone metastases: a systematic review. J Clin Oncol. 2007;25(11):1423–36. https://doi.org/10.1200/JCO.2006.09.5281.
34. Coleman RE. Clinical features of metastatic bone disease and risk of skeletal morbidity. Clin Cancer Res. 2006;12(20 Pt 2):6243s–9s. https://doi.org/10.1158/1078-0432.CCR-06-0931.
35. Lehrer EJ, Singh R, Wang M, et al. Safety and survival rates associated with ablative stereotactic radiotherapy for patients with Oligometastatic cancer: a systematic review and meta-analysis. JAMA Oncol. 2021;7(1):92–106. https://doi.org/10.1001/jamaoncol.2020.6146.
36. Timmerman RD, Herman J, Cho LC. Emergence of stereotactic body radiation therapy and its impact on current and future clinical practice. J Clin Oncol. 2014;32(26):2847–54. https://doi.org/10.1200/JCO.2014.55.4675.

37. Lievens Y, Guckenberger M, Gomez D, et al. Defining oligometastatic disease from a radiation oncology perspective: an ESTRO-ASTRO consensus document. Radiother Oncol. 2020;148:157–66. https://doi.org/10.1016/j.radonc.2020.04.003.
38. Guckenberger M, Lievens Y, Bouma AB, et al. Characterisation and classification of oligometastatic disease: a European Society for Radiotherapy and Oncology and European organisation for research and treatment of Cancer consensus recommendation. Lancet Oncol. 2020;21(1):e18–28. https://doi.org/10.1016/S1470-2045(19)30718-1.
39. Oldenburger E, Brown S, Willmann J, et al. ESTRO ACROP guidelines for external beam radiotherapy of patients with complicated bone metastases. Radiother Oncol. 2022;173:240–53. https://doi.org/10.1016/j.radonc.2022.06.002.
40. Husain ZA, Sahgal A, De Salles A, et al. Stereotactic body radiotherapy for de novo spinal metastases: systematic review. J Neurosurg Spine. 2017;27(3):295–302. https://doi.org/10.3171/2017.1.SPINE16684.
41. Palma DA, Olson R, Harrow S, et al. Stereotactic ablative radiotherapy versus standard of care palliative treatment in patients with oligometastatic cancers (SABR-COMET): a randomised, phase 2, open-label trial. Lancet. 2019;393(10185):2051–8. https://doi.org/10.1016/S0140-6736(18)32487-5.
42. Palma DA, Olson R, Harrow S, et al. Stereotactic ablative radiotherapy for the comprehensive treatment of Oligometastatic cancers: long-term results of the SABR-COMET phase II randomized trial. J Clin Oncol. 2020;38(25):2830–8. https://doi.org/10.1200/JCO.20.00818.
43. Sahgal A, Myrehaug SD, Siva S, et al. CCTG SC.24/TROG 17.06: a randomized phase II/III study comparing 24Gy in 2 stereotactic body radiotherapy (SBRT) fractions versus 20Gy in 5 conventional palliative radiotherapy (CRT) fractions for patients with painful spinal metastases. Int J Radiat Oncol Biol Phys. 2020;108(5):1397–8.
44. Sprave T, Verma V, Förster R, et al. Randomized phase II trial evaluating pain response in patients with spinal metastases following stereotactic body radiotherapy versus three-dimensional conformal radiotherapy. Radiother Oncol. 2018;128(2):274–82. https://doi.org/10.1016/j.radonc.2018.04.030.
45. Tubin S, Ashdown M, Jeremic B. Time-synchronized immune-guided SBRT partial bulky tumor irradiation targeting hypoxic segment while sparing the peritumoral immune microenvironment. Radiat Oncol. 2019;14(1):220. Published 2019 Dec 4. https://doi.org/10.1186/s13014-019-1423-9.
46. Lee JH, Shi DD, Shin KY, et al. A prospective study assessing the efficacy and toxicity of stereotactic body radiation therapy for Oligometastatic bone metastases. Adv Radiat Oncol. 2023;9(4):101411. Published 2023 Dec 6. https://doi.org/10.1016/j.adro.2023.101411.
47. Nguyen TK, Louie AV, Kotecha R, et al. Stereotactic body radiotherapy for non-spine bone metastases: a meta-analysis and international stereotactic radiosurgery society (ISRS) clinical practice guidelines. Radiother Oncol. 2025;205:110717. https://doi.org/10.1016/j.radonc.2025.110717.
48. Lopez-Campos F, Cacicedo J, Couñago F, et al. SEOR SBRT-SG stereotactic body radiation therapy consensus guidelines for non-spine bone metastasis. Clin Transl Oncol. 2022;24(2):215–26. https://doi.org/10.1007/s12094-021-02695-6.
49. Zelefsky MJ, Yamada Y, Greco C, et al. Phase 3 Multi-Center, Prospective, Randomized Trial ComparingSingle-Dose 24 Gy Radiation Therapy to a 3-Fraction SBRT Regimen in the Treatment of Oligometastatic Cancer. Int J Radiat Oncol Biol Phys. 2021;110(3):672–79. https://doi.org/10.1016/j.ijrobp.2021.01.004.
50. Chen H, Ghia AJ, Maralani PJ, et al. Advanced Radiotherapy Technologies in Spine Tumors: What the Surgeon Needs to Know. Global Spine J. 2025;15(1_suppl):104S–119S. https://doi.org/10.1177/21925682241229665.
51. Yadav P, Musunuru HB, Witt JS, Bassetti M, Bayouth J, Baschnagel AM. Dosimetric study for spine stereotactic body radiation therapy: magnetic resonance guided linear accelerator versus volumetric modulated arc therapy. Radiol Oncol. 2022;56(4):553. Published 2022 Dec 13. https://doi.org/10.2478/raon-2022-0044.

12 Complex Cases: Tips and Tricks and Combined Approaches

Salvatore Marsico, Flavio Zuccarino,
Ana Rodríguez Troyano, and Claudio Pusceddu

12.1 Introduction

The field of interventional musculoskeletal oncology has evolved to address increasingly complex clinical situations involving malignant bone lesions. While standard techniques such as thermal ablation, cementoplasty, and percutaneous fixation are effective in many cases, complex lesions often necessitate a combination of strategies, creative adaptations, and advanced procedural planning.

In this chapter, we focus on eight selected complex cases that required innovative and combined approaches to achieve the therapeutic goals. For each case, we describe the clinical context, imaging findings, procedural details, technical

S. Marsico (✉)
Department of Radiology, Hospital del Mar, Barcelona, Spain

Interventional Oncology Institute, Barcelona, Spain

F. Zuccarino
Department of Radiology, Hospital del Mar, Barcelona, Spain

Department of Diagnostic Imaging, Hospital Sant Joan de Déu, Esplugues de Llobregat, Barcelona, Spain
e-mail: fzuccarino@hmar.cat

A. R. Troyano
Department of Radiology, Hospital del Mar, Barcelona, Spain
e-mail: arodrigueztroyano@hmar.cat

C. Pusceddu

Department of Radiology, Mater Olbia Hospital, Olbia, Cagliari, Italy

Interventional Oncology Institute, Barcelona, Spain

C. Pusceddu, S. Marsico (eds.), *Malignant Bone Lesions and Beyond*,
https://doi.org/10.1007/978-3-032-00018-7_12

challenges, and outcomes. Particular attention is given to the practical aspects—what worked, what required adjustment, and what key lessons were learned.

The goal is to share not only the success stories but also the technical nuances that are critical when dealing with complex or borderline cases, providing readers with immediately applicable knowledge for their clinical practice.

12.2 Case 1: Multilevel Acetabular and Pubic Metastasis Treated with Curved Needle Radiofrequency Ablation and Cementoplasty in a Palliative Setting

12.2.1 Clinical Background

A 65-year-old male diagnosed with stage IV lung adenocarcinoma, with bone and cerebral metastases.

The patient had previously received palliative radiotherapy to the right coxofemoral joint, left iliac bone, and T10 vertebra. Despite these measures, he continued to experience severe pain (VAS 9) and was referred to the pain unit.

Following discussion in a multidisciplinary tumor board, an interventional radiology approach was indicated due to:

Ineffectiveness of prior radiotherapy
Contraindication to surgery owing to poor functional status
The proposed strategy included radiofrequency ablation (RFA) and cementoplasty of the symptomatic right acetabular lesion.

12.2.2 Imaging Findings

Figure 12.1: Coronal CT scan (bone filter) demonstrates a lytic metastasis involving the right supraacetabular, anterior acetabular, and ipsilateral pubic regions, with signs of mechanical instability

12.2.3 Procedure

12.2.3.1 Preprocedural Planning

CT imaging was used to define the lesion extension and access trajectories. Given the multifocal involvement and complex anatomy, a strategy using curved ablation needles was planned.

12.2.3.2 Sedation and Positioning

The patient was placed in left lateral decubitus and underwent conscious sedation with remifentanil. During needle mobilization, ketamine boluses were administered due to poor pain control.

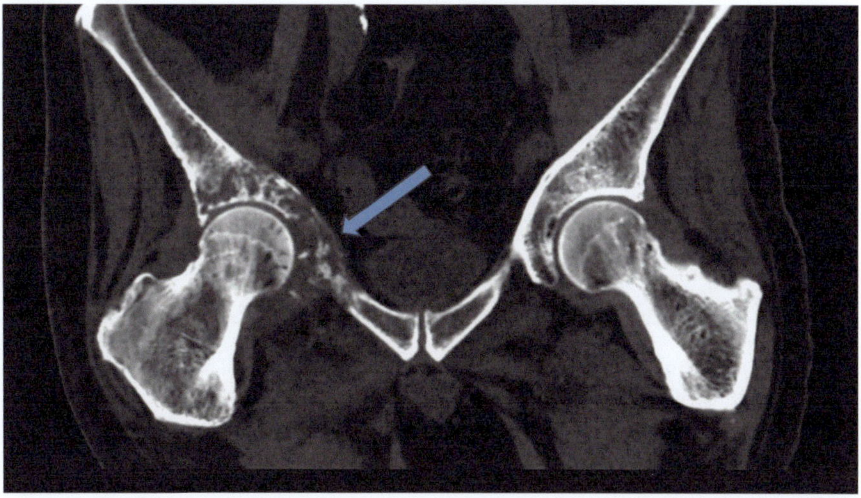

Fig. 12.1 In this coronal plane, with bone filter, performed prior to ablation demonstrates the lytic appearance of the right acetabular lesion, and the component of joint instability

12.2.3.3 Ablation Technique

A left lateral approach was chosen to access all three lesion sites.

Three curvable STAR® ablation needles (Merit Medical) were used to reach:

- The right supraacetabular lesion
- The anterior-inferior acetabular lesion
- The ipsilateral pubic symphysis

The curved needle configuration was essential to reach the deep pubic lesion, which would have been difficult to target with straight instruments due to its internal and anterior location.

Figure 12.2: Axial CT images show step-by-step needle placement under combined CT and fluoroscopic guidance

12.2.3.4 Ablation Parameters

Once the needle positions were confirmed, RFA was performed using tailored power and duration (90 degrees during 9 min).

12.2.3.5 Cementoplasty

After ablation, cement was delivered through a second coaxial cannula.

Figure 12.3: CT images with maximal intensity projection (MIP) illustrate the position of the radiofrequency needle, precisely located, using a combination of devices in order to achieve complete ablation

Figure 12.4: Coronal and sagittal CT (MIP) images demonstrate optimal cement distribution within the ablated zones

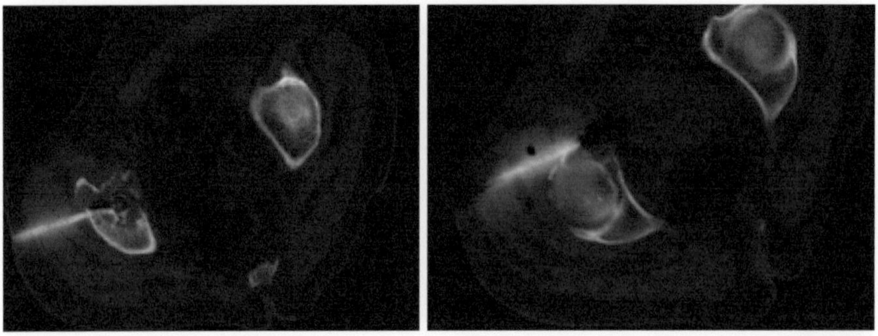

Fig. 12.2 Axial CT images with bone window demonstrating sequential needle placement during radiofrequency ablation. On the left, the curvable needle is positioned in the supraacetabular region. On the right, a second curvable probe is advanced to target the anterior-middle acetabular lesion. Both trajectories were planned under combined CT and fluoroscopic guidance, using an 11-gauge bone trocar as a coaxial introducer. Once the positioning was verified, an ablation was performed sequentially at each site

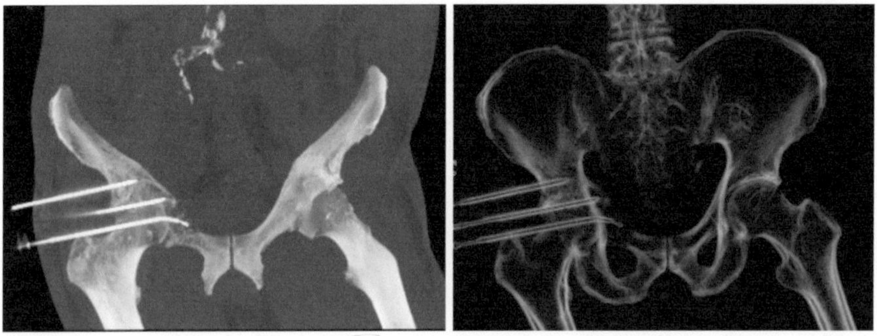

Fig. 12.3 These coronal CT images with maximal intensity projection (MIP) illustrate the position of the radiofrequency needle, precisely located, using a combination of devices in order to achieve complete ablation

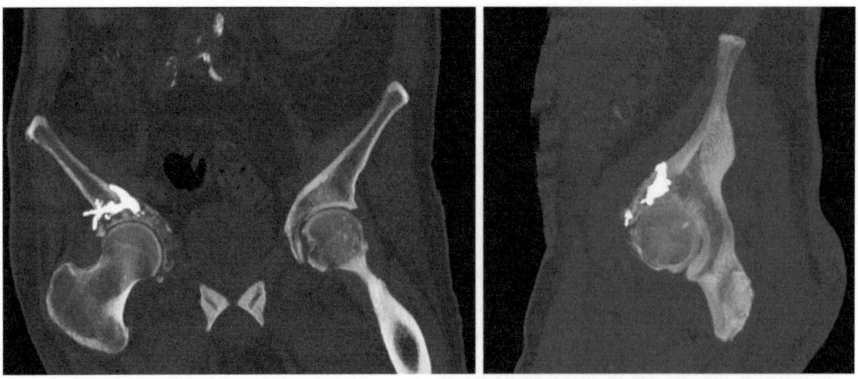

Fig. 12.4 Coronal and sagittal CT (MIP) images demonstrate optimal cement distribution within the ablated zones

12.2.4 Tips and Tricks

In complex pelvic lesions, particularly those anterior or medial to the acetabulum, curvable needles enable effective access and coverage.

Combining CT and fluoroscopy allows real-time needle trajectory confirmation in three planes.

Conscious sedation with remifentanil is effective but may require adjunct ketamine during high-manipulation phases.

A lateral approach permits access to both acetabular and pubic lesions with a single patient position.

12.2.5 Follow-Up

12.2.5.1 Clinical Evolution

The next day, the patient reported no pain in the right hip joint and walked with a walker without increased discomfort showing good tolerance and functional improvement.

12.3 Case 2: Cryoablation with EMG Monitoring of a Supraclavicular Metastasis Adjacent to the Brachial Plexus

12.3.1 Clinical Background

A 67-year-old male with metastatic urothelial carcinoma, stage IV (M1: pleural, pulmonary, and supra/infradiaphragmatic lymph node involvement).

The patient had previously received chemotherapy and radiotherapy, followed by weekly methotrexate (4 L protocol) started on March 2024. The best overall response was stable disease (SD) as of May 2024.

He presented with a progressively enlarging right supraclavicular mass, causing:

Local discomfort and pressure in the neck, especially in the supine position.
Cosmetic deformity, perceived by the patient as distressing.
Mild sensory and motor symptoms in the ipsilateral upper limb.
However, baseline EMG was negative for plexopathy or peripheral nerve involvement.
Given the lack of systemic options and increasing symptoms, a multidisciplinary tumor board indicated image-guided cryoablation as a palliative treatment.

12.3.2 Imaging Findings

Figure 12.5: Multiplanar CT scan shows a well-defined supraclavicular lytic mass in close contact with the brachial plexus, without osseous erosion

12.3.3 Procedure

12.3.3.1 Planning and Anesthesia

The procedure was performed under general anesthesia to ensure immobilization and optimal comfort.

Due to the proximity of the brachial plexus, continuous intraoperative EMG monitoring was used to minimize neurological risk.

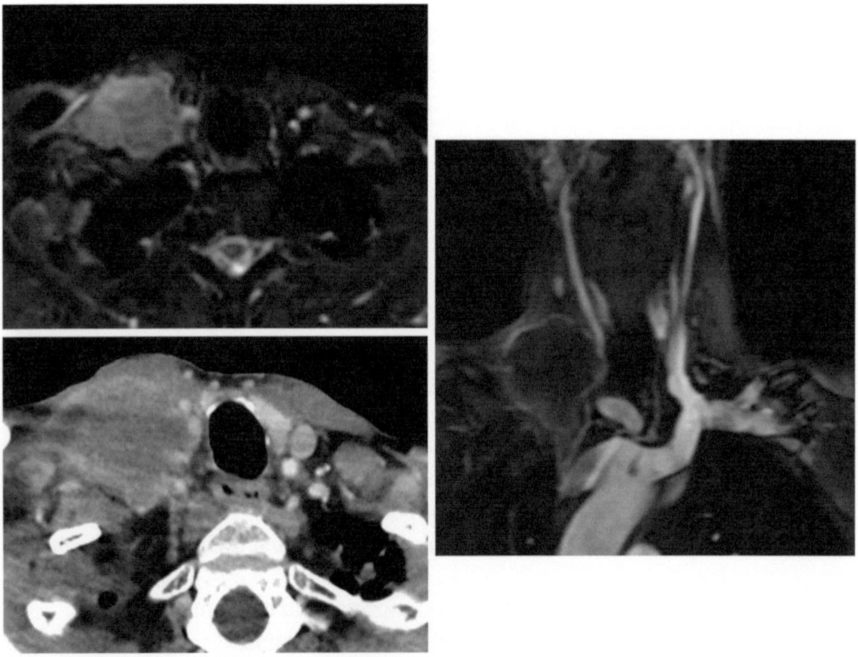

Fig. 12.5 Preprocedural CT–MRI correlation of a right supraclavicular metastatic lesion in proximity to the brachial plexus. Top left: Axial fat-suppressed T2-weighted MRI image demonstrates a hyperintense soft tissue lesion in the right supraclavicular fossa, closely abutting the brachial plexus neurovascular bundle without a clear fat plane. Bottom left: Axial contrast-enhanced portal phase CT image confirms the presence of a well-defined, mildly enhancing soft tissue mass adjacent to the subclavian vessels, with no osseous erosion. Right: Coronal DP fat-suppressed MRI shows the cranio-caudal extent of the lesion, which spans the lower neck and upper thorax, with moderate mass effect and deviation of adjacent structures, but no evidence of bone invasion

12.3.3.2 Positioning and Access

Patient was kept in supine position with a slight shoulder elevation to facilitate anterolateral probe trajectory.

12.3.3.3 Ablation Technique

Two IceSphere® cryoprobes (Boston Scientific) were inserted under CT guidance.

A double freeze–thaw cycle was applied with continuous EMG monitoring to detect early signs of nerve irritation.

Figure 12.6: Axial CT images illustrate optimal probe placement and the formation of a controlled overlapping ice ball that avoided direct contact with the neurovascular bundle

12.3.4 Tips and Tricks

In lesions adjacent to major nerves, cryoablation is preferred over heat-based techniques due to the predictable ice ball formation and visualization under CT.

General anesthesia improves patient compliance and allows better control of respiratory motion.

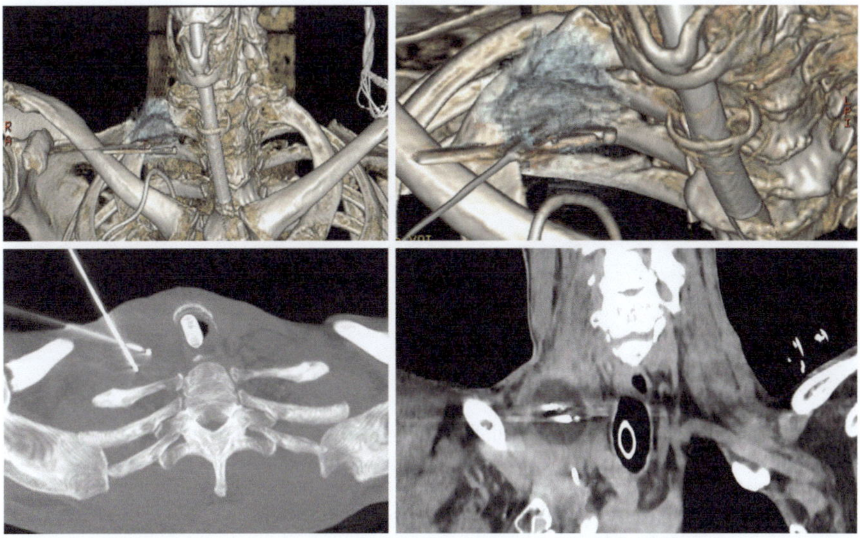

Fig. 12.6 Cryoprobe positioning and iceball formation. The image includes: A volume rendering (VR) reconstruction showing both IceSphere® probes positioned within the lesion, entering from inferolateral to superomedial, with their tips in the lower medial quadrant of the tumor. In the bottom left, an axial CT image shows the coaxial insertion of both probes. In the bottom right, a coronal CT reconstruction demonstrates the developing iceball encompassing the lesion while sparing the neurovascular bundle

EMG monitoring is a valuable adjunct to detect subclinical nerve stress and adjust ablation margins in real time.

Using two cryoprobes ensures a more complete and uniform ablation zone in larger or irregularly shaped lesions.

12.3.5 Follow-Up

12.3.5.1 Immediate Recovery

The patient awoke from anesthesia without complications.

No neurological deficits were observed post-procedure.

24 h: Full shoulder range of motion preserved; no increase in upper limb symptoms.

One-month post-procedural axial T1-weighted fat-suppressed post-contrast MRI reveals a marked decrease in enhancement, with an estimated 70% central necrosis, consistent with treatment response. The lesion shows reduced vascularity and volume, with no signs of progression or new invasion (Fig. 12.7).

There was complete resolution of neck discomfort, no further cosmetic complaint, and stabilization of sensory symptoms.

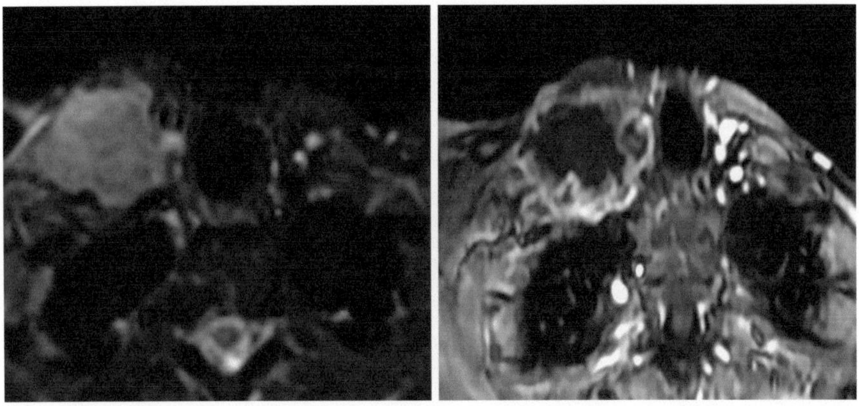

Fig. 12.7 Pre- and postprocedural axial MRI (T1-weighted fat-suppressed post-contrast) of a right supraclavicular metastatic lesion adjacent to the brachial plexus. Left: Preprocedural axial T1-weighted fat-suppressed post-contrast MRI shows a solid, heterogeneously enhancing mass in the right supraclavicular fossa, in direct contact with the brachial plexus, with obliteration of the normal fat plane and mass effect on adjacent vascular structures. Right: One-month postprocedural axial T1-weighted fat-suppressed post-contrast MRI reveals a marked decrease in enhancement, with an estimated 70% central necrosis, consistent with treatment response. The lesion shows reduced vascularity and volume, with no signs of progression or new invasion.

12.4 Case 3: Percutaneous Cryoablation of Pleurocostal Metastasis in a Patient with Pulmonary Leiomyomatosis

12.4.1 Clinical Background

A 37-year-old woman was incidentally diagnosed in 2021 with a pulmonary mass detected during a thoracic CT angiography (Fig. 12.8, black arrows) performed to rule out a pulmonary embolism in the context of a SARS-CoV-2 infection. Initially suspected to be a neuroendocrine tumor, the lesion was biopsied and diagnosed as metastatic leiomyomatosis. The patient underwent a left lower lobe lobectomy, which was complicated by postoperative hepatic hemorrhage.

12.4.2 Imaging Findings

In December 2023, a control PET-CT scan showed a hypermetabolic subcentimetric pleurocostal lesion (Fig. 12.8, yellow arrows).

Spectral thoracic CT with IV contrast allowed better distinction between soft tissue and bone, confirming the extraosseous origin of the lesion (Fig. 12.8, yellow arrows).

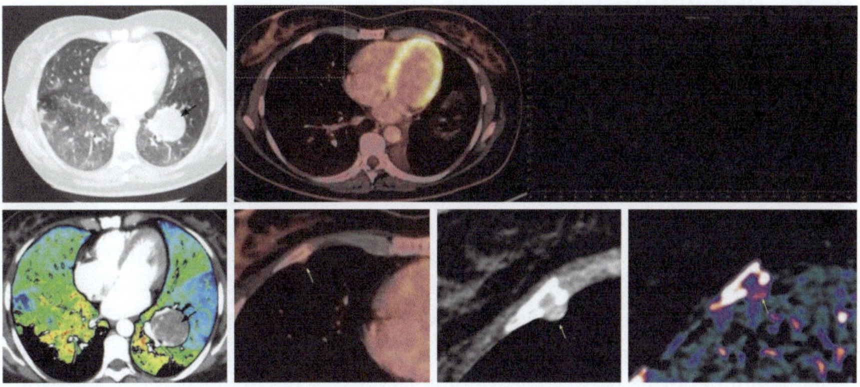

Fig. 12.8 2021 CT angiography detecting left lower lobe leiomyoma (black arrows). 2023 PET-CT and spectral CT confirming the presence of a focal tumoral lesion in soft tissues overlying a right anterior rib. The spectral curve of the lesion was suspicious for a tumor lesion

12.4.3 Procedure

The initial biopsy attempt was nondiagnostic due to limited access and insufficient material.Following a multidisciplinary review, curative cryoablation was proposed and accepted by the patient, who refused surgical resection.

The main technical challenge was the difficult access due to rib obstruction directly over the lesion.

To overcome this:

A 16 G percutaneous biopsy introducer needle was first used to “dock” against the rib surface.

Once stable contact was achieved, a coaxial technique was used to introduce the IceSphere® cryoprobe (Boston Scientific) by navigating around the rib into the target lesion.

This approach allowed precise positioning of the cryoprobe without traversing bone, minimizing trauma and avoiding pleural injury (Fig. 12.9).

Post-ablation CT showed typical ground-glass changes representing the ablation zone (Fig. 12.10).

12.4.4 Tips and Tricks

Use bone as a docking platform: In cases where the lesion is directly beneath the rib, use the rib surface as a stable anchor point to guide the introducer needle and maintain control during trajectory redirection.

Coaxial navigation around osseous barriers: Employ the angled coaxial technique to bypass bone obstructions while preserving access accuracy. This minimizes trauma and prevents pleural penetration.

Spectral CT enhances lesion characterization: Use spectral CT imaging when standard imaging does not clearly differentiate soft tissue from bone. It improves confidence in preprocedural planning and prevents misinterpretation of extraosseous metastases.

Ice-ball monitoring for safety: Continuous CT-based monitoring of the cryoablation halo allows real-time confirmation of adequate ablation margins while avoiding injury to adjacent pleura or ribs.

Minimize procedural invasiveness in a surgical refusal: When patients are not surgical candidates or decline surgery, cryoablation offers a curative-intent, minimally invasive alternative with high precision and low complication rates.

Soft tissue access planning is critical: In extraosseous lesions located in anatomically complex areas (e.g., pleurocostal region), dedicate time to preprocedural 3D planning to define the safest and most direct access route.

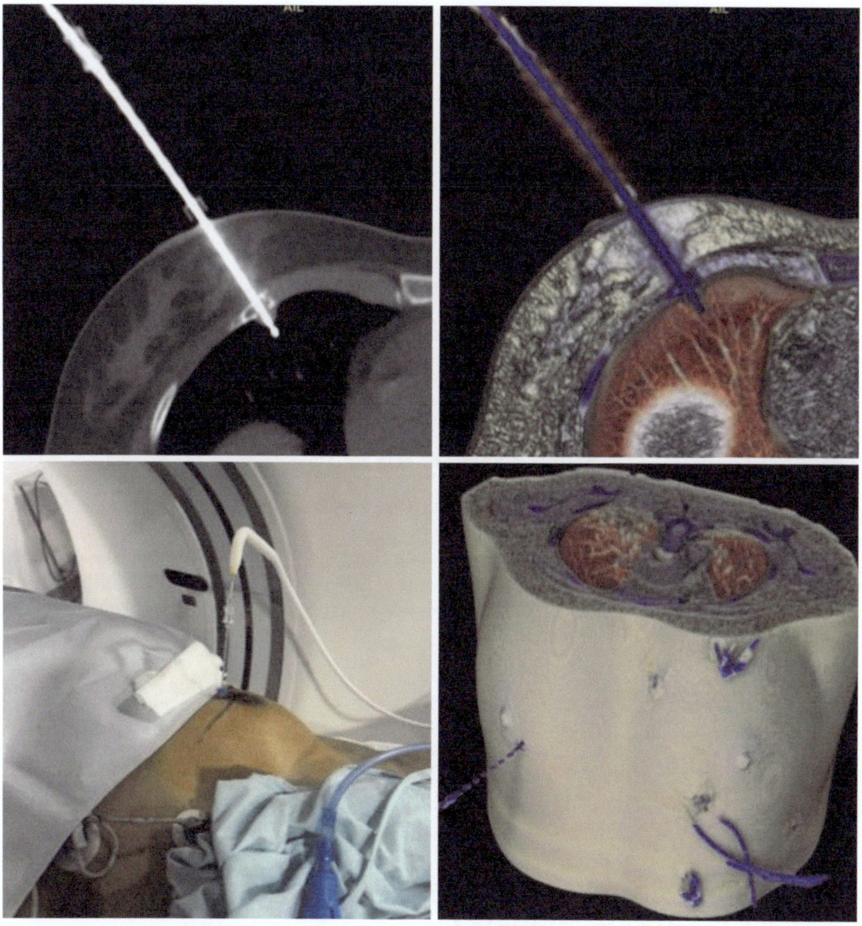

Fig. 12.9 3D planning and CT guidance demonstrating trajectory adjustment around the rib. Intraoperative photos showing probe manipulation and placement

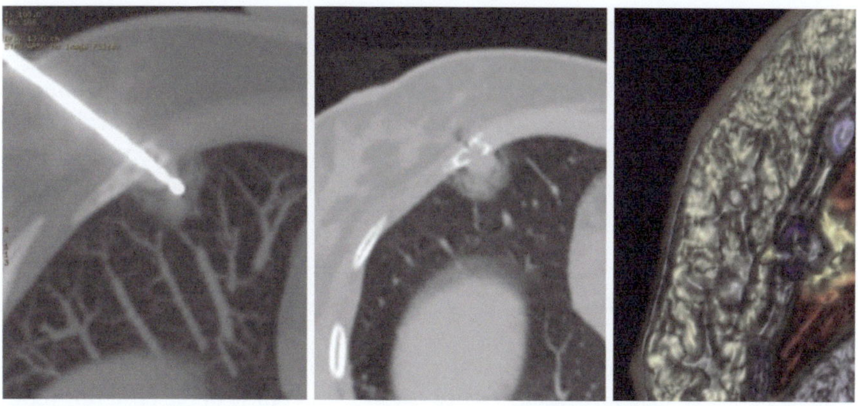

Fig. 12.10 CT and 3D images showing post-treatment halo of ground-glass opacity, confirming adequate ablation margins

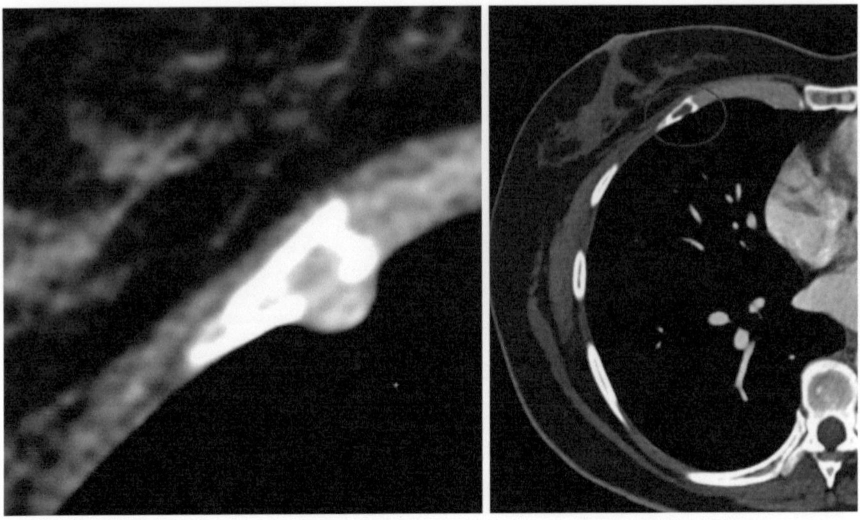

Fig. 12.11 Left: Preprocedural CT image showing the pleurocostal nodular metastasis located beneath the rib, prior to cryoablation. Right: One-month follow-up CT image demonstrating the complete resolution of the nodular lesion, with a stable residual lytic defect in the subcostal region. Red circles highlight the treated area

12.4.5 Follow-Up

At the 1-month CT follow-up, the lesion appeared fully treated with no enhancement or signs of recurrence (Fig. 12.11).

12.5 Case 4: A Multimodal Approach to Treating Pathological L5 Fracture in Multiple Myeloma: Combining Radiofrequency, Microwave Ablation, SpineJack Vertebroplasty, and Radiotherapy

12.5.1 Clinical Background

A 67-year-old female presented with severe low back pain (VAS 9), inability to ambulate, and significant functional limitation. PET-CT imaging revealed hypermetabolic osteolytic lesions involving the L5 vertebral body and proximal third of the left femur. Biopsy confirmed a solitary bone plasmacytoma, consistent with an early presentation of multiple myeloma (MM).

12.5.2 Imaging Findings

Radiological assessment demonstrated a pathological compression fracture at L5 with bilateral endplate involvement and a partial compromise of the posterior vertebral wall (Fig. 12.12).

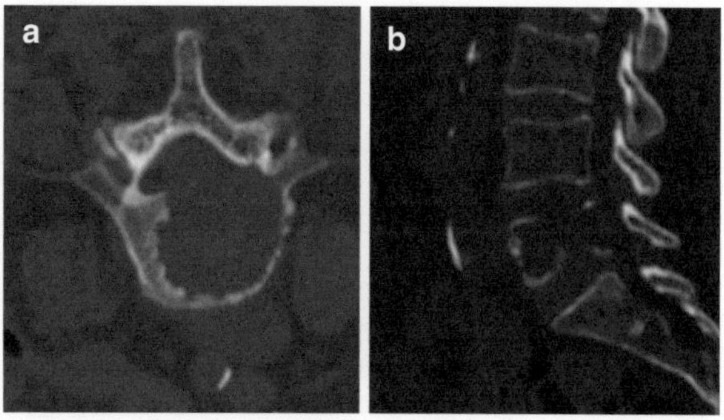

Fig. 12.12 Axial (**a**) and sagittal (**b**) CT images reveal a pathological fracture of L5 due to osteolytic infiltration, with collapse of both superior and inferior endplates and partial extension into the posterior cortical wall

Despite the presence of neuropathic pain corresponding to the L5 dermatome, no significant motor deficit was observed. Surgical decompression or fixation was considered disproportionate to the patient's functional condition and overall health status. A multidisciplinary tumor board—including interventional radiology, oncology, radiation oncology, and pain management—opted for a non-surgical, image-guided, percutaneous approach aimed at relieving pain, stabilizing the vertebra, and reducing local tumor burden.

12.5.3 Procedure (Fig. 12.13)

12.5.3.1 Preprocedural Preparation

The patient received prophylactic cefazolin (2 g IV) 30 min before the procedure.

Baseline CT was obtained with the patient in the prone position using laser guidance to ensure optimal trajectory planning and precise anatomical localization.

12.5.3.2 Pulsed Radiofrequency (PRF)

A 22G curved PRF probe was advanced under CT guidance to the right L5 dorsal root ganglion (DRG).

PRF settings: 45 volts for 6 min.

Adjunctive injection: 8 mg dexamethasone and 3 mg bupivacaine (5 mL total) for periradicular anti-inflammatory effect.

This step aimed to modulate the neuropathic component of pain due to foraminal involvement and early DRG irritation, without producing neuroablative injury.

12.5.4 Microwave Ablation (MWA)

Conscious sedation was induced using IV midazolam and alfentanil, with oxygen support via a nasal cannula.

A 14 G, 20 cm microwave antenna (AMICA-GEN, HS Hospital Service) was inserted via a transpedicular coaxial route through a bone access cannula.

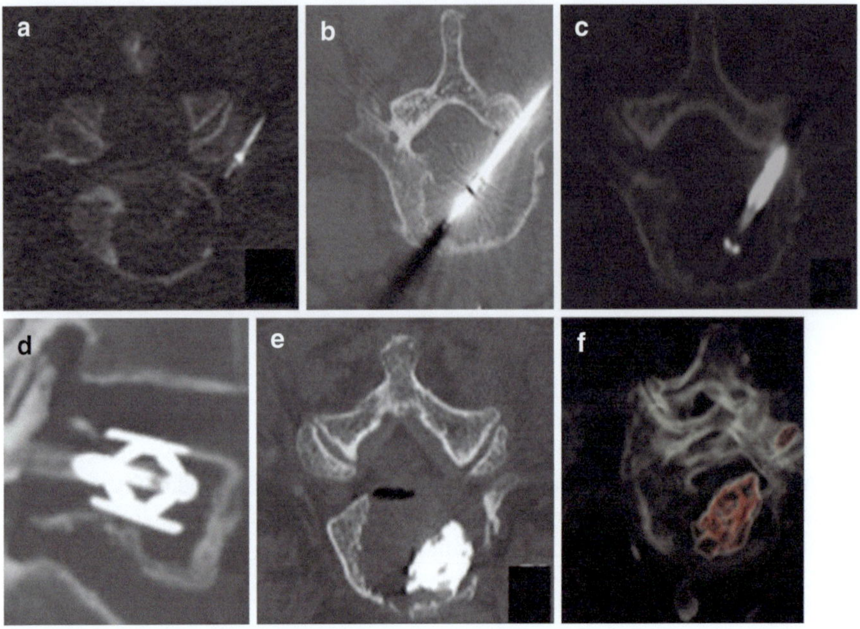

Fig. 12.13 Procedural steps: (**a**) PRF probe placed at L5 dorsal root ganglion; (**b**) transpedicular MWA antenna insertion; (**c–d**) SpineJack® deployment; (**e**) post-procedural CT showing vertebral stabilization; (**f**) 3D-VR post-processing reconstruction

Once proper positioning was confirmed on CT, the introducer was retracted to prevent overheating and ensure direct energy delivery to the osteolytic lesion.

Ablation was performed using 20 W for 3 mins. The objective was local debulking—thermal destruction of myelomatous tissue—to reduce mechanical pressure on cortical structures and adjacent neural elements, and to prepare the bone matrix for cementoplasty.

12.5.5 SpineJack® Vertebroplasty

Under general anesthesia with spontaneous ventilation (IV propofol and alfentanil), a right transpedicular approach was used.

A 5 mm expandable titanium SpineJack® implant (Stryker Corp.) was deployed through a working cannula and expanded under fluoroscopy (13 full clockwise turns).

Once height restoration was achieved, PMMA cement was injected using the Autoplex system, ensuring homogenous filling and minimizing the risk of cement extravasation.

Fluoroscopy and CT confirmed proper device expansion and cement distribution within the cavity.

12.5.6 Radiotherapy

One week after the procedure, the patient underwent five sessions of radiotherapy (total 20 Gy), directed to the L5 vertebral lesion. This timing allowed for initial mechanical stabilization and reduced the risk of vertebral collapse due to ablation-induced weakening.

12.5.7 Tips and Tricks

Combine therapeutic goals in a single session: Addressing neuropathic, mechanical, and oncologic pain simultaneously improves patient outcomes and avoids multiple interventions.

MWA before cementoplasty enhances efficacy: Thermal ablation decreases tumor volume, reduces intralesional pressure, and creates a more stable cavity for cement filling.

SpineJack® for structural reconstruction: This expandable implant not only restores vertebral height but also redistributes axial load, reduces kyphosis, and minimizes adjacent vertebral fractures.

Careful trajectory planning: Use preprocedural CT and laser alignment for safe and accurate access, particularly in fractured or infiltrated vertebrae.

PRF as a neuromodulatory bridge: This is particularly useful in cases with radicular pain not requiring decompression surgery. It reduces DRG sensitivity without causing thermal damage.

Delay radiotherapy until after mechanical stabilization: Prevents collapse or worsening of structural integrity due to early irradiation of thermally and mechanically altered bone.

12.5.8 Follow-Up

The patient experienced rapid pain relief, with the VAS score decreasing from 9 to 4 within 48 h postprocedure.

By one week, the patient was ambulatory with the aid of a walker.

At one month, VAS further improved to 3 with no radicular symptoms and cessation of rescue analgesics.

Three- and six-month follow-up CT scans confirmed stable cement position, intact vertebral architecture, and no evidence of disease progression at the treated site.

12.6 Case 5: Image-Guided Ablation, Screw Fixation, and Cementoplasty for Distal Femoral Metastasis in Renal Cell Carcinoma

12.6.1 Clinical Background

A 49-year-old woman with a known history of metastatic renal cell carcinoma (RCC) presented with severe right thigh pain (VAS 9) and severely compromised ambulation. Imaging revealed a large, osteolytic metastasis of the distal right femur involving both the metaphysis and diaphysis. The lesion extended circumferentially around the femoral cortex, indicating a high risk of pathological fracture.

The patient had previously undergone high-dose external beam radiotherapy, with no improvement in symptoms. Surgical intervention was deemed unfeasible due to the extent of disease and overall patient condition. The case was reviewed by the multidisciplinary tumor board, and a percutaneous interventional radiology approach was selected to achieve local tumor control, mechanical stabilization, and pain relief.

12.6.2 Imaging Findings

MRI multiplanar images (Fig. 12.14) demonstrate a large, aggressive-appearing lytic lesion involving the distal right femoral metaphysis and diaphysis.

No evidence of extraosseous soft tissue extension or neurovascular bundle invasion was observed, suggesting the lesion remained confined to bone.

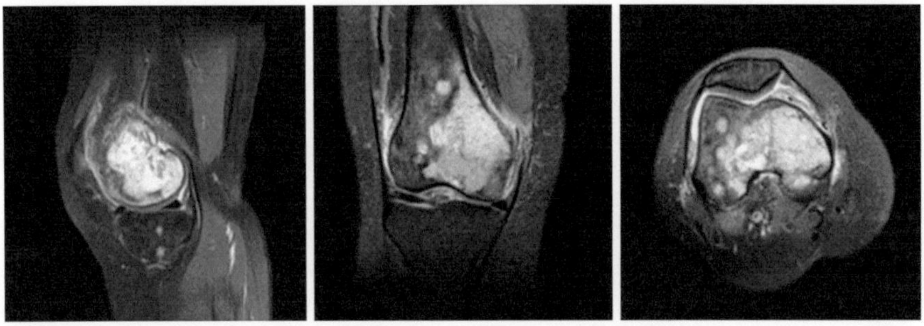

Fig. 12.14 MRI multiplanar images (sagittal, coronal, and axial planes) demonstrate a large, aggressive-appearing lytic lesion involving the distal right femoral metaphysis and diaphysis. The lesion is heterogeneously hyperintense on fat-suppressed sequences and shows cortical thinning and partial destruction, centered at the diaphyseal-metaphyseal junction

12.6.3 Procedure (Figs.12.15 and 12.16).

12.6.3.1 Preprocedural Planning

CT imaging was used for planning the ablation trajectory and screw positioning.

Conscious sedation was induced with remifentanil and midazolam, ensuring adequate patient comfort and preserving neurological monitoring during the intervention.

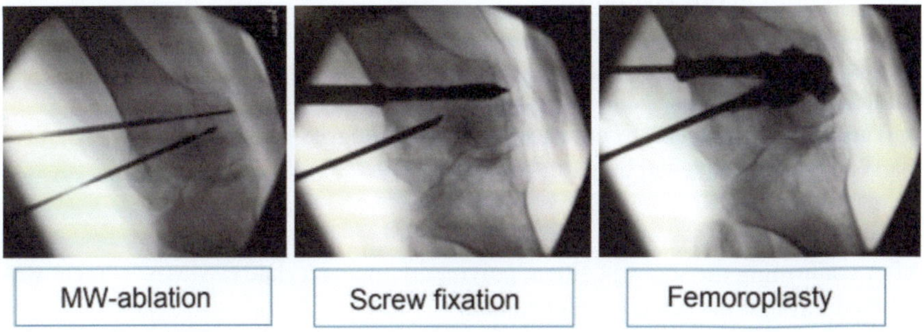

Fig. 12.15 Stepwise fluoroscopic images showing the following: (left) microwave antenna placement within the femoral metastasis for thermal ablation; (center) insertion of a cannulated screw for internal fixation; (right) injection of PMMA cement around the screw to achieve mechanical stabilization (femoroplasty)

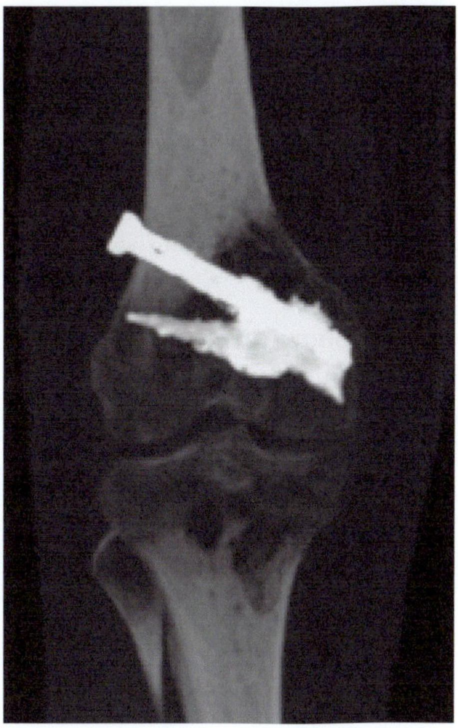

Fig. 12.16 Postprocedural coronal CT image with MIP reconstruction showing the final result of the combined treatment: successful internal stabilization with screw fixation and adequate cement distribution within the distal femur (femoroplasty), ensuring structural reinforcement

Microwave Ablation

Under CT guidance, a 14-G, 20 cm microwave antenna was introduced coaxially into the center of the lesion.

Ablation was performed at 60 W for 4 min, using the AMICA-GEN system with internal cooling.

The goal was to thermally debulk the lesion and induce tumor necrosis, reducing intraosseous pressure and pain.

Percutaneous Screw Fixation

A large-caliber cannulated screw (9.5 mm × 8 cm length) was placed under fluoroscopic and CT guidance to traverse the femoral metaphysis and provide internal fixation.

This step was critical to enhance structural integrity and distribute mechanical load across the weakened bone.

Cementoplasty

After confirming the screw position, polymethylmethacrylate (PMMA) cement was injected through the same access cannula.

The cement permeated the ablation zone and around the screw threads, anchoring the construct and preventing further collapse.

12.6.4 Tips and Tricks

Multistep approach for combined efficacy: Debulking with MWA reduces tumor mass and pressure, while fixation and cement provide immediate stability.

Screw placement prior to cement injection ensures that the implant is well-anchored and that the cement acts to lock the screw in position.

Conscious sedation allows procedural tolerance and immediate feedback if neurological symptoms arise.

Careful trajectory planning ensures protection of neurovascular structures and optimizes screw purchase in viable bone.

12.6.5 Follow-Up

At the 24-h follow-up, the patient reported a dramatic reduction in pain (VAS 2) and was able to walk with full weight-bearing using a walker.

At the one-month evaluation, she was ambulating independently with a stable gait, and imaging confirmed maintained alignment and stable cement distribution without complication.

12.7 Case 6: Multimodal Management of Thoracic Plasmacytoma with Laminectomy, Microwave Ablation, Screw Fixation, Vertebroplasty, and Radiotherapy

12.7.1 Clinical Background

A 67-year-old female presented with severe mid-thoracic pain, progressive lower limb weakness, and complete loss of ambulation over several weeks. She had a known diagnosis of solitary thoracic plasmacytoma confirmed by biopsy six months earlier and had already undergone systemic chemotherapy with partial hematologic response but persistent symptomatic disease.

Despite the indication for radiotherapy, it was deemed high-risk due to the mass's close proximity to the spinal cord. Surgical resection was ruled out due to the lesion's size and the impossibility of en bloc removal without significant morbidity. The clinical picture was dominated by a mixed mechanical and compressive syndrome with neurological impairment and severe functional decline.

A multidisciplinary tumor board, including hematology, neurosurgery, interventional radiology, and radiation oncology, agreed on a combined, staged treatment strategy. The goal was to achieve:

Urgent decompression of the spinal cord to prevent permanent neurological damage.

Cytoreduction of the soft tissue mass to allow for eventual radiotherapy.

Stabilization of the structurally compromised vertebral segment through a percutaneous approach.

12.7.2 Imaging Findings

MRI and CT scans revealed a voluminous paravertebral mass centered at the T8 level, extending into the spinal canal with compression of the spinal cord. The lesion infiltrated the posterior wall of the vertebral body and was associated with lytic destruction of the T8 vertebra. No distant metastases were identified (Fig. 12.17). The imaging raised concern for both neural compromise and mechanical instability.

This tailored approach was aimed at maximizing therapeutic efficacy while minimizing procedural morbidity in a patient with limited surgical options.

12.7.3 Procedure

The treatment was executed in the following sequential steps:

12.7.3.1 T7–T8 Laminectomy

Performed to decompress the spinal canal and relieve pressure on the spinal cord.

Partial resection of the epidural portion of the paravertebral mass was achieved during this step.

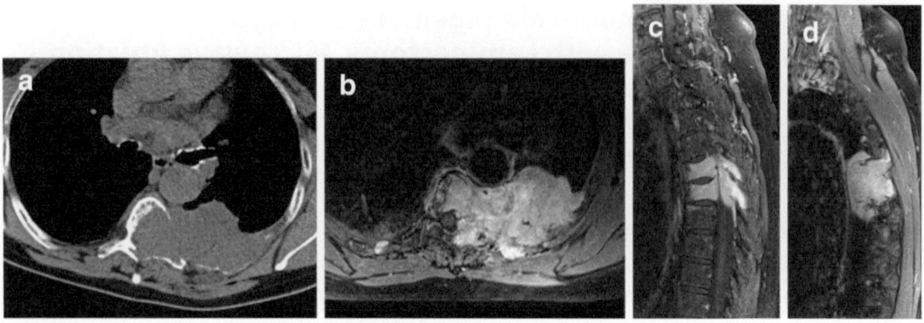

Fig. 12.17 Imaging findings of thoracic plasmacytoma.(A) Axial no contrast CT image showing a voluminous soft tissue mass centered at the T8 vertebral level, with erosion of the posterior vertebral body wall and extension into the spinal canal. (B) Axial T1-weighted fat-suppressed contrast-enhanced MRI demonstrating a large paravertebral enhancing lesion with involvement of the posterior elements and epidural extension. (C) Sagittal T1-weighted contrast-enhanced MRI highlighting the vertical extent of the lesion, with spinal canal narrowing and compression of the thoracic spinal cord. (D) Sagittal T2-weighted fat-suppressed MRI confirming the hyperintense signal of the lesion, with signs of marrow replacement and adjacent soft tissue involvement

12.7.3.2 Microwave Ablation (MWA) of the Paravertebral Mass (Fig. 12.18)

Intraoperative MWA was applied to the residual paravertebral soft tissue component using a 14-G microwave antenna.

CT and intraoperative navigation were used to ensure precise probe placement and safety margins relative to neural elements.

12.7.3.3 MWA of the Vertebral Body (T8) (Fig. 12.19)

Performed during a second session under CT guidance.

A coaxial transpedicular left approach allowed safe antenna insertion into the center of the T8 vertebral body. Ablation (60 W × 3 min) aimed to reduce tumor burden and prepare the site for mechanical stabilization.

12.7.3.4 Percutaneous Cannulated Screw Fixation and Vertebroplasty (Fig. 12.19)

Bilateral transpedicular 6.5 mm × 50 mm cannulated screws were placed under fluoroscopic control.

PMMA cement was injected through the screw cannulas to provide mechanical support and anchor the screws within the ablated vertebra.

Cement permeated both the vertebral body and the screw interface, creating a reinforced construct.

12.7.3.5 Delayed Radiotherapy

Following initial recovery and stabilization, adjuvant external beam radiotherapy (20 Gy in 5 fractions) was delivered to consolidate local disease control.

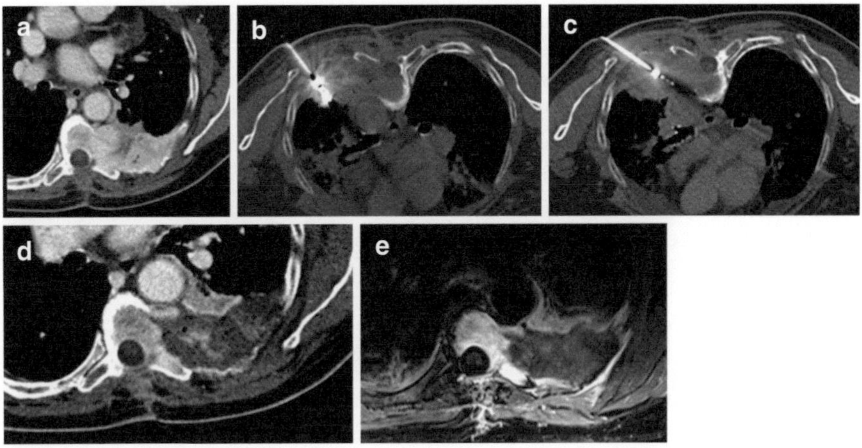

Fig. 12.18 (**a**) Preprocedural axial CT image showing the residual paravertebral mass after laminectomy, with erosion of the posterior vertebral body and epidural extension. (**b–c**) Intraoperative CT-guided placement of a 14-G microwave antenna into the paravertebral lesion; probe positioning was planned to optimize tumor coverage while preserving adjacent neural structures. (**d**) Post-ablation axial CT confirms correct ablation zone with expected hypoattenuating changes and absence of immediate complications. (**e**) Post-procedural axial T1-weighted fat-suppressed contrast-enhanced MRI demonstrates devascularization of the lesion, consistent with effective thermal ablation margins

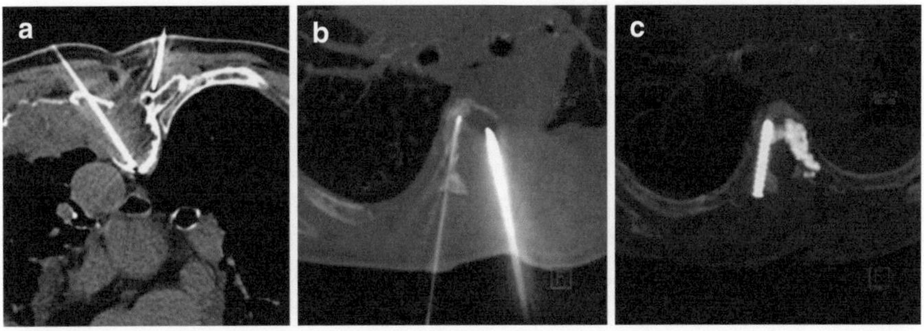

Fig. 12.19 (**a**) Axial CT image showing the coaxial left transpedicular insertion of a 14-G microwave antenna into the T8 vertebral body during the second treatment session. (**b**) Ablation was performed with 60 W of energy for 3 min to achieve tumor debulking and prepare the bone matrix for stabilization. (**c**) Postprocedural CT demonstrating right transpedicular screw fixation and PMMA cement distribution around the screws and within the ablated vertebral body, confirming mechanical reinforcement and proper construct integration

12.7.4 Tips and Tricks

Combine decompression and ablation when feasible: Laminectomy permits safe access to intraspinal disease, while MWA complements the cytoreduction of residual mass in the same session.

MWA before cementoplasty improves mechanical outcomes: Ablation reduces tumor burden and allows for uniform cement distribution around screws.
Screw fixation provides immediate stability: Cannulated screws are ideal for anchoring in ablated vertebral bodies, especially in cases with posterior wall erosion.
Sequential staging increases safety: Spacing the intervention into surgical and percutaneous phases allows for tailored monitoring and complication mitigation.
Multidisciplinary planning is essential: Optimal results were achieved through close coordination between surgical and interventional teams.

12.7.5 Follow-Up

At the 2-month follow-up, CT showed stable hardware, optimal cement distribution, and no evidence of residual epidural mass. The patient reported significant pain relief (VAS reduced from 9 to 2), partial neurological recovery, and was able to ambulate with assistance.

At 12 months, clinical and imaging evaluation confirmed disease control at the treated level, with a well-maintained spinal alignment, no hardware failure, and no need for additional interventions (Fig. 12.20).

12.8 Final Considerations and Key Messages from Complex Cases

These complex oncologic cases underscore the increasing need for advanced interventional strategies capable of achieving multiple therapeutic goals:

1. Pain control, by directly targeting neuropathic and somatic components through thermal ablation and neuromodulation
2. Local disease control, through effective tumor debulking techniques such as MWA
3. Mechanical stabilization, using cementoplasty and expandable implants such as SpineJack® to restore vertebral height and prevent further structural collapse

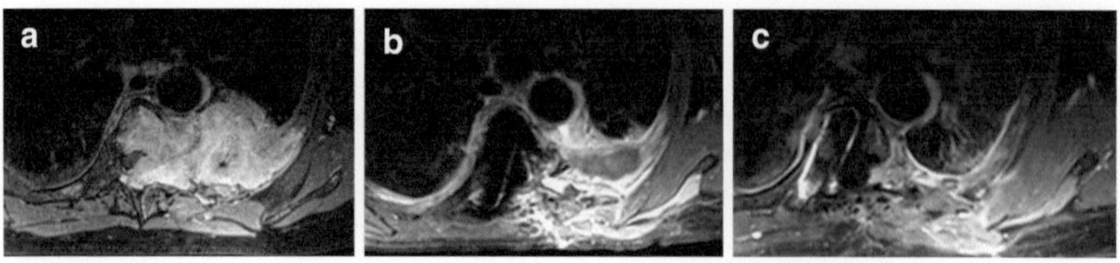

Fig. 12.20 (**a**) Preprocedural axial T1-weighted fat-suppressed contrast-enhanced MRI shows a large enhancing paravertebral mass centered at T8 with epidural extension and spinal cord compression. (**b**) Two-month follow-up MRI demonstrates a significant reduction in lesion size and enhancement, with the resolution of epidural compression and signal changes consistent with postablation necrosis. (**c**) At 12 months, MRI confirms complete lesion devascularization and stable posttreatment changes, with preserved vertebral alignment and no evidence of disease recurrence

The cases presented in this chapter illustrate how thoughtful integration of multiple percutaneous techniques—tailored to each anatomical and clinical scenario—can dramatically improve patient quality of life, even in advanced disease settings. The technical tips and tricks reported here are intended to support interventional radiologists when facing challenges in musculoskeletal oncology, particularly where anatomical complexity, limited access, or proximity to neurovascular structures require adaptation beyond standard procedures.

Ultimately, these experiences emphasize the dual role of interventional oncology: providing palliative benefit while also pursuing curative intent where feasible. Leveraging image-guided precision, real-time planning, and multidisciplinary collaboration remains essential in delivering optimal care for patients with a malignant bone disease.

The cases presented in this chapter illustrate how complex malignant bone lesions, especially those involving weight-bearing structures, challenging access routes, or proximity to critical neurovascular elements, can be successfully managed through strategic combinations of image-guided interventions and surgical collaboration. The inclusion of case 6 underscores the relevance of integrating open surgery with percutaneous therapies in anatomically delicate or neurologically compromised situations.

The key takeaways from this multimodal interventional experience include:

- Multidisciplinary decision-making is essential to balance palliative and curative intent, particularly in fragile patients or those with limited therapeutic alternatives.
- Technical adaptability—including the use of curved or coaxial needles, angulated trajectories, and intraoperative navigation—is crucial when addressing anatomically complex or surgically inaccessible lesions.
- Debulking techniques like microwave ablation not only relieve pain but also achieve local tumor control, creating a favorable environment for subsequent structural consolidation with cement or hardware.
- Combined mechanical reinforcement strategies (SpineJack®, screw fixation, and PMMA cementoplasty) ensure stabilization, recovery of vertebral alignment, and resistance to progressive collapse—even in previously irradiated or structurally fragile bone.
- Surgical decompression integrated with ablative therapy allows for the safe management of spinal lesions with epidural extension, as shown in case 6, highlighting the importance of staging and hybrid approaches.
- Neuromodulation strategies such as pulsed radiofrequency (PRF) are effective for managing radicular pain without thermal injury to neural structures.
- Cryoablation with EMG monitoring enables precise and safe treatment of lesions near critical nerves, expanding the scope of thermal therapies to anatomically sensitive regions.
- Early patient mobilization remains a key marker of procedural success, directly impacting recovery time, morbidity, and quality of life (Table 12.1).

Table 12.1 Interventional strategies employed across the complex cases described in this chapter

Technique	Indication	Purpose	Clinical benefit	Case
Pulsed radiofrequency (PRF)	Neuropathic radicular pain	Neuromodulation	Pain reduction without neuroablation	Case 4
Microwave ablation (MWA)	Lytic bone lesions/tumor debulking	Tumor necrosis, volume reduction	Facilitates cement fill, reduces pain, improves oncologic control	Cases 4, 5, 6
Cryoablation + EMG monitoring	Lesions near critical nerves (e.g., brachial plexus)	Controlled ablation with safety	Avoids nerve injury, preserves function	Case 2
SpineJack® vertebroplasty	Vertebral compression fracture/ instability	Height restoration and stabilization	Improved alignment, pain relief, and early mobility	Case 4
Cementoplasty	Mechanical support in lytic bone destruction	Load redistribution and reinforcement	Pain relief, prevents collapse, stabilizes the lesion	Cases 1, 4, 5, 6
Screw fixation + cementoplasty	Long bone or vertebral metastasis with instability	Internal stabilization	Enables weight-bearing, prevents fracture progression or collapse	Cases 5, 6
Curved or coaxial needle access	Deep or difficult anatomical access (pelvis, pubis)	Lesion access/ navigation	Expands treatable zones, avoids injury to surrounding critical structures	Case 1
Biopsy introducer "docking" trick	Subpleural/ rib-obstructed lesions	Overcomes bony obstacle	Allows coaxial access without rib penetration or pleural violation	Case 3
Surgical decompression + MWA	Spinal lesions with epidural involvement	Cord decompression and tumor control	Safe ablation in neurologically compromised patients	Case 6

This table synthesizes the core interventional strategies employed across the complex cases described in this chapter. Each technique is matched with its primary indication, therapeutic goal, resulting benefit for the patient, and the clinical case in which it was applied. The table highlights the breadth of available tools and the need for personalized, anatomy-driven procedural planning in musculoskeletal interventional oncology

12.9 Conclusion

The management of malignant bone lesions in anatomically challenging or surgically inoperable scenarios has evolved significantly, thanks to the advancement and integration of image-guided interventional techniques. The six complex cases presented in this chapter underscore the pivotal role of technical adaptability, multimodal planning, and precise execution in achieving both palliative and functional goals—even in patients with advanced diseases.

Each case illustrates how the tailored combinations of thermal ablation, mechanical stabilization (e.g., cementoplasty, screws, or expandable implants), and neuromodulatory techniques can not only control pain but also restore mobility, enhance local tumor control, and improve overall quality of life. Importantly, these outcomes were achieved with minimal morbidity and rapid recovery, emphasizing the value of minimally invasive, percutaneous solutions within a multidisciplinary framework.

Beyond the individual outcomes, the chapter reinforces several universal principles:

The importance of case selection and real-time imaging in planning.

The necessity of customized procedural strategies for each anatomical site and lesion type.

The power of combining oncologic debulking with mechanical stabilization to maximize benefit.

The value of innovative technical solutions—like curved needle paths, docking maneuvers, and integrated cement-screw systems—to overcome anatomical limitations.

These insights reflect the growing maturity and complexity of interventional musculoskeletal oncology. As the field continues to evolve, so does the responsibility to standardize techniques, share technical knowledge, and document outcomes, so that these life-improving procedures can be safely and effectively replicated across centers and patient populations.

Interventional radiologists, as procedural architects, and collaborators in cancer care, are uniquely positioned to lead this transition—combining imaging, technology, and clinical acumen to redefine the care of patients with malignant bone disease.

MIX
Papier aus verantwortungsvollen Quellen
Paper from responsible sources
FSC® C105338

If you have any concerns about our products,
you can contact us on
ProductSafety@springernature.com

In case Publisher is established outside the EU,
the EU authorized representative is:
Springer Nature Customer Service Center GmbH
Europaplatz 3, 69115 Heidelberg, Germany

Printed by Libri Plureos GmbH
in Hamburg, Germany